The
COMPLETE
KĀMA SŪTRA

Also by Alain Daniélou
(in English)

**Gods of Love and Ecstasy: The Traditions of Shiva
and Dionysus**
Inner Traditions International, Rochester, Vermont, 1992

Manimekhalai: The Dancer with the Magic Bowl
Merchant-Prince Shattan, translated from the Tamil by Alain
Daniélou and T. V. Gopala Iyer, New Directions, New York, 1989

Myths and Gods of India
Inner Traditions International, Rochester, Vermont, 1991

The Ragas of Northern Indian Music
Reprint, Munshiram Manoharlal, New Delhi, 1980

Shilappadikaram (The Ankle Bracelet)
Prince Ilango Adigal, translated from the Tamil,
New Directions, New York, 1965

**Virtue, Success, Pleasure, and Liberation:
The Four Aims of Life in the Tradition of Ancient India**
Inner Traditions International, Rochester, Vermont, 1993

The Way to the Labyrinth: Memories of East and West
New Directions, New York, 1987

**While the Gods Play: Shaiva Oracles and Predictions on the
Cycles of History and the Destiny of Mankind**
Inner Traditions International, Rochester, Vermont, 1987

Yoga: Mastering the Secrets of Matter and the Universe
Inner Traditions International, Rochester, Vermont, 1991

The

COMPLETE

KĀMA SŪTRA

*The First Unabridged Modern Translation
of the Classic Indian Text by Vātsyāyana*

including the *Jayamangalā* commentary
from the Sanskrit by Yashodhara
and extracts from the Hindi commentary
by Devadatta Shāstrā

Translated by

ALAIN DANIÉLOU

Prepared with the help of Kenneth Hurry

Park Street Press
Rochester, Vermont

Park Street Press
One Park Street
Rochester, Vermont 05767

Library of Congress Cataloging-in-Publication Data

Vātsyāyana.
[Kāmasutra. English]
The complete Kāmā Sūtra: the first unabridged modern translation of the
classic Indian text / translated by Alain Daniélou.
p. cm.
Includes index.
ISBN 0-89281-492-6
1. Love. 2. Sex. I. Daniélou, Alain. II. Title.
HQ470.S3V313 1993b
306.7—dc20   93-31474
                                                            CIP

Printed and bound in the United States

10 9 8 7 6 5 4 3 2 1

Text design by Charlotte Tyler

Park Street Press is a division of Inner Traditions International

Distributed to the book trade in the United States by American
International Distribution Corporation (AIDC)

Distributed to the book trade in Canada by Publishers Group West, Montreal
West, Quebec

Distributed to the book trade in the United Kingdom by
Deep Books, London

Distributed to the book trade in Australia by
Millennium Books, Newtown, N. S. W.

CONTENTS

Editor's Note

As Alain Daniélou observes in his Introduction, the Sanskrit text of the *Kāma Sūtra* and its commentaries frequently use familiar terms, like *yoga*, *tantra*, and *upanishad*, in highly unusual and technical senses. Because of the inherent interest of this terminology and because of the *Kāma Sūtra*'s rich vocabulary, this edition cites an extensive list of Sanskrit words and phrases and features several appendices, which we hope will be of use to specialist and nonspecialist alike.

Since this edition is intended to be accessible to all readers, we have adopted an informal Sanskrit transcription style. Except for the use of the macron to mark long vowels, we have avoided the use of diacritical marks. Thus, we have preferred *kshīra*, *rishi*, or *shruti*, which seem more easily recognizable for an English-speaking audience than their more technical equivalents. For the same reason, we have chosen to use *āchāra* and *āchārya* to indicate pronunciation, instead of the alternate spellings *ācāra* and *ācārya*. We also have not distinguished between dental and retroflex consonants, for the sake of simplicity and with the nonspecialist reader in mind.

Many hands helped make this edition of *The Complete Kāma Sūtra* possible. Special thanks go to George Thompson, a Sanskritist from the University of California, Berkeley, for his assistance with the Sanskrit terminology and to Charlotte Tyler for her care and diligence with the diacritics in the typesetting and design of this book.

INTRODUCTION

The Aims of Life

Since very ancient times, sometimes going back as far as what we term prehistory, Indian thinkers have asked themselves questions about the nature of the world and the position of man in creation. They considered matter as being formed of atoms, cells constituted by energetic elements, organized according to mathematical formulas that define the various elements under relatively stable and permanent forms. Life presents a different problem. Being based on formulas, codes defining the peculiarities of the various species, it only exists by transmitting itself through temporary links. The species is permanent, but each link has only a limited existence. Once it has transmitted the code that defines its nature, it is itself destroyed. During its brief existence, each link needs, for its own subsistence and self-transmission, to consume energy, to nourish and protect itself. Furthermore, existing only as a species, beings form interdependent communities and must observe rules of social behavior. They therefore possess obligations—ethics— that form part of their nature. This is particularly important for the human species.

Life thus necessitates three kinds of activity: to assure its survival, its means of existence, and its nourishment; to realize its reproduction

1

according to forms of activity generally connected with sexuality; and, lastly, to establish rules of behavior that allow different individuals to perform their roles within the framework of the species. In human society, this is represented as three necessities, three aims of life: material goods (artha) assure survival; erotic practice (kāma) assures the transmission of life; and rules of behavior, a moral nature (dharma), assure the cohesion and duration of the species. An ethical or social nature forms part of the genetic code of the species whose collective consciousness functions as it does in the individual. The various organs play a different, although coordinated, role. This can be easily observed in animal society, and in particular among insects.

The various members of society have distinct roles, and the ethical duties of individuals differ according to their function. This is what is known as svadharma, the ethical duty peculiar to each individual. In Hindu society, function is considered in most cases as being hereditary, whence the caste institution. Cases do exist, however, in which a function is acquired. This problem is raised by Vātsyāyana in connection with the moral code, or dharma, as applied to prostitutes.

Vātsyāyana considers that individual ethics, meaning the accomplishing of one's individual social duty, are essential for success in the domain of prosperity and love. He mentions belief in a future life as a kind of wager, whether as transmigration or heaven, but on the whole sides with the materialists who, without denying the possibility, deem it too problematical for consideration. The commentators, Yashodhara and Devadatta Shāstrī, on the other hand, side with the believers.

A fourth aim represents perception of the supernatural and the continued existence of certain acquirements of the mind beyond life's limits, and is called liberation (moksha). This aspect is contemplated by what is called religion, but remains a separate domain, considered as peculiar to mankind, even though a perception of the supernatural probably exists among other species.

As far as the necessities of life are concerned, only the first three aims are therefore considered.

These aims are mentioned in the most ancient texts, the *Vedas*, the *Purānas*, the *Laws of Manu*, the *Mahābhārata*, and so forth, but their practical definition is mainly known through the codes established during what is called the period of the Sūtras which, according to Max Muller, runs from the birth of Buddha (500 B.C.) to the accession of Ashoka (270 B.C.).

Writing disappeared in India during the second millennium before our era, as a result of the Aryan invasions, and only reappeared toward the eighth century B.C., in new forms—first Brāhmī, which was of Phoenician origin, followed in the seventh century by Kharoshti, of Aramaean origin. Although their antiquity is unquestioned, the *Vedas* as well as all the other forms of ancient knowledge were only put into written form starting from this period. Knowledge, which had been previously transmitted orally, was then codified in Sanskrit, which had become the instrument of culture. It is not certain whether even Panini's famous grammar was originally a written text. Thus it was that, starting from the seventh century B.C., the basic texts concerning the aims of life were transcribed in the *Artha Shāstra, Dharma Shāstra,* and *Kāma Shāstra.*

The Predecessors of Vātsyāyana

The first formulation of the *Kāma Shāstra*, or rules of love, is attributed to Nandi, Shiva's companion.

During the eighth century B.C., Shvetaketu, son of Uddalaka, undertook the summary of Nandi's work. The date is known, since Uddālaki and Shvetaketu are the protagonists of the *Brihat Āranyaka Upanishad* and *Chandogya Upanishad*, which are usually dated to this period and contain important passages connected with erotic science.

A man of letters called Babhru, together with his sons or disciples, known as the Bābhravya, made an important written work, summarizing the too-vast work of Shvetaketu. The Bābhravya came originally from Panchāla, a region located between the Ganges and the Yamuna, to the south of present-day Delhi, but most probably lived in the city of Pātaliputra, the great center of the kingdom of Chandragupta, which resisted Alexander's invasion in the fourth century and became the seat of the Ashoka empire a century later.

Between the third and first centuries B.C., several authors took up parts of the Bābhravya work in various treatises. The said authors are Chārāyana, Suvarnanābha, Ghotakamukha, Gonardīya, Gonikāputra, and more especially Dattaka who, with the aid of a famous courtesan of Pātaliputra, composed a work on courtesans which Vātsyāyana reproduces almost entirely.

The text of Suvarnanābha must date from the first century B.C., since it mentions a king of Kuntala (to the south of Pātaliputra), named

Shātakarni Shātavāhana, who reigned at this time and who killed his wife accidentally in the course of sadistic practices.

On the other hand, Yashodhara, at the beginning of his commentary, attributes the origin of erotic science to Mallanāga, the "prophet of the Asuras" (the ancient gods), meaning to prehistoric times. Nandi, Shiva's companion, is then said to have transcribed it for mankind today. The attribution of the first name Mallanāga to Vātsyāyana is due to the confusion of his role as editor of the *Kāma Sūtra* with that of the mythical creator of erotic science.

The Author of the Kāma Sūtra

Vātsyāyana appears to have been a Brahman and a great man of letters, residing in the city of Pātaliputra around the fourth century A.D., at a time of widespread cultural effervescence known as the Gupta period. The fact that Varāha Mihira in his *Brihad Samhitā*, dating from the sixth century, draws his inspiration from the *Kāma Sūtra*, and the mention of King Shātakarni Shātavāhana, who lived in the first century B.C., determines the limits for the possible dates of the *Kāma Sūtra*.

According to Vātsyāyana, the various works belonging to the *Kāma Shāstra* had become difficult to access. For this reason, he undertook to collect them and summarize them in his *Kāma Sūtra*, which thus became the classic work on the subject.

It was while staying in the city of Benares for purposes of religious study that he managed to collect the works from which he drew his inspiration and from which he quotes important passages. The *Kāma Sūtra* thus describes the customs of the Maurya period (fourth century B.C.), reviewed during the Gupta period (fourth century A.D.). The fact that the *Kāma Sūtra* is a compilation of works of the Maurya period explains the similarities in composition and style with the *Artha Shāstra* of Kautilya, the minister of Chandragupta, as well as the numerous references to this work.

The *Kāma Sūtra* does not claim to be an original work, but a compilation. Vātsyāyana states, on the other hand, that he himself had checked through personal experience the practices he describes.

The *Kāma Sūtra* is not a pornographic work. It is merely an impartial and systematic study of one of the essential aspects of existence. First and foremost, it is a picture of the art of living for the civilized and refined citizen, completing in the sphere of love, eroticism, and the pleasures of life, those parallel treatises of politics and economy and ethics, the *Artha Shāstra* and *Dharma Shāstra*, to which it makes constant reference.

Eroticism is firstly a search for pleasure, and the goal of the techniques of love is to attain a paroxysm considered by the *Upanishads* as a perception of the divine state, which is infinite delight. The refinements of love and the pleasures that include music and other arts are only possible in a prosperous civilization, which is why the *Kāma Shāstra*, the art of love, is linked to the *Artha Shāstra*, the rules of prosperity and the art of making money. Poverty is not a virtue. According to Vātsyāyana, indeed, it is an obstacle, not only to pleasure, but also to ethics and virtue. Morality is a luxury which very poor people can rarely afford.

Tradition and Commentaries

As is the custom in all Hindu technical works, including the dictionary, grammar, and scientific treatises, the text of the *Kāma Sūtra* is written in a condensed, versified form (sūtra), meant to be memorized with explanations provided by a teacher. The commentaries are thus an integral part of the teaching. Those transcribed at any given period are not therefore new interpretations, but represent tradition, without which the text would be incomplete. The *Kāma Shāstra* is a typical example of this. Considered as a supplementary science to religious tradition, it forms part of the traditional teaching to be studied by children and adolescents.

The texts that have come down to us, often purely by chance, are never presented as original works. Nevertheless, it is sometimes possible, according to certain indications, to have an approximate idea of the period in which they were composed or edited. The *Kāma Sūtra*, its sources and commentaries, represent a continuous tradition. Vātsyāyana declares that he only quotes and condenses previous works, and modestly speaks of himself in the third person, "Vātsyāyana's opinion is that . . . ," when he adds an opinion of his own.

Around the twelfth century, at the time when the Shaivite renewal gave rise to a considerable development in sacred architecture, of which the temples of Khajuraho with their innumerable erotic sculptures are the best-known example, a great scholar, Yashodhara, wrote the highly important commentary on Vātsyāyana's text, called the *Jayamangalā*, which is included here. The text of Yashodhara's commentary, rendered in italics in the text, does not present a new interpretation, but is an integral part of tradition. The same is true for the modern Hindi commentary by Devadatta Shāstrī, (rendered in roman type in the text), whose quotations from parallel sources earlier or later than Vātsyāyana's *Kāma Sūtra* represent a precious contribution to our knowledge of the concepts of eroticism. Shāstrī's modern commentary shows the continuity of concept and teaching of the *Kāma Sūtra* down to our own times.

Other Sanskrit commentaries also exist, but those which have come down to us are later and less important, such as the *Sūtra Vritti* by Narsingha Shāstrī in the eighteenth century.

It would clearly be possible to consider only Vātsyāyana's condensed text, as has already been done, and translate it, despite its difficulty and the problems raised by the interpretation of technical terms. In order to reach an exact interpretation of the Hindu concept of the art of love, however, it cannot be separated from its commentaries and its teaching tradition.

Considered as one of the supplementary texts to the sacred books of Hinduism, the *Kāma Sūtra* retains a surprising topicality. It is a breviary of love valid for all times and places.

The Translation

The full translation of the commentaries inevitably gives rise to repetition, while deference to the text causes a stylistic maladroitness for which I apologize. I have, first and foremost, sought not to transpose it into modern language and run the risk of detracting from the authors' thought in a text that is considered sacred.

Terminology often presents problems, since dictionaries do not give the meaning of technical terms, thus adding confusion. Thus, the word *yoga* means "sexual intercourse," *tantra* means "technique," *upanishad* "occult and magical practices." For *svairinī* (lesbians), the dictionary gives "corrupt woman," neither does it give the meaning of *adhorata* "anal coition," and so forth.

The terminology is often allusive and humorous: When the lesbian kisses her partner's goatee and, seizing her chin, slips her finger in the slit, the pubis is clearly meant; the instrument, *yantra*, or the phallus, *linga*, in some places signify the male organ and sometimes the dildo; and some of the rather tedious ways of enumerating all the situations possible are more an exercise in logic for the student than true descriptions.

Society

Society is the hierarchical society of India, with its castes—Brahmans, warrior-princes, merchants, monks, and workers' corporations—which collaborate without any problem. Marriage and procreation between different social groups is not recommended in the children's interests, although amorous relations are very free. Buddhist monks are mentioned.

The Citizen

The work is essentially addressed to the citizen (nāgaraka), meaning a wealthy, cultivated bourgeois male who is an art-lover and either a merchant or civil servant living in a large city.

The citizen is first and foremost a merchant or landed proprietor, awaiting the arrival of ships laden with goods, or the harvest of his crops. The arts play an important role in his life, especially music, dancing, painting, the theater, and literature. The list of arts given in the *Kāma Sūtra* has often been reproduced in other works.

Although erotic techniques concern all men, the refinements of the art of love are only possible if one possesses a pleasant dwelling with comfortable beds, bathrooms, reception rooms, gardens, flowers, and scents.

The citizen was not a vegetarian. He ate all kinds of meat and drank wine and strong spirits whether at receptions or while making love. A beverage based on Indian hemp, nowadays called bhang, was also widely used.

The City

For Vātsyāyana, as for his predecessors, the "great city" is Pāṭaliputra, an immense town and river port, situated on the Ganges between Benares and Calcutta. It could be compared to present-day Calcutta, itself a river port and great commercial and cultural center.

The town still exists and has retained its popular name Patna, an abbreviation of Pāṭaliputra Nāgara, but the sinking of the water level has reduced its role as a port. In Vātsyāyana's day, sea transport extended to Southeast Asia, Africa, and even Europe. At that time, the Romans had important entrepots in the south of India. Ptolemy's geography mentions the main cities of the Indian subcontinent.

The *Kāma Sūtra* describes the customs of various regions of India, whose territory included Gandhara (present-day Afghanistan) and Bactria (Tadjikistan).

Women

At the time of the Bābhravyas, as in Vātsyāyana's own time, women enjoyed great freedom. The *Kāma Sūtra* obviously describes the duties of the faithful wife attending solely to her family and her household, but, at the same time, it also indicates all the ways of seducing her and inviting her to deceive her husband. For form's sake, it cites the various kinds of marriage mentioned in the books of law, but recommends the love-marriage, or gāndharva marriage, and explains how to seduce the girl—who often appears to have been merely a child—with gifts of dolls and toys.

The remarriage of widows, later forbidden, was accepted. Although polygamy was widespread, Vātsyāyana extols the advantages of having a single wife. It is, above all, in speaking of the royal harem that he describes, not without humor, the sometimes wearisome side of the sovereign's obligation to satisfy numerous wives and deal with the intrigues of the seraglio.

Suttee, the widow's sacrifice on her husband's pyre, is only mentioned in the modern commentary.

Courtesans

Courtesans played an important role in urban society. They were the ornaments of the city. Familiar with the arts, it is through them that the refined techniques of music and dance were transmitted, a role they continue to play even nowadays.

Some of the most famous female dancers and musicians at the beginning of the twentieth century still belonged to this corporation. The nobility and purity of style of the arts has seen a marked decline since women of the rich bourgeoisie have begun to take their place in the artistic world.

A remarkable picture of the life and role of courtesans is given in *Manimekhalaï*, a Tamil novel written by the merchant-prince Shattan, a contemporary of Vātsyāyana's.

Courtesans could command a considerable fee and made generous contributions to social and religious works, such as the building of temples and pools for ritual baths.

During the Dattaka period, when the *Artha Shāstra* was composed and from which Vātsyāyana quotes, the fee for prostitutes of lower rank was fixed by the government, and they paid taxes. In Vātsyāyana's own time, they were free to negotiate the price of their services. The institution of the devadāsī, female dancers attached to the temples, does not appear and is not even referred to in Yashodhara's commentary, although it must have existed at his time.

It was as a result of the Shaivite renewal between the ninth and fourteenth centuries that the great temples were built. These were vast religious precincts comprising numerous sanctuaries, pools for ablutions, booths supplying flowers, and other accessories necessary for the rites, as well as a theater called the dance hall, in which plays of a religious nature were given. Each temple possessed groups of dancers, forming an important corps de ballet. Professional female dancers and musicians by definition belonged to the social category of courtesans, whether or not they sold their charms, a commerce which did not take place within the sacred precinct.

The Muslim conquerors captured hundreds of these women as booty of war and, later on, the British authorities, with puritanical indignation, forbade the association of "prostitutes" with the Hindus' sacred places, to the great detriment of artistic tradition which, secularized, still exists in the Bharata Nātyam. I knew Bālā Sarasvati, the last of the great dancers belonging to that profession, very well. With her unrivalled talent and without any accessories, she could, by her gestures, evoke the beauty of a garden, the surprise of a flower opening out, the anguish of a woman in love, a hero scaling a mountain. I also knew well Siddheshvari Devi, the famous singer of Benares, who still lived in the special district of the town. Both were incomparable artists, wholly dedicated to their art and their inner vision, which they expressed by gesture and word, without any trace of the vulgar winks and smiles to the audience that are too often a feature of those artists belonging to the bourgeoisie who have succeeded them.

The association of prostitution with the theatrical profession is not peculiar to India. In the West, dancers and famous actresses were "kept" women, or else practised serial marriage. The Ouled Nail dancers in North Africa belonged to a caste of courtesans.

Sacred prostitution has never existed in India, even though temple dancers belonged to the caste of courtesans, whose profession was dancing. Furthermore, the rare hierogamies of Vedic ritual did not take place in the temples and public women were not used for the mystical couplings of tantric rites except in modern times, as mentioned by Devadatta Shāstrī's commentary.

Troupes of male dancers also existed, for the staging of religious legends. This tradition has survived in the Katha Kali. I lived for a long period at the school created by the great poet Vallathol in order to preserve the tradition of theater art, the aim of which was to make known to the public the sacred legends concerning the gods and the mighty deeds of the heroes. Moreover, in the spectacles known as Rāma Līlā and Krishna Līlā, all the roles are played by boys dressed as women.

Sexual Variants

Lesbianism is described in detail, as well as the inversion of roles by a dominating female. Male homosexuality forms an integral part of sexual life and various homosexual practices are described in detail. Transvestite prostitutes play a role in public life, and their presence at weddings and religious ceremonies was considered a symbol of good luck down to our own times.

All sexual variations, including relations with animals, are mentioned in the *Kāma Sūtra* and are represented with great emphasis on the façades of great temples, such as those at Khajuraho, as well as many others abandoned in the jungle, which I have been able to visit.

Puritanism in Modern India

In the country of the *Kāma Sūtra*, where amorous ecstasy is assimilated to mystic experience, to that perception of the divine that is supreme enjoyment, the puritanism of modern India, arising from Islamic and Anglo-Saxon prejudice, is all the more stupefying, although it largely only concerns the managerial classes with English education.

Mahatma Gandhi, educated in England, sent squads of his disciples to smash the erotic representations on the temples. It was the poet Rabindranath Tagore who managed to halt this iconoclastic massacre. Pandit Nehru was irritated by my having photographed and published the photographs of sculptures showing homosexual relations, dating from the eleventh century, when he claimed that such vices in India were due to Western influence. The blossoming of sexuality and all its variants has never formerly been persecuted in India. It was only starting with the new penal code promulgated by Nehru's socialist government that, for the first time, article 377 punished "sexual relations against nature with a man, woman or animal, whether the intercourse is anal or oral."

The country of the *Kāma Sūtra* had thus been relegated to the level of the most backward countries in the sphere of liberty.

The intelligent traveler can, however, outside official circles, find amorous adventures that show that the people of India have forgotten nothing of the teachings of the *Kāma Sūtra*.

Erotic Sculpture and Painting

Indian sculptures representing the various sexual positions, group sex, homosexual practices, and relations with animals are justly famous. Photographs of the same can be found in my book *Erotisme divinisé*. According to legend, they protect the temples from lightning.

Paintings representing intercourse have always formed part of popular art. They are still to be seen today on the earth walls of village homes, or on the pottery used for weddings for which they are deemed of good omen.

At the same time, it seemed to me to be a mistake to illustrate the *Kāma Sūtra* with pornographic drawings from the Muslim period, and in particular with miniatures which, whatever their artistic merits, evidence a state of mind that is completely foreign to that of the sacred text.

Texts Quoted in the Commentaries

The first commentary, the *Jayamangalā* by Yashodhara, over and above the works mentioned by Vātsyāyana, also quotes from:

The *Manu Smriti*
The *Nyāya Sūtra* by Gautama
The *Markandeya Purāna*, attributed to Bhargava
The *Nātya Shāstra* by Bharata
The *Nīti Shāstra* by Shukra.

The modern commentary in Hindi by Devadatta Shāstrī takes into account a great number of works prior to the *Kāma Sūtra*, starting with the *Atharva Veda* and the *Upanishads* influenced by Shaivite tradition.

He also quotes from the *Mahābhārata*, the *Purānas*, the *Nātya Shāstra*, the *Nīti Shāstra* and the various works on eroticism sometimes edited later than the *Kāma Sūtra*, but deriving from the same sources and showing numerous parallels, such as:

The *Kuchumāra Tantra*

The *Rati Rahasya* by Kokkoka

The *Panchashāyaka* or *Dashashāyaka* by Jyotirīshvara

The *Smara Pradīpika* by Gunākara, son of Vāchaspati

The *Rati Manjari* by Jayadeva

The *Rasa Manjari* by Bhānudatta

The *Ananga Ranga* by Kalyānamalla (around 1500)

The *Kuttinīmata* by Damodara Gupta.

The literary and historical works, codes of ethics and politics mentioned are:

The *Nāgarsarvasva* by Padmashrī

The *Ujjvala Nīlamani* by Rūpagoswāmī and its commentary by Jīvagoswāmī

The *Naishadīya Charita* by Harsha

The *Brihad Samhitā* by Varāhamihira

The *Gītā Govinda* by Jayadeva

The *Harsha Charita* by Bāna

The *Mālatī Mādhava* by Bhavabhūti

The *Svapna Vāsavādatta* by Bhāsa

The *Mricchakatikā* by Shudraka

The *Kādambarī* by Bāna

The *Sarasvatī Kanthābharana*

The *Dashakumāra Charita* by Dandin

The *Sāhitya Darpana*, history of literature

The *Kāvya Prakāsha* by Mammata

The *Kāla Vilāsa* by Kshemendra

The *Lalita Vistara*

The *Shishupālavadha* by Māgha

The *Kirātārjuna* by Bhāravi

The *Shakuntalā* by Kālīdāsa

The *Bhoja Prabandha* by Vallabha.

Part One
General Remarks

Chapter One

CONTENTS OF
THE BOOK

- *Invocation*
- *Origin and development of erotic science, or Kāma Shāstra*
- *Summary of subjects dealt with in the Kāma Sūtra*

1–2 Praised be the three aims of life, virtue [dharma], prosperity [artha], and love [kāma], which are the subject of this work.

Why does Vātsyāyana begin his work thus, without invoking other gods? It is in order to explain this that I have written this commentary.

There are four social functions in this world, namely the priest's, the warrior's, the merchant's, and the artisan's, as well as four stages of life, that of the student, the married man, withdrawal into the forest, and the mendicant monk. For Brahmans and others, so long as they are heads of a family, the search for spiritual realization is not practicable, and the aims of life are limited to three. The advocates of eroticism consider that love, given its results, is the most important inasmuch as virtue and prosperity both depend on it and without it they would not exist. According to the most ancient scholars, the prophet of the Asuras, Mallanāga, created this science after studying its means of accomplishment. Treatises have been written on the ways to acquire

15

virtue and wealth, but love, being practiced with another person, requires other methods, methods concerning mutual relations. Such methods are expounded in the Kāma Shāstra, *and not in works on economy* [Artha Shāstra] *or ethics* [Dharma Shāstra]. *Because it depends on relations with another, because it deals with men and women, love requires a know-how that is explained only in the* Kāma Sūtra.

The methods indicated by erotic science are easy to put into practice, but are difficult for those who act alone or who follow the opinions of someone who does not know the Kāma Sūtra. *Inventing procedures one knows nothing about is like trying to read a text from the channels traced in wood by worms: its accomplishment is absolutely impossible for the ignorant.*

Since there are so many ways of doing things, townsmen cannot without instruction behave like men of culture. That is the reason for the saying, "Those that claim to accomplish something without knowing its theory are like those who read texts traced by worms."

Although those that know the texts may make mistakes if they are clumsy in putting them into practice, it is not the fault of the texts. The texts are valid for all cases. Not everyone follows the same rules of eating and drinking, laid down in medical books. First of all, one must respect and venerate the Scriptures and try to understand their meaning, before putting them into practice.

This is why, before bowing down before the gods, Vātsyāyana first invokes the Scriptures, in order to remove any obstacles that may hinder the composition of his work, hence the opening invocation, "I bow before virtue, wealth, and love," since the aim of this work is to teach virtue, prosperity, and eroticism, which are mutually interdependent.

"The first things mentioned are those to which one wishes to give importance," says the proverb. This treatise begins by mentioning love, together with virtue and wealth, which are the three aims of life, and it teaches the means of attaining them.

"The three aims must be pursued simultaneously, since they are connected to each other and are of the same nature." Although procreation is connected to ethics and material goods, however, erotic desire (rati) is an instinctive impulse, and is not tied to the pursuit of an aim.

In considering the order of values, the gods are the most important, but their worship depends on speech. Virtue and prosperity are defined by words. The gods cannot be greeted without using words. The gods' supremacy, moreover, depends on their worshipers.

Love is necessary to satisfy the mind, ethics to satisfy the conscience, and spiritual seeking for peace of soul. Without food and clothes, the body becomes thin and weak. Without eroticism, the mind becomes restless and unsatisfied. Without virtue (ethics), the conscience goes astray. Without spirituality, the soul is degraded.

This is why, even with the spiritual life in view, it is necessary to earn money and enjoy women. Whoever seeks money and pleasure without taking spiritual values into account is a materialist and sensualist. When people are only attached to money and pleasure, the decadence of their country is inevitable. Only when profit and pleasure are controlled by ethics can they become instruments of spiritual progress, but not if they are contrary to ethics. That is why Master Vātsyāyana, in his *Kāma Sūtra*, describes a moral eroticism leading to spiritual realization, and not the sating of the passions or the encouragement of pleasure seekers.

3–4 I also salute the sages of old, who expounded the concepts of their own time concerning our subject.

"I bow before the wise men who have taught us the concepts of ethics, prosperity, and love of their own time, since such concepts are not permanent, but change according to custom. I therefore bow before the writings representing the values of a certain epoch, and not before others."

The masters of old were wont to say that ethics are based on knowledge. Prosperity and ethics are the cornerstones of civilization. Without satisfaction of a material kind, no interest is felt for the spiritual life. Just as the soul needs the spiritual life, the conscience needs ethics, the mind love, and the body requires well-being. Without well-being and sexuality, no form of life can exist.

Like ethics and prosperity, sexuality is one of the bases of civilization. Eroticism, like ethics and money, is an aid to spiritual realization.

The fundamental aspirations of the individual are of three kinds: alimentary, sexual, and social. To fulfill the desire for wealth, procreation, and reputation is the very source of happiness.

The *Taittirīya Upanishad* says that "beings issued forth from bliss (ānanda). Born of bliss, all things and all living creatures live in bliss and dissolve in bliss. Bliss is everything."

The instrument for measuring success or failure in life is happiness. If something is lacking, it is considered an injustice.

Man derives happiness from his relationship to or with things.

In his commentary on the *Brahma Sūtra*, Shankarāchārya says, "In every misfortune to my wife or children, I see a personal injury."

The coupling of one being with another is called Eros, uniting the object of desire with its possessor. Primeval energy is compared to erotic desire, "He was alone and became aware of it" (*Brihad Āranyaka*, 1.4.1). The spirit was alone. He knew he was male, but knew no one beside himself. His first word was "I am," but it did not give him pleasure. That is why he desired to be two. The second was the object of his desire, which, gradually, took on multiple forms.

This desire, which is the origin of everything, is the procreative Eros. But, with the manifestation of duality, fear also appeared in his mind. Fear begot rejection and then attachment manifested itself once more, since alone there is no enjoyment.

Fear comes from difference and, where difference exists, the desire for possession becomes manifest in order to destroy fear. Thus are established the dualities of attraction/repulsion, attachment/detachment, love/hate, desire/fear, which are manifestations of the creative illusion (māyā).

In the *Shiva Purāna*, it is said that "the power to create comes from Eros." Vātsyāyana defines Eros as the tendency to seek to satisfy hearing, touch, sight, taste, and smell, which are mental activities. The Shaivas like the Shaktas consider creation as copulation. "Nāda, primordial sound, represents the copulation of Shiva and Shakti. The idea is that duality precedes the birth of the Word (shabda) and that duality implies a relation, or copulation, between two principles. Respect, devotion, love, affection, sympathy, friendship, courtship, embraces, kisses are all manifestations of attraction, of relations of an erotic kind. Eros inflames the mind. All philosophical systems consider that "the principle of Kāma precedes the creative word" (*Rig Veda*).

Indeed, desire is the seed of thought, the first thing that appears in a child's mind. Eros is an immense force, manifest in the feelings, emotions, and impulses of human beings. It is the first of the gods, the prime force that activates the mechanism of the mind.

In his *Kāma Sūtra*, Vātsyāyana has summarized the works of ancient authors. In acknowledgement of his debt, he bows before them.

5　Prajāpati, the Lord of the Creatures, after creating man, composed a treatise of one hundred thousand verses, defining the rules of social life at the triple level of civic virtue, prosperity, and sexuality.

6 Manu, the son of the god born of himself, set aside the aphorisms concerning civic virtues and ethics in his *Dharma Shāstra.*

7 Brihaspati set aside the aphorisms concerning politics, economy, and prosperity in his *Artha Shāstra.*

8 Shiva's companion, Nandi, set aside the one thousand chapters concerning sexuality, thus creating the *Kāma Shāstra.*

9 Shvetaketu, the son of Uddalaka, summarized Nandi's *Kāma Shāstra* in five hundred chapters.

10 Later on, the sons of Babhru, of the country of Panchāla, reduced the five hundred chapters of Shvetaketu to one hundred and fifty, grouped in seven parts, under the titles General Remarks, Amorous Advances, The Choice of a Wife, A Wife's Duties and Rights, Relations with Other Men's Wives, On Courtesans, Occult Practices.

11 Dattaka, after consulting the courtesans of Pātaliputra, summarized the sixth chapter on prostitutes in a separate work, called *Kāma Shāstra.*

12 Similarly, Chārāyana set forth separately the chapter of general remarks [sadharana], Suvarnanābha the chapter on erotic approaches [samprayoga], Ghotakamukha the one on the art of seducing girls [kanyāsamprayukta], Gonardīya the one on the wife's duties and rights [bhāryād hikarikā], Gonikāputra the one on relations with other men's women [paradārikā], Kuchumāra on occult practices (aupanishadika).

13 Thus it came about that, divided by different authors into separate works, this science had almost vanished.

14 By publishing the various chapters separately, Dattaka and the others had lost the overall concept and, due to its length, the text of the Bābhravyas [the sons of Babhru] was difficult to study, which is why Vātsyāyana summarized the great work of the sons of Babhru and [correcting some lacunae] composed the *Kāma Sūtra.*

15 The contents of the various chapters are as follows:

16 The first part, "General Remarks," comprises five chapters dealing with five subjects:

Contents of the book

The realization of the three aims of life

The counsels of common sense

Behavior of the educated man

Reflections on the use of intermediaries to assist the
lover

17   The second part, "Amorous Advances," comprises ten
chapters dealing with seventeen subjects:

The possibilities of the moment and of the feelings

Various manifestations of love

Embraces and caresses

Kisses

The art of scratching

Biting

Behavior in various countries

Matters of intercourse

Peculiar tastes

Of slaps and accompanying sighs

Mannish women

Sodomization of boys

Buccal coition

Behavior before and after the act

Variations on the sexual act

Lovers' quarrels

18   The third part, "Acquiring a Wife," comprises five chapters dealing with nine subjects:

Questions of choice

Decision to unite

Inspiring confidence in the girl

First overtures to the girl

Interpretation of her behavior

Union with one man only

Arousing the girl's desire

Persuading the girl thus prepared to unite

Marriage

19   The fourth part, "Duties and Privileges of the Wife,"
comprises two chapters dealing with eight subjects:

The wife must love none but her husband

Living in his place of residence
Respect for the chief wife
Behavior toward younger wives
Accepting the arrival of a new wife
Behavior of the repudiated wife
Final duty
The husband's behavior toward many wives

20 The fifth part, "Relations with Other Men's Wives," comprises six chapters dealing with ten subjects:

The establishment of a mutual attachment between man and woman
Obstacles
Men that please women
Women able to free themselves
Opportunities for getting to know each other
Meetings
Examination of feelings
The procurer's role
The rich lover
The guards at the entry to the harem

21 The sixth part, "About Courtesans," comprises six chapters dealing with twelve subjects:

Reflections on prospective customers
Reasons in favor of sexual relations
The means of seduction
Behaving like a lover
Means of achieving one's aims
Signs of detachment
How to get back a man who breaks away
How to get rid of a lover
Restarting an old affair
Special profits
Reflections on the advantages and disadvantages of a relationship
Various kinds of courtesan

This chapter describes the conduct (charitra) of prostitutes and the ways of sleeping with them. Vātsyāyana deems that keeping company with prostitutes is a bad thing in itself, harmful to ethics and health, but that prostitutes belong to society and society uses them. For this reason, in the interest of both prostitutes and society, their characteristics are studied in this chapter.

Experience shows that eroticism is a powerful, but highly unstable, force. This power grows according to the development of the feelings and impulses. Each amatory desire (vāsanā) is matched by an emotional experience. When our longings form a knot, it is called vāsanā. The intensity of amatory desire is manifest in the sexual impulse. An emotional state consists of favorable, or contrary, feelings rising in a man's heart.

An attachment that grows gradually takes the form of a sexual impulse or erotic excitement. The presence or remembrance of a person, or love (premā) for an imaginary person, arouses the sexual impulse. The presence of a sexual object, in one way or the other, causes a state of excitement (samvega). The *Bhagavad Gītā* says, "Kāma (sexual attraction) is born from contact, and from attraction is born excitement. All amatory desire causes excitement."

The attachments of the mind (chittavritti) are made up of knowledge, feeling (bhāva), and action (kriyā). Perception (jñāna) awakens feeling (bhāva) and sexual impulse. Innumerable sparks accumulate in the mind's whirl, stimulating erotic energy.

Every individual seeks variations of feeling: change, novelty, the taste for beauty, are all part of man's nature. According to the *Yoga Vasishtha*, "at the moment at which it is obtained, a thing gives you immediate satisfaction, but if you do not obtain it at once, you tend to idealize it."

Novelty is another name for desire (abhiruchi). We always take pleasure in whatever is new. The sexual impulse makes our actions unpredictable. Commencing out of mere curiosity, the thirst for satisfaction (trishna) soon appears.

Once the sexual impulse is fully awakened, a day waiting for one's lover seems an eternity.

When the presence of the object provoking our passion is denied, our heart is in pain, our spirit fettered, and our mind troubled. A great effort is needed to behave according to the dictates of society. Thus, from age to age, society has experienced the impossibility of controlling erotic impulses. Society's control is limited to the physical deeds resulting from passion, but the rebellion of the mind is still very powerful. One of the principles of this experience is that, in not allowing the passions to surface, they can be checked, but not rooted out.

When we repress our desires, they do not disappear but stay beneath the surface and continue to exert their influence. Prohibition arouses desire and suggests stratagems for satisfying it. From an ethical and social point of view, relations with other men's wives are to be condemned. Copulation with them is forbidden. The result is that other men's wives are considered to be the most piquant. This is taken into account by Vātsyāyana in composing the chapter on courtesans, in considering the good of society.

22   The seventh part concerning occult media [aupanisha-dika] comprises two chapters dealing with six subjects:

Means for becoming attractive

How to infatuate

How to increase sexual drive and achieve multiple coition

How to develop the sexual organ

Reviving a failing impulse

Unusual copulation

Becoming attractive means improving one's appearance and qualities.

To infatuate signifies taking control over someone by means of words, diagrams, and magic rites.

Sexual drive can be increased thanks to aphrodisiacs.

Methods exist for increasing the size of the penis, as well as for reviving the ardor of one who has become impotent.

This text has a double basis, since it is connected with Tantrism.

Excitation caused by magic involves sexual practices of a Tantric nature, which is why a chapter has been set apart to deal with magic practices. Such practices are not, however, very widespread. In sexual relations, magic practices also give results, which is why they are dealt with, since magical practices and their results form part of the subject.

23   Thus terminates the summary of the thirty-six chapters dealing with sixty-four subjects in seven parts and 1250 verses of these teachings based on earlier works.

24   Having established the plan in summary form, it will be reexamined in detail, since in this world, men of culture need to study matters both as a summary and in detail.

Vātsyāyana has called this seventh chapter "aupanishadika," a word with the popular meaning of "magic." This chapter examines in detail the means of achieving sexual inclinations (kāma vāsanā), with a view to success in the life of this world. What is written concerning magical practices in the form of drugs, etc., involves procedures that are effective, but not without risk, and are antisocial and unethical. They imply a form of risk, which must be clearly borne in mind.

Magical practices, diagrams, formulas, and rites are part of Indian culture. In all its literature, beginning with the *Rig Veda* and *Atharva Veda* down to our own days, they have always been a part of everyday life in India. For this reason, careful attention should be paid to Vātsyāyana's words, since his aim is the pleasure and happiness of mankind. In reading it, ordinary people should neither be upset nor misled, since he refers constantly to the virtues of chastity and nonviolence.

End of the First Chapter
Contents of the Book
of the First Part entitled General Remarks

Chapter Two

THE THREE AIMS OF LIFE

1 During the one hundred years of his life, a man must pursue the three aims successively, without one being prejudicial to another.

During the first three periods of his life, a man must realize himself on three interdependent levels, which are virtue [dharma], wealth [artha], and love [kāma], harmonizing them in such a way that none is prejudicial to the others.

Holy scripture describes the three aims that women, notwithstanding their dependence on men, must also achieve on their side. For the man who wishes to have progeny, the sexual relations without desire that he must have with his legitimate wife concern virtue and interest; if desire exists, then virtue and eroticism are involved.

Approaches to a girl of a good family, made with marriage in mind, are a matter of self-interest and virtue. On the other hand, approaches made to a married woman or a girl of low social level in order to gain her favors are a question of money and eroticism. Approaches to one's wife for nonprocreative loveplay involve eroticism and virtue.

Approaches toward a married woman of whatever social condition in return for money are tied to eroticism and money. Approaches made for the purpose of sexual relations to an unmarried girl who is a virgin concern ethics, society, and eroticism. If the girl to be seduced comes from a good family, the social aspect is the most important, although tied to eroticism and ethics. Due to its social consequences, mutual desire concerns ethics, society, and eroticism.

All men desire long life, knowledge, fame, love, justice, and final salvation. Living beings other than man seek only survival.

Only the teaching of the *Vedas*, while giving due importance to longevity, the satisfaction of all human desires, and the equal rights of all, leads to liberation. For long life, pure food (sāttvika) is most important. Those who are careful about food avoid sickness, and are always happy and cheerful. Moreover, they acquire qualities connected with good luck, such as strength, beauty, intelligence, memory, and patience. Apart from food, air, water, and exercise are factors of a long life. Beside these, anxiety must be avoided. "Just as fire burns the dead, so anxiety burns the living and reduces them to ashes." Another element of long life is continence. The yoga texts speak of chastity as a "gain of sperm" (vīryalābha). The wise man who controls his sperm is death's conqueror.

2 Childhood must be dedicated to acquiring knowledge.

This period lasts up to the age of sixteen.

3 Eroticism predominates in adulthood.

4 Old age must be dedicated to the practice of virtue and spiritual pursuit [moksha].

Although a certain period of life is attributed to the practice of each of the three aims, they are interdependent and present at all ages.

5 Since life's duration is uncertain, all opportunities must be taken advantage of.

6 Celibacy is recommended during the period of study, for the acquiring of knowledge.

7 Discernment concerns apparent as well as invisible things. Due to their supernatural and invisible results, the practice of yajña and other ritual ceremonies can only be

known through the sacred texts. Since their nature is material and visible, actions such as abstaining from meat, because forbidden by the texts, are a matter of morality or dharma.

Since life's duration is uncertain, must a child be deprived of erotic realization? Vātsyāyana endeavors to answer this question by quoting: "Knowledge must be acquired while living chastely."

According to Vātsyāyana, after the rite of shaving the head, one should learn to read and count. After the rite of the sacred string, one should study the three sciences (traya vidyā) with respected masters and scholars. Up to sixteen years of age, one should remain chaste. Then, having accomplished the rite of the gift of a cow, one should marry. Once married, one should keep contact with persons of culture, since contact with well-informed people is the basis of progress and the increase of knowledge. Vātsyāyana and Kautilya insist on the importance of study and chastity in youth, inasmuch as control over the senses is necessary for progress in learning. It is by dominating eroticism, anger, envy, vanity, excitement, and exhilaration that the senses can be kept under control.

Virtue is of two kinds, inclination toward certain actions and detachment from others.

According to the *Mahābhārata*, the word *dharma* has a very wide meaning. It comes from the root *dhārana*: "support." The various meanings of the word are:

Good deed (sukriyā), merit (pūjya)
Accomplishment of the rites (vaidika vidhi, yajña, etc.)
Dharma-rājā, "The Judge," is the name of the regent of
    the infernal world
Law (nyāya)
The underlying nature (svabhāva) of beings
Conduct (āchāra)
The drinker of soma (the elixir of immortality)
Dharma also refers to:
The means of attaining future results by conduct required
    by the Scriptures
The behavior taught by Vedic or traditional texts
The invisible results of prescribed conduct
The individual or universal soul (ātman)

Proper conduct (sadāchāra)
The qualities (guna) of the individual
The relative value (upamā) of things
Ritual sacrifices (yajña)
Nonviolence
Keeping good company (satsangha)
Magical practices (upanishad)
Archery (dhanusha)
The ninth lunar house (in astrology)
Charity (dāna), etc.

According to the symbolic etymologies (*Nirukta*), the root of the word *dharma* means "that which supports the world." For the *Kāma Sūtra*, it means "rules of conduct." Virtue (dharma) is the source of happiness (sukha), which is of two kinds, in this world, or the next.

8 One must behave according to the instructions of those who know the Scriptures.

"The Veda is the basis of dharma" (Manu); eroticism (kāma) is the touchstone of virtue.

9 Artha signifies material goods, wealth. Artha consists of acquiring and increasing, within the limits of dharma, knowledge, land, gold, cattle, patrimony, crockery, furniture, friends, clothing, etc.

According to the Artha Shāstra *of Kautilya, Artha is the "means of existence of mankind" [manushya vritti].*

Dharma applies to the spirit, artha to the body. Without sexuality [kāma], the body would not be born at all, and without a body there is no future life.

10 It is from those that know their subject that one can decide the time for sowing or the methods for raising cattle.

The Artha Shāstra *explains all the techniques of economy and government, but there is a great difference between true knowledge and the texts that teach it.*

11 Kāma signifies the mental inclination [pravritti] to-

ward the pleasures of touch, sight, taste, and smell, to the extent that the practitioner derives satisfaction from it.

Kāma is the perception of the power of illusion [avidyā] materialized in an object, since from perception is born desire, attraction [ākarshana], ardor [samvega]. The tendency to possess oneself of these objects of the senses is eroticism [kāma].

Eroticism is of two kinds, general [pradhāna] or specific.

12 Particularly concerned with touch, closely connected to selfish pleasure, eroticism is an experience that finds its finality in itself. This is the most general aspect of Eros [prādhānya kāma].

The organs of action are the tongue, the hand, the foot, the anus, and the sexual organ. Of these, leaving aside the pleasures deriving from speech, the highest pleasure is the reciprocal discovery by man and woman of the natural differences of the lower part of their bodies, which are the vulva and the penis. This pleasure is connected with the sense of touch, seated particularly in the organ known as upastha [the sexual organ], which, in the act of procreation, causes wonderful bliss [ānanda].

This experience is essentially connected with the sense of touch.

A whirl of pleasurable sensations is connected with the perception of the organ of touch. The desire for such experience is the cause of the state of erotic excitement in both man and woman. In the woman, it manifests itself as a diffuse desire for contact with the man, while for the latter, it is desire of the pleasure of touching, especially the thighs and center of the body.

A specific desire [vishesha] is the urge to achieve a result [phala]. Seeking for sexual relations has its aim in the pleasure experienced at the moment sperm is emitted. This enjoyment is called the result [phala]. From the point of view of touch, this moment is a special experience, because the previous pleasurable sensations did not bear fruit.

Since this experience is oriented toward a goal, the sensation of touch is not its essence. The achievement of a goal is therefore distinct from eroticism.

Kissing, biting, and scratching with the nails, which serve to augment the erotic charge of both men and women, belong to general eroticism. They are not considered forms of possession.

The fact that the sexual act has a goal poses a difficult problem. Yashodhara considers as a whole the continuity of pleasure, starting from kisses and caresses up to the emission of sperm. Vātsyāyana, however, differs from Yashodhara since he considers procreation as the real goal. According to the Atharva Veda *[14.1 and 14.2], "Wife! Stretch yourself with pleasure on this bed and procreate sons for your husband. You will be blessed like the Queen of Heaven. You shall awake at dawn, before the rising of the sun."*

"Prudent men take a wife early, intermingling their bodies as they must. O thou astonishing creature, able to procreate children, unite with your husband!"

"O Supreme God that protectest this woman in whom I have today planted my seed, inspire her so that she realizes my wish, full of desire as I am, and that, opening her thighs, she allows my penis to assail her vagina." "Wife! I made my penis slide effortlessly along the path of your vagina, between your thighs. I marked with red this sublime union connected with the sun."

"Man! With your hand, stroke the virginal thighs of your wife and joyfully both beget a son so that the sun god will prolong your life."

"Let us throw into the fire, together with the blanket, the defilements we have left in the marriage act."

The meaning of these Vedic texts suggests that:

Love must be made at night so as to avoid fear, doubt, or inconvenience. Before copulating, embraces and caresses must be exchanged so that man and woman experience feelings of pleasure. Once the light is extinguished, caresses are not only made without shyness, but the pleasure is greater. Man and woman must take pleasure in the act with satisfaction and they must both take care not to injure the fetus. At the entry to the vagina, there is a delicate membrane that breaks at the first union. This is why the man must take care not to hurt the girl.

The act must be performed in the normal position, since children begotten in an abnormal posture are deformed. For reasons of hygiene and cleanliness, a bath must be taken after making love.

The *Chandogya Upanishad* compares the sexual act to the ritual of the *Sāma Veda*, "The message to the girl is the spark . . . ," etc.

13 Sexual behavior is to be learned with the aid of the Kāma Sūtra and the counsel of worthy men, experts in the arts of pleasure.

Without knowing the technical texts, a man who follows only his own fantasy knows neither success, happiness, nor supreme bliss. A master is one whose teachings lead to the achievement of virtue, success, and pleasure. In the *Upanishads*, after educating his disciple as well as he can, the master says, "Tell the truth, live honestly, never boast of your knowledge, do not fail to beget a son" (*Taittirīya Upanishad*).

In order not to break the ancestral line, it is important to have studied erotic arts before marriage, during one's period of study.

14   The relative importance and value of things must be taken into account. Money is more important than love, social success more important than success in love, and virtue is more important than success and fortune.

The ordinary virtues [sāmānya dharma] are nonviolence, honesty, chastity, avoiding anger and envy, striving to love all living beings equally. Vātsyāyana is in favor of the social hierarchy [varnāshrama], which is why he insists on the importance of equal feelings toward all beings.

15   Money is the basis of royal power. Life's journey is based on it. It is the means of realizing the three aims of life, even in the case of prostitutes.

Money is the basis of material life, which is why it is more important for a king than virtue or pleasure. For prostitutes, money and pleasure are closely connected. It is a king's duty to accumulate money, inasmuch as it is an instrument of power. For a prostitute, money is essential. She exchanges her body for money. She is an object of desire for the lustful Brahman as well as for the sensual citizen, but she is indifferent to love and ethics. Later on, when she gives up her trade, she lives as she wishes with the money she has put aside.

According to Kautilya, author of the *Artha Shāstra*, without money there is no virtue, without money, there can be no power. Uncontrolled eroticism leads to failure.

Vātsyāyana mentions both favorable and contrary opinions to the theses of the *Kāma Sūtra*.

16   The rules of virtue, which are connected with the spiritual life, can only be known through authoritative texts.

The secrets of material success, on the other hand, are a matter of experience, and the texts merely indicate how such experience should be put into practice.

Material success is a matter of accumulating goods. To start with, mistakes may be made, which is why it is useful to have a treatise on economy when in doubt.

As far as moral behavior is concerned, the *Taittirīya Aranyaka* defines the virtues connected with supernatural aims, which are:

Courage
The search for truth
Frankness
Listening to religious teachings
Serenity
Self-control
Clemency
Charity
Practicing the rites and worship of the Immense Being, present on earth, in the intermediate world, and in heaven

According to the *Smriti* of Yājñavalkya, the principles of ethical behavior are expounded in the fourteen annexes to the *Vedas*, which are: the ancient chronicles (*Purānas*), the historical narratives (*Itihāsa*), logic (*Nyāya*), Yoga, cosmology (*Sāmkhya*), ritual (*Mīmāmsā*), the moral codes (*Dharma Shāstra*), medicine (*Ayurveda*), the analysis of the texts (*Shikshā*), ritual (*Kalpa*), grammar (*Vyākarana*), etymologies (*Nirukta*), astrology (*Jyotisha*), and poetics (*Chanda*).

The field of material success is much wider than that of virtue. Final salvation concerns the soul. Virtue is a matter of discernment (buddhi). Eroticism is connected with the mind (manas). The means of existence are essential for bodily survival. Spirituality and virtue are the privilege of mankind, but no being can live without the means of existence and sexuality, whether man, animal, wild beast, bird, insect, or even plants and trees. For a short time, one can live without erotic practice, but not without the means of subsistence. This predominance of material goods forms part of the divine plan and should be carefully reflected on, since riches acquired dishonestly are an obstacle to spiritual realization. This is the reason for composing treatises regulating the material life. Rules of ethics concern all life's aspects. With regard to landed property and its upkeep, ancient authors have composed numerous treatises, which have been summarized by Kautilya in his *Artha Shāstra*, from which Vātsyāyana took his inspiration. The principal scope of the *Artha Shāstra* is the art of government (rājanīti), describing all man's material satisfactions. Economic problems find their solution in the *Artha Shāstra*.

17 Since eroticism is a universal natural phenomenon, common to all animals, certain authors ask why a treatise on eroticism is needed.

Having demonstrated the usefulness of the texts concerning material success and moral virtues, certain authors raise doubts about the utility of a treatise on eroticism.

They remark that, without having learned it, animals and birds incline to sexuality, which is thus a universal phenomenon. What need is there for directives in such a case?

Since it can be seen that cattle and other animals devoid of discernment have an inclination to eroticism without having received any instruction, is it not the same among mankind in all countries? For this reason, it is said, "Love is learned alone, without being taught by anyone. What teacher do the beasts need to give enjoyment to their partner? Given the compatibility of the partner's secretions, erotic desire is universal. It is said that those who want to succeed in life consider incompatibilities before making love. Even when his desire has a particular object, the wise man forgoes becoming attached. Even in the case of affection, the texts warn against realizing an attachment. The sages deem that virtue, interest, and pleasure must be coordinated.

The question of amorous advances will now be dealt with.

18 Given the importance of the preliminary acts [samprayoga], man and woman need rules of conduct.

The preliminaries of love often depend on convention. These amorous approaches are of two kinds, according to whether they take place inside the house [āyatana] or outside [anga]. Amorous approaches inside the house take place in the woman's residence, while those outside take place in the countryside [malya].

"Love is easy in gardens, stimulated by beautiful ornaments and beauty products. It takes place within nature, beneath arbors, to the

sound of the lute, and so on. It is better for young people, who fear the constrictions of the home and desire to amuse themselves without interruptions or problems."

Loveplay in the home is of two kinds: before witnesses and in private. Loveplay practiced in secret permits varied kinds of expression, while the forms practiced in front of witnesses will be described in dealing with lovemaking.

Love in the garden [anga samprayoga] is when one decides to utilize the garden for sensual pleasures. If the aim is merely to bring together the organs of the senses, the amatory practices are classified as ordinary. If both parties have already had erotic experience, they do as explained above, otherwise nothing happens.

The characteristics of amorous behavior during a first meeting are as follows: If the man and the woman do not desire each other, they are both on the defensive and, from modesty or fear, they do not give themselves to each other. Expedients must then be found. What means has a man ignorant of the sixty-four positions of copulation of achieving the act? If he does not know how to perform, he will not achieve anything with his partner, whether occasional or permanent. It is necessary to know about foreplay.

Those who do not seek to understand the profound mystery of a universal law, present in all things, contest the value of a sacred treatise on eroticism.

Considering that eroticism, copulation (maithuna), is an end in itself, alike for man and beast, certain lawgivers do not see the utility of an erotic treatise. They claim that the *Kāma Sūtra* only gives rise to ill conduct. This shows that their mind is not very alert and that they seek to impose their own prejudices.

Vātsyāyana's opinion is that knowledge of the *Kāma Shāstra* is necessary for those that are paralyzed by modesty or fear, or who are dependent on others. To make the couple's life happy, the sixty-four forms of sexual amusement are necessary. Practice of the arts, which are a means of seduction, is not described in treatises on ethics or politics. This is why Vātsyāyana explains that the *Kāma Shāstra* is essential in making marriage agreeable, fruitful, and happy. The aim of the couple's mating is the highest achievement of pleasure, as well as mutual progress, which is not the case for animals.

The *Kāma Shāstra* teaches that the final aim of sexual pleasure is spiritual. The development of the transcendent aspect of human love in the couple, together with mutual progress, is not possible for animals, birds, or insects. Men who do not understand the ultimate meaning of sexual pleasure behave like animals.

The *Kama Shāstra* teaches respect for the union of the sexes. Procreation and problems connected with the sexual organ and copulation merit respect, since they concern the evolution of the human species and cause esteem and affection for the partner, as well as the pursuit of his or her well-being. Without spiritual union between spouses or partners, marriage and love have no meaning. Ignorance of, or scorn for, the rules of the *Kama Shāstra* is a source of quarrels, incomprehension, break-up, unfaithfulness, frequenting prostitutes, rape, practices against nature, and bad morals.

19 Through the *Kama Sūtra*, Vātsyāyana defines the approaches to erotic practice.

Among the means taught by the Kama Sūtra, *Vātsyāyana suggests an exchange of letters, if the girl is of the same caste and well educated.*

The *Kama Shāstra* defines moral and social rules for the couple. If the couple's conduct is in accordance with the teachings of the *Kama Sūtra*, their life will be a success from an erotic point of view. The partners will always be satisfied with each other and their spirit will not be touched by any desire to be unfaithful.

The *Kama Sūtra* teaches that sighs, flirtation, and foreplay are three important elements in amorous relations. There are: three kinds of boy; three classes (jāti) of girl; three sorts of equal copulation (sama); six sorts of unequal copulation; three modes of copulation; nine ways of copulating according to the different modes; nine sorts of copulation according to different moments; making a total of twenty-seven modes of copulation (sambhoga).

During copulation, at what moment and in what way do the man and the woman reach enjoyment?

What problems are faced in a first sexual relation?

What effect does ejaculation have on the woman?

What use are the various positions at the moment of union?

What illness can beset a woman after copulating with an inexpert man?

The *Kama Shāstra* gives the answer to all questions that may arise when man and woman unite like milk and water.

This is why the Master explains that an erotic treatise is as important as a treatise on morals or politics.

20   Among animal species with a relatively low level of consciousness, the females, urged on by an unconscious instinct, behave according to their desire when the season arrives.

Female animals are free. Nothing restrains their liberty. They are satisfied in due season. Animals are entirely free to satisfy their erotic desires. However, once their desire is sated, the animals do not begin again. In this, they differ from mankind.

If they have no guardian or protective barrier, women are free. In what way then can a relationship be preserved, since promises serve no purpose. As far as amorous behavior is concerned, the question of trust depends on love, or opportunity. The sages explain that, where there is no protection, there is no other means of controlling sexual relations.

All things arrive in due season. Animals mate when the season comes. Men, too, if they wish for children, wait for the women's period, allowing their seed to accumulate. It is said, one's seed must be used at the proper time, otherwise it is wasted. Even when there are clear signs of satiety, people continue to make love. They do not refuse to do it a second time, as though they were not satisfied, and they do not behave in such a way as to indicate that their loveplay has finished.

Love born of a common aim requires that the woman be protected, since otherwise, her inclinations will incite her to frequent various men. Since, however, she cannot find this unity of aim elsewhere, the wife who goes with another man can in no way realize her life's aim. In this connection, it is said, "Happy is the possessor of a single lover. He whose heart goes after other loves kills his family, destroys virtue, loses his fortune, and drifts away from happiness."

This is why love born from a common aim is a source of happiness for women. The means indicated by Manu for protecting girls from a very young age are housework, the pounding of wheat, etc. By these means, their sexual impulses are kept under control.

Manu recommends that, for their protection, girls should be made to work from their tenderest years. This tames them, like the rope that attaches the elephant to its stake. The author does not mention the lover's infidelities, which must not be taught by holy writ.

As far as increasing the household with progeny is concerned, questions of ethics and material resources are important. It is not simply a matter of animal nature [pashudharma]. The goal is different.

Without some system of control, it is chance that determines attraction to whomever it may be. Animals do not conform to specified rules, and the same goes for men. On the other hand, it is because they know the goal that they bow down before the scriptures.

Vātsyāyana considers that there is a great difference between a woman of the human species and birds born of animal species. The woman is not free like the birds, nor devoid of discernment. She is tied by the restrictions of family and society. She prizes her reputation and fears moral law. This is why all kinds of obstacles are set to prevent any man in the street from having relations with just any woman.

Man's nature is not only animal, and he may not follow his desires at will, like a beast. Man must keep his aims before him: virtue, material success, the begetting of sons, and the growth of his family.

Furthermore, animals and birds make no difference between brother and sister, mother and father, etc., and their life as a couple is not for life. For the couple to enjoy a continual life of bliss together, the moral laws laid down in the texts are of great importance.

Those who do not believe in ethics say:

21 Of what use is it to practice virtue, when its results are uncertain?

Doubts arise as to the necessity of ethical behavior [āchārana] in matters of virtue, wealth, and love.

There is no good ground for virtuous behavior, since the benefits that might be obtained by it in the future are uncertain. It is doubtful whether they will be obtained. It is said that the results of sacrifices and other rites are not to be had in this world, but in the next. One does not let go what one holds in one's hand in the hope of having it in the future. Whoever in the world, neglecting the experience of tradition, would eat the fruits of the harvest before they are ripe, because the results of the harvest are doubtful.

In preparing for the yajña and other rites, the efforts required for the preparations are arduous if their goal is not clear. He who hesitates because he does not believe in benefits such as paradise sees no reason to perform these actions and gives it up, uncertain of the result.

Here we have two different points of view, according to whether the benefits involved are in this world or in another.

22 Who, in his right mind, lets drop what he holds in his hand in order to catch a dubious object?

What one holds in one's own hand is better than what is in someone else's hand. When the time comes for action, if one enters the forest, one eats whatever is to be found, without postponing it till later. The same goes for the yajña, etc. In saying, "I shall enjoy these fruits in another life," one postpones one's enjoyment till later.

23 A pigeon to eat is worth more than a peacock in the sky.

If the pleasure is certain, the dictum indicates the appropriate conduct.

For anyone who wishes to eat meat, the pigeon he already possesses is worth more than the peacock he hopes to snare the next day. In this connection, there is another proverb.

24 According to the materialists [laukāyatika], an authentic copper coin is better than a false gold coin.

25 Some people doubt the Scriptures, while they note that magical practices and words sometimes give results. This is why they carefully study the constellations and the movements of the sun, moon, and planets in the hope of obtaining profits of a material order.

Others, however, more inclined to philosophy, whose behavior conforms to the rules of society [varnāshrama], during the pilgrimage of this life behave like one who sows the seed he holds in his hand, with a view to a future harvest. Such is the opinion of Vātsyāyana.

It is not stupid to scatter the seed one holds in one's hand, in the hope of a future harvest. In the same way, to practice virtuous actions in the hope of heavenly bliss is reasonable, and not useless.

Good conduct concerns the supernatural world, and its practice is defined in the holy books that deal with human values and transcendental realities. But, as we have seen in the case of those that doubt and consider the reality of the invisible world to be an illusion, men, blinded by their desires, are victims of enormous untruths. Men without character, whose perverse spirit chooses doubt, wish to believe that, whatever their virtues or vices, everyone attains the same result. For them, not acting according to the Vedas poses no problem. For them, spiritual realization is a field apart, and nothing proves there is any advantage in behaving according to moral law during this life.

Magic is an act of violence. A curse may cause misfortune. However, rites that use magic, such as agnihotra, demonstrate that violence, war, etc., although contrary to dharma theories, are also connected with supernatural powers and can lead to heaven. Whatever their efficaciousness, the various schools differ in considering whether or not they are an integral part of the sacred texts.

The signs of the zodiac, the moon, the sun, and the planets, five of which are beneficent, are invisible means of realization. Their influence, which is material and not spiritual, depends on the proximity of their orbits in the constellations. Experts observe the movements of the sun and the planets and note their influence. Their importance must not be exaggerated, however, nor should it be thought that every action in this world depends on them.

Besides religious texts, there are many codes of behavior based on philosophical systems [darshana], tradition, or experience. Their influence on people gives good or bad results in the material or immaterial fields. The material field refers to the abundance or poorness of the harvest, which is evident from the movements of the planets. Immaterial influences concern mishaps, gain and loss, pleasure and pain. Although such influences are evident, their secret cause remains mysterious. Those who, in their business, are always asking themselves, "Must I do this in such a way; do it or leave it?," live in continual indecision. Unlucky predictions should always be ignored. Virtue averts them and allows them to be rectified. It is said that, "Those who keep themselves prisoners in the cage of the signs of the zodiac and the planets err in their human tasks, since everything that appears good or bad is in reality the result of their former lives."

Behavior according to function and age is governed by svadharma, the code of individual conduct. The realization of what one is is the goal of life's journey. The rules of behavior are composed with a view to future life. Three notions should be contemplated:

He who envisages life as a journey has nothing to lose in following the rules of ethics.

Those who seek material well-being find nothing contrary in them. He who vows not to follow the rules of ethics also meets with difficulties. Not all people have the same way of seeing things and results are therefore often unexpected. This is quite normal, inasmuch as what can be proved and what cannot are closely intermingled.

Vātsyāyana believes that the holy scriptures transmitted by the sages of old are of divine origin and represent the truth. This is why the reality of ethical law is evident to him.

The influence of the zodiac and the planets is beneficent. In the part of the *Vedas* dealing with mantras, or magic formulas, we find that: "The sun is the principle of life (prāna) for all living beings. All beings are born of the sun." The cycle of the equinoxes (vishuvat) and the ecliptic cycle (krānti) have much to do with the body's structures. In this connection, the *Aitareya Brāhmana* says, "Man is like the equinox, one right half and one left half. He has an upper north side (uttara) just as the equinox has a north side. It is the upper part that speaks, and is the seat of speech. Man's head forms a whole like the equinox. Individual characteristics are to be found within."

This text implies that man is only half of his being. Incomplete, he seeks to be whole, to unite with his other half. Alone, man finds no pleasure. "Because alone he had no pleasure at all, he desired to be two." To play, a partner is needed. This is the law of life. The sacred texts say that so long as a man is not married, he is not complete. So long as the man is not united with the brood female, the transmission of life is impossible.

Human society is based on a functional hierarchy (varnāshrama). Vātsyāyana sees it from a general point of view. He considers that this kind of social division is not peculiar to mankind, but is found everywhere, in everything that exists, whether or not it has consciousness. Whatever is fiery is priest. Whatever is power is warrior. The regents of the world (vishvadeva) are merchants. The solar divinities [nourishers (pusha)] are artisans (shūdras). It is these divinities that determine the differences of nature in men and women, and it is according to the same differences of nature that Vātsyāyana classifies loveplay and, to the contrary of what has been said, he denies the importance of material goods.

26　Riches should not be pursued. They do not come to those who make proper effort, but to those who do not deserve them.

Effort does not bring riches. Rites and regular work bring nothing, but fortune comes by chance, without logic. Fortune depends on destiny. Since it is without logic, effort serves no purpose. It follows its whim. It appears unexpectedly. This is why the texts that explain the means to acquire it are useless.

27 Everything in this world depends on destiny (kāla).

It is destiny that gives material goods. In judging human attempts, it is said:

28 Man's fortune and ill-fortune depend on destiny, his successes and his reverses, his joys and his sorrows.

29 Destiny made Bali the king of Heaven, destiny was the cause of his downfall: destiny gave him back his place: destiny is the cause of everything that happens.

Time devours all that exists; time destroys peoples; time awakens that which slept. None can escape destiny. Everything is the work of destiny. Destiny is the cause of everything. Even the gods are under its sway. The means of living depend on destiny. Expressing the contrary opinion, Vātsyāyana says:

30 To succeed in an enterprise, a man needs to make great effort.

Since success in any enterprise is the fruit of hard work, it must be understood that the means employed are the basis of success. Certain men, however, tend to believe that success depends solely on destiny, or perhaps on both. They never succeed in their enterprises, because they forget that means are indispensable. In the final analysis, wealth is the basis of success for any enterprise.

31 Vātsyāyana says: In order to live, the use of material goods is indispensable. The sluggard will never prosper.

But do the actions of past lives have no influence? It can be seen that both the one and the other bear fruit. However, it is said that, "It is destiny that fructifies man's actions. Destiny is thus sufficient."
Vātsyāyana quotes the legend of Shunahshepa, according to the

Aitareya Brāhmana: Having taken on human form, Indra made the gift of long life to Rohita, the son of Harishchandra, who would have died young. This shows that fortune can smile on him who makes no effort. Nevertheless, Indra is the friend of him who is always active. "He who is always in movement sees his thighs develop."

"Heaven does not belong to the weak" (*Mundaka Upanishad*).

32 One cannot give oneself over to pleasure without restrictions. One's activities must be coordinated taking due account of the importance of virtue and material goods.

Eroticism puts man in contact with disreputable people and leads to evil deeds, defilement, ill-fated results.

33 The lewd man is vain. He undergoes humiliations, does not inspire trust, and attracts people's scorn.

34 It can be observed that those who give themselves over to an exaggerated sexual life destroy themselves as well as their relations.

35 Thus King Dāndakya of the line of the Bhojas ruined his life, his family and his kingdom, for having raped the daughter of a Brahman.

36 Those that reflect on the consequences of our actions remind us that the king of Heaven was destroyed for being enamored of Ahalyā, and so it was too for the most powerful Kichaka because of Draupadī, and for Rāvana because of Sītā. Many others have been destroyed for letting themselves be possessed by Eros.

37 Sexuality is essential for the survival of man, just as food is necessary for bodily health, and on them depend both virtue and wealth.

Having himself posed the questions, Vātsyāyana also proposes the answer. Since bodily survival depends on it, eroticism is indispensable, like food. Virtue and prosperity depend on them.

Although it can cause indigestion, food must, however, be consumed daily to preserve the body. The same goes for sexuality. The survival of the species cannot be neglected because of errors committed in the madness of erotic excitement.

Virtue and prosperity are the fruit of love. To be happy, virtue and wealth must be sought. Being related, they only give results at the price of great effort. It is said that, "Being the source of virtue, woman is the best means of reaching heaven. Man's efforts to be virtuous are impossible outside conjugal virtue. If she is able to have sons, a woman brings bliss to this world and the next. There is no doubt but that women are a source of happiness."

In the preceeding verses, Vātsyāyana presents arguments suggesting that eroticism degrades man, makes him dependent and pitiful, and finally destroys him entirely. The examples given to support this point of view refer only to material goods. Preoccupations of this kind are also expressed by the authors of the *Artha Shāstra*. Kautilya advises the king to control his impulses and adds that control over feelings is the basis of wisdom and piety. Control over the senses also refers to contacts, odors, tastes. In his exposition, Kautilya gives the example of King Dāndakya of the Bhoja dynasty. Vātsyāyana takes up the same example. In his reply to the argument, he compares sexuality to food. Although gluttony makes a person sick, food is essential to life. In the same way, although sexuality troubles the mind and poses social problems, it cannot be renounced since it is a natural instinct. Without sexuality, life would disappear.

38 Vātsyāyana says, "One must put up with risks. But one does not forgo cooking one's food, fearing that a beggar might come and claim his part, and one does not forgo sowing wheat for fear of wild beasts."

If one has digestive problems, one seeks a remedy. Inevitably, there are mistakes in erotic practice that one must also try to remedy. This law is valid at all times. One should not deprive oneself of the joys of life for the sake of insignificant details. "Defects must be eliminated," is the sages' point of view.

39 It has been said that, "The man accomplished in riches, love, and virtue effortlessly attains the maximum of bliss in this world and the next."

In this connection, he quotes the words of the ancients.

The behavior established according to the rules described by the ancients should be followed in all matters of money, virtue, and love.

Certain men would like to attain bliss in this world and the next without effort. In saying, "I wish to achieve painlessly all the aims of life," the mind is satisfied. But if we do not seek to achieve the three aims, it will be impossible to achieve even one of them in this world or the next, because we are bound by actions performed previously in former lives, or because of stupidity, and we are thus incapable of following the rules of virtue.

In his indifference, the unbeliever (nāstika) does not see that failure in a single sector may create obstacles to the attainment of happiness.

40 Another quotation:

"Wise men choose ways of acting that allow them to achieve the three aims of life without letting the pursuit of pleasure lead them to ruin.

"Whether one pursues the three aims, or two, or even one, the achievement of one of them must not be prejudicial to the other two."

An excess of charity is an obstacle to the fulfilment of duty, to achieving prosperity, and also to erotic realization. An excess of asceticism, which suppresses eroticism by weakening the body, destroys material success. By an exaggerated pursuit of riches, even Pururava came to grief in virtue and love. In the same way, the abuse of erotic practices is prejudicial to the achievement of the other two aims of life.

End of the Second Chapter
The Three Aims of Life
of the First Part entitled General Remarks

Chapter Three

THE ACQUISITION OF KNOWLEDGE

[Vidyāsamuddesha]

To succeed in the three aims of life, the first means is the acquisition of knowledge. Without knowledge, almost any achievement is impossible. A brief summary is given below of the teachings dealt with fully in other works.

1 **Without curtailing the time dedicated to studying spiritual and material subjects and related sciences, a man should also study erotic science, the Kāma Shāstra and its annexes.**

Spiritual subjects include revealed scripture [shruti] and the traditional books [smriti]. The art of governing [artha vidyā], includes economy [varta shāstra], the criminal code [danda vidhi], profits and losses [yogakshema], and investigation [anvīkshikī], so as to give an understanding of the real nature of things. These subjects are of prime importance. In the time left free, one should study the Kāma Shāstra and its related sciences, such as instrumental music and singing, which should be both practiced and listened to.

Traditional teaching is based on fourteen sciences belonging to seven disciplines (siddhānta). The first of all the sciences is the study of the sacred scriptures, the *Vedas*, and their annexes, forming a series of works on fundamental subjects, classified in order of importance. The *Smriti* of Yājñavalkya numbers fourteen sciences, which are:

The four *Vedas*
The six *Vedāngas* (annexes to the *Vedas*)
The *Mīmāmsā* (theology and ritual)
The *Nyāya* (logic)
The *Purānas* (ancient traditions)
And the *Dharma Shāstra* (ethical rules)

to which are added seven *Siddhāntas*, or [non-Vedic] religious traditions, which are:

Pāncharātra (the five nights, Genesis of Creation)
Kāpila (cosmology)
Aparāntaratam (foreign religions)
Brahmishtha (devotional cults)
Hairanyagarbha (theory of the golden egg)
Pāshupata (cult of the Lord of the Animals)
Shaiva (Shivaism)

On the fourteen schools there exist three hundred basic texts and seventy *Mahā Tantras*, embodying the religious traditions of Shivaism.

According to the *Mahābhārata*, numerous sciences coming from Shivaism deal with subjects that, among others, concern politics and economy. Some of the subjects dealt with are:

Materialistic philosophy (lokāyata shāstra)
Archery
Strategy
Chariots
Horses
Elephants
Elephant medicine
Veterinary science
War machines (yantra)
Trade (vanijya)
Alliances (gandha shāstra)
Agriculture
Zoology

Cattle medicine
Arboriculture
Carpentry
Athletics (malla); development of the body
Interior decoration (vāstu)
Eloquence (vākovākya)
Drawing (chitra)
Writing (lipi)
Measurements (māna)
Mineralogy; the science of metals (dhātu)
Mathematics (sāmkhya)
The science of precious stones
Fortifications (atta shāstra)
Tantrism (tāntrika shruti)
Architecture (shilpa shāstra)
Magic (mahāyoga)
Anthropology (mānavavidyā)
Executions (suda shāstra)
Chemistry (dravya shāstra)
Ichthyology
Ornithology
Herpetology
Languages (bhāshya)
Treatise on the art of thieving (chaura shāstra)
Midwifery (mātri tantra)

These thirty-eight subjects form part of the *Artha Shāstra*. Economics are explained in detail in the *Artha Shāstra* of Kautilya.

The *Kalpa* is one of the six texts annexed to the *Vedas*. It explains the meaning of words, and the rules and practice of the rites. The *Kalpa Sūtras*, which are divided into three parts, deal with Vedic (shruta), domestic (grihya), and social (dharma) ceremonies. The religious part explains social and moral duties and rights, which are dealt with in detail in numerous treatises, such as those of Manu, Yājñavalkya, Gautama, Vasishtha, Purushara, and Shankha.

Besides eroticism, Vātsyāyana's teaching also covers important subjects concerning ethics and economy, as well as sciences connected with the *Kāma Sūtra*, such as music.

Like the *Dharma Shāstra* and the *Artha Shāstra*, the *Kāma Shāstra* is a wonderful guide to life's feelings and actions. By calling his work *Kāma Sūtra* and not *Kāma Shāstra*, Vātsyāyana indicates that his work takes the place of ancient treatises that are no longer accessible.

While studying sexuality, it is essential to study music (sangīta), which belongs to the art of love. Just as eroticism is related to procreation, music is connected with the science of sounds (nāda vidyā), which is one of the basic elements in understanding the creation of the world. The relation of the notes (svara) with divinities, prophets (rishi), the planets, constellations, colors, and rhythms is not mere speculation, but has a profound meaning, corresponding to a reality. To this should be added the study of instruments, which are of four kinds: strings, parchment (drums), wind, and percussion, comprising innumerable instruments. Music contributes to the experience of divine bliss (brahmānanda).

2 A woman should study even before reaching adolescence, and then, once married, should continue her studies with her husband.

The study of the sciences also concerns women. During her tender years under her father's roof, a girl should study religion and economy, as well as erotic science and music.

While under the paternal roof, from their earliest years, girls should study the Kāma Sūtra *and the sciences that form part of it. Certain people object, "But, being deprived of their freedom, how can such girls study? Do they have the opportunity to do so? Later on, once married, they are subject in thought, word, and deed to their husband's instructions." Only lesbians [svairinī] have no problems.*

3 The ancient authors consider that since women are incapable of understanding the sciences, it is useless to teach them such things.

4 Vātsyāyana notes that they can understand practical science and that practice depends entirely on theory.

Women are capable of putting into practice the theories of the *Kāma Shāstra*, and putting into practice cannot be easily separated from theory. The study of the *Kāma Sūtra* is therefore of value.

The aim of sexual union is not merely the satisfaction of a need (vāsanā), but also has social and spiritual significance. Women have a natural and undeniable inclination for sexual union, an inclination that forms part of their physical being. All animals, birds, and fish practice the sexual act (maithuna). The only difference between man and other creatures is his discernment (viveka). A man without common sense (vivekashunya) who practices coition is in no way different from an animal. The *Kāma Sūtra* is essential for man and woman to distinguish themselves from animals in becoming aware of the final aim of the sexual act. When doubts arise, and we ask ourselves, "Shall we do it or not, this way or that?," the answer is found in the *Kāma Sūtra*. If a girl has studied erotic science, she will know how to behave in her married life, as well as in her youth, and will not fall into the snare of ignorance.

According to the *Mīmāmsā*, in the beginning there existed an independent male current and an independent female current, which can be compared to the two poles of electric power (vidyutashakti), attracting and repulsing each other, whose union gives light and energy. Creation is born of the union of the two energies, male and female, and everything disappears when they separate. According to the *Mīmāmsā*, it is only when the female current is impregnated by the male that it can reach the highest levels.

By studying the *Kāma Shāstra*, man and woman united in their desire for sexual enjoyment form a whole, and together achieve material and spiritual progress. When the man and woman are of very different races, their nature and inclination differ. By studying the *Kāma Shāstra*, they manage to understand each other and, although different, they mingle like milk and water.

5   In all fields, and not only as concerns sexual relations, few know the theoretical aspect of things.

This is the case for both grammar and astrology.

Although they know the practical side, they are poorly informed about the texts on the subject.

6   Theory is always the basis, even if it is divorced from practice.

Knowledge of theory, transmitted by tradition, is the basis, even when the connection is not apparent. A person who knew the theory established the practice, which was subsequently transmitted to another and then to another.

7   An illiterate priest, with no knowledge of grammar, still pours the offerings onto the altar fire.

Although the priest may understand nothing of the meaning of the formulas he utters in accomplishing the rites, they are based on grammar, and he knows them by tradition. "It is while invoking the eight guardian divinities that the offering is poured."

8   Astrology defines the dates of the feasts.

People observe feastdays and fasts, etc., although they are ignorant of astrology.

9   People ride horses and elephants although knowing nothing of the sciences concerning these animals.

10   Although for them the king is an inaccessible personage, the lower classes observe the laws he enacts.

Similarly, although the rules of the *Kāma Shāstra* are not known, they are observed in practice. Vātsyāyana explains the hidden influence and importance of the *Kāma Shāstra*, whose rules are transmitted by tradition.

11   The principles of erotic art concern the daughters of kings and ministers as well as courtesans, even if they have no chance to study the relative theory.

For all girls, whatever their social standing, the teaching of the *Kāma Shāstra* and the arts, such as music, etc., which are part of it, is a very ancient principle of Indian civilization. This is why, in Indian society, courtesans have always been respected, not only for their beauty, their way of life, and their attraction, but also for their knowledge, their usefulness, and their social role.

In the histories of the Buddhist Jātakas and in Bhāsa's play *Daridrachārudatta*, the beauty and qualities of the courtesan Vasantasenā are quoted as models of feminine behavior. Powerful kings and holy men came to visit her. In ancient times, princes and princesses were sent to courtesans to learn the arts and good manners. Not only were the courtesans respected, but their presence brought good luck. They were known as the "faces of fortune" (mangalamukhi).

According to treatises on astrology, seeing a courtesan before leaving for a journey brings good luck. The yajña, or great ritual sacrifices, require the presence of a courtesan beside the officiant. Courtesans are an important element in society, respected both by the people and the establishment. They are teachers of the arts of pleasure and music for the children of kings and nobles.

12 This is why, in good society, women must secretly study the theory and practice of the *Kāma Sūtra*.

And particularly, music and other related sciences.

13 A young girl should take herself off to an isolated spot to practice the sixty-four arts.

14 The sexual instructress of young girls should be independent and know the meaning of the words. She may be of six kinds:

A woman used to sleeping with men
A girlfriend who has already been initiated
A maternal aunt of her own age
An old confidential servant woman, treated like an aunt
A mendicant nun known for a long time
An older sister whom she trusts and who has had experience with men

Together with these women, the additional accomplishments known as the sixty-four arts [kalā] should also be studied.

It is always easy to find male instructors, but in the case of girls, it is not at all easy to find one for erotic arts. This is why Vātsyāyana finds it simpler to advise that women should teach this subject, so long as they are trustworthy and wellborn. In such a case, no question of sexual modesty arises, and thus is of help in forming character. Vātsyāyana includes the sixty-four arts, considered as accomplishments in the teaching of erotic techniques. Even in cases where it is not possible to study them all, at least some of them should be practiced.

15 The sixty-four arts considered as accomplishments are:

1 Vocal music (notes, modes, rhythms, tempo)
2 Instruments (percussion, strings, drums, flutes)
3 Dance (hand and body movements, expression, emotion, feeling)
4 Drawing (various styles and techniques, feeling and charm, likeness)
5 Cutouts

Cutting out small stencils from paper or peel for marking the forehead or other parts of the body with patterns.

6 Carpets of flowers or colored grains of rice

To decorate the temple of the goddess or the temple of love.

7 Flower bouquets

Of various colors, in vases, to decorate the apartments and meeting places.

8 Dyes and colorants for the body and the teeth

9 Mosaics

To decorate the floor with small chips of emerald or other stones.

10 Bed arrangement

Covered with colored fabrics, placed in the center of the room, for taking meals.

11 Musical instrument made of bowls filled with water

12 Water-spewing games

13 The use of charms, drugs, magic words [chitrā yogā]

As used in anger, they will be explained together with occult practices, but do not include black magic.

14 Garland making

Strung without their leaves, to venerate the gods or decorate the house.

15 Crowns and head ornaments

Headbands or circlets of flowers of all colors, used especially by townspeople.

16 The art of dressing

To choose garments and jewels to embellish the body, according to place and circumstances.

17 Ivory or mother-of-pearl ear ornaments

18 The preparation of perfumes

See the special treatise on this subject.

19 Jewelry

These are of two kinds: necklaces ornamented with jewels or ornaments worn around the hips, used mostly for the theater.

20 Conjuring (indrajāla)

To hypnotize and make people see armies or heavenly dwellings.

21 Magic (kuchumāra)

Methods taught in the Kuchumāra Tantra *to increase sexual prowess and to enhance beauty.*

22 Manicure

To soften hands spoiled by work or age, or products.

23 The art of cooking
24 The preparation of drinks

Cooking is the art of transforming various vegetables into soups and dishes. Food is of four kinds: bitten, eaten, licked, or drunk. The food is cooked with condiments to give it a pleasant flavor. Vegetables that are unpleasant to the taste without condiments often become acceptable thanks to the latter. Vegetables are of ten kinds: roots, leaves, seeds, buds, fruits, tubers, stalks, peels, flowers, bamboos. Drinks are of two kinds, distilled or not. The latter may be fermented or not. Unfermented drinks are made by squeezing mudga beans [Phaseolus mungo], mango, or mulberry fruit, and adding sugar or tamarind fruit. Fermented drinks are made with palm wine [toddy], or wild fig wine [mahua]. When distilled, a liqueur is obtained that may be mild, medium, or strong.

Products that are pleasant to lick are made of powdered aphrodisiacs mixed with honey, which may be sweet, salty, sour, or bitter according to choice, which are chosen at the right moment to reinvigorate the body or stimulate amorous ardor. Food and drinks are thus prepared, either uncooked, or else cooked to improve their flavor. Although different, these processes all indicate ways of satisfying taste.

25 Needlework

This comprises sewing together, weaving, manufacturing clothes, bodices, and costumes, and darning.

26 Lacemaking

Crocheting thread or vegetable fibers to create a net, showing, with holes and crocheted areas, patterns of birds, animals, temples, houses, etc.

27 Art of playing the vīnā and the damaru (drum)

Stringed instruments are the most important, particularly the vina. The drum is indispensable. Both are difficult and need to be practiced from childhood if the various notes are to be clearly distinguished.

28 Conundrums

Presented as a game or as the subject for a discussion.

29 The art of completing a quotation (pratimālā)

30 Riddles

Utilizing formulas in which the sound and meaning of the words are uncertain.

31 Bookbinding

32 The art of telling stories

33 Quoting the classics in answering questions

34 Plaiting cane baskets, etc.

Making solid seats with dry canes.

35 Woodwork

Using a lathe and other tools.

36 Carpentry

Sawing planks to make seats and beds.

37 House furnishing and decoration

38 Expert knowledge of stones and gems

39 Mixing and polishing metals

40 Valuing the shape and color of stones

41 Arboriculture, the care of trees

For the house or garden.

42 Stockbreeding

Raising and training rams, cocks, fighting partridges, and organizing battles, as for an army.

43 Teaching parrots and mynah birds to talk

44 Massage and care of the body and hair

Vigorous massage using the feet or hands, delicately on the hair giving it an aesthetic set.

45 Sign language

Utilizing the mudrā, or symbolic gestures of the theater.

46 Understanding barbarous foreign languages (mleccha)

Or by inverting syllables, being understood only by the initiated.

47 Speaking regional languages

48 Decorating chariots with flowers

49 Observing the omens

Observing the favorable or unfavorable signs before any enterprise.

50 Fabricating machines

Either hand-operated or automatic, for raising water, measuring time, etc.

51 Developing the memory

Remembering words and works read, dictionaries, subjects, ephemeris.

52 Alternate reciting of texts

53 Puns

Changing a letter or accent to change the meaning of a sentence.

54 Knowledge of the dictionary

Giving the Sanskrit equivalent of local dialects and popular jargon.

55 Poetic meter

56 Versification and literary forms

57 The art of cheating

58 The art of disguise (vastragopanam)

The wearing of local costume, whether or not made up, for amusement or in order not to be recognized.

59 The art of gaming, the game of dice

For amusement or gain.

60 The game of chess

61 Children's games

Dolls' houses, toys, dolls.

62 Good manners

The manner of greeting and returning greetings.

63 The rules for success (for military success, see the Artha Shāstra)

Even when conquered by fate, man wins by a battle.

64 Physical culture

A vigorous man defends himself against ferocious animals, protecting his chattels and his life.

Singing, instruments, dancing, and writing are each dealt with in separate texts. Music is based on notes, poems, tempo (laya), and rhythm.

Both the *Shukranīti* and the *Tantras* mention the sixty-four arts. Others are sometimes added. The *Lalitavistara* counts eighty-six. According to the *Kalāvilāsa*, thirty-two conform to the three aims of life and thirty-two have a bad influence on character, thirty-four concern goldsmiths, sixty-four serve prostitutes for seducing citizens, ten concern medicine, sixteen the kāyasthas (scribes), who take fees for writing messages and, by knowing the art of writing, are able to deceive the people and the authorities. The arts mentioned by astrologers number more than one hundred different kinds.

16 Besides the sixty-four arts described, a further sixty-four come from Panchala country. Since they form part of the techniques of love, they will be described below.

17 Prostitutes (veshyā) who are beautiful, intelligent, and well educated have an honored place in society and are known as courtesans (ganikā).

18 They are respected by kings; respectable people sing their praises; respected for their art, they live in the sight of all.

19 They associate with the daughters of kings and ministers and can get themselves married to a man who owns a thousand dwellings.

20 Then, divorcing their husband, or if a misfortune should happen to him, they go to another country and live comfortably on their savings.

21 A man who is expert in the arts, even though suffering a certain contempt, has success with women, if he is a good talker.

22 Fortunes can be acquired by practicing the arts, but they can only be practiced when the conditions of the country and the period are favorable.

End of the Third Chapter
The Acquisition of Knowledge
of the First Part entitled General Remarks

Chapter Four

THE CONDUCT
OF THE
WELL-BRED TOWNSMAN

1 Having completed his studies and acquired the means of livelihood by gifts received, conquest, trade, and work, or else by inheritance, or both and, having married, the well-bred townsman [nāgaraka] must settle down in a refined manner.

In order to establish himself, a Brahman acquires assets through gifts; a noble [kshatriya] by arms and conquest; a merchant [vaishya] by trade; a worker [shūdra] by hard work and service. The way of life recommended by Vātsyāyana is not for the penniless and applies to all four castes.

2 He must establish himself in a big city, a town, or even a large village, near the mountains, where a decent number of persons of good society are living. He may also, for a time, go journeying.

3 He must build himself a house with two separate apartments, on a site near water, with trees and a garden and a separate place of work.

4   The antechamber, outside the private apartments, must be vast, pleasant, with a wide divan in the center covered with a white cloth. Close to this great bed, another similar one shall be placed, for the games of love.

At the head of this bed, on a table only slightly taller, are placed a bunch of sacred herbs to attract the gods' protection, beauty products, ointments, flower necklaces, incense sticks, pots of scent, and citrus and betel leaves.

On the floor, close to the couch, a spittoon must be placed for betel and, on a cushion, an ivory-encrusted vīnā, drawing materials and accessories, illustrated books, and necklaces of yellow amaranth flowers, which do not fade quickly. Not far, on the ground, is spread a pretty round rug, behind which are cushions and large bolsters to support the head and back, which is practical for playing at dice and other gambling games. Outside the antechamber cages of tame birds are fixed to the walls, and a little way off, a place for urinating and other needs. Swings are installed in the garden and flowery arbors, in which benches are placed.

This completes the appointments of the antechamber of the house.

Those who frequent prostitutes must have two beds. Respectable people and scholars must not be made to sit where the master of the house amuses himself with girls.

At the head of the bed there should be a mirror and, on shelves, sandalwood, flowers, necklaces, and ointments should be arranged, as well as the ingredients for preparing betel. Sometimes, during the night, the woman lying in one's arms emits a smell of sweat and does not hold her evil-smelling wind. Cardamom and citron peel should be pounded to combat bad smells. Nearby, covered with a cloth, a vīnā, encrusted with ivory, and colors and tools for drawing, as well as necklaces of kurantaka flowers, which have no scent but are useful for decoration, since they do not fade quickly. On the veranda facing the courtyard are placed cages with parrots, quails, partridges, and fighting cocks.

The description of the inner courtyard is similar to the one described in the *Mrichakatika*. When the thief Charvilaka breaks into Chārudatta's house, he thinks he has entered a theater. Scattered all around are vinas, drums, percussion instruments, here and there books, pictures, drawings. For the townsman with a sensitive heart, the vina and drawing implements are as precious as life itself.

Vātsyāyana gives an extremely vivid description of the entrance hall, but does not describe the inner apartments. He only speaks of the lianas, arbors, and swings of the inner garden, which belongs to the harem.

In poems like *Kādambarī*, wonderful descriptions are given of the inner rooms. Rājā Chandrapīda, when he penetrated into the inner apartment, was dumbfounded by the realism of the frescos covering the walls, depicting imaginary landscapes. The ceiling was covered with representations of the genies of knowledge, the Vidyādhāras. White cushions were lying on the blue-draped bed. Painters were highly honored, and frescos in houses were considered to bring good luck. At the same time, the house contained all the implements, colors, etc., for drawing, practiced by the women on ivory, wood, or cloth.

5   A well-bred townsman gets up very early in the morning, performs his natural functions, and cleans his teeth. Having carefully washed his face, he rubs it with ointment and marks the sacred signs on his brow, using sandalwood. He dyes his hair, using wax and lacquer, while looking at himself in a mirror. Then, having eaten some betel, he places a necklace of scented flowers around his neck, after which he begins his daily routine.

6   He must bathe every day, have a massage every two days, soap himself every three days. Every four days, he must trim his beard and moustache, on the fifth or tenth day shave his pubic hair and armpits and, always, scent himself to disguise the smell of sweat from the armpits and be pleasant to contact.

One must bathe every day before taking food. The lower part of the body must be washed with soap, otherwise the skin is not soft.

A beard should be cut into three points. It is not fitting to separate it in two. However, some citizens do otherwise, according to fashion. Body hair should be shaved by a barber. The pubic area should always be free, since sexual activity causes sweat. The piece of cloth [cache-sexe] should also be changed frequently to avoid bad odor and irritation.

It appears that, according to the *Kāma Sūtra*, the townsmen were not parsimonious as concerns knowledge and the arts. With regard to daily routine, the townsman had his servants prepare a mixture of scented ingredients, a week in advance, for washing his teeth. First sandalwood powder was mixed with cow urine, in which the sticks used for brushing the teeth were soaked for seven days. They were then dipped in a paste made of cardamom, cinnamon, anjana (*Hardwickia binata*) honey, and black pepper. These sticks, used to clean the teeth, were also considered lucky. Great care was taken in utilizing sticks from a special tree, gathered according to the days of the moon. The priests and servants would keep the master informed about it.

Massage is usually performed with sandalwood. Other products used are musk, saffron, and aloes, mixed with cream. According to the medical treatises, these ointments make the skin supple and luminous.

For the hair, lotions are used to keep it in place, to disguise white hairs, and make the hair shiny and soft.

Varāhamihira, in his *Grihya Samhitā*, says that "even dressed with sumptuous garments, wearing scented necklaces, and covering the limbs with sparkling jewels, if the hair is white, all these ornaments lose their attraction." For hair treatment, the hair is smeared with camphor, saffron, and musk for a few moments, after which a bath is taken. Once his hair is done, the townsman puts on a necklace of flowers, which he chooses carefully according to season, but most often of yellow champa flowers (*Michelia champaka*), of jasmine (mālati), and of juhi (white ixora). For moments of amorous dalliance, garlands of yellow amaranth flowers are recommended, since they do not fall during caressing, kissing, or hugging.

He cleans his feet with a damp cloth, and then puts red lacquer on the soles of his feet and around the nails. He then looks at himself in a polished mirror and chews betel. Betel is the hallmark of a civilized person. It is also a sign of welcome, when offered, even to the gods. After taking betel, the townsman attends to his daily business.

Vātsyāyana does not describe how to take a bath, but a description is to be found in the *Kādambarī:* "Having finished his business, a little before noon, before taking his bath, the townsman chats for a few moments with his friends, then, having performed a little exercise, he enters the bathroom where there is a marble table-seat with gold or silver vessels nearby filled with water scented with various ingredients. First, the townsman sits on a soft towel and his servants perfume him and massage his head. Then his body is massaged for several moments with scented oil, after which he plunges into the pool. He then sits on the marble table to wash himself and his assistants pour the scented water over him. The townsman is then soaped, after which he dresses again, winding a thin muslin strip like a snake's skin around his hair. Then he goes to the domestic shrine for the daily rites.

"Nails may be cut to a point or in a half-moon shape. The people of Gaura keep their nails very long, those in the south short and square, while in the north people consider nails of a medium length to be more elegant."

Vātsyāyana recommends cutting the hair every four days. The *Atharva Veda* recommends knotting the hair. The sages of old wore their hair long. Some knot it at the back of the head, others on the forehead, others on top. These texts mention various hairstyles for women, parrot-style, four plaits, with a fringe, etc.

In the *Rig Veda*, the sages wear their hair knotted on the right. The gods Indra and Pūshan have moustaches.

The *Taittirīya Samhitā* considers that beard and moustache are signs of virility.

Varāhamihira explains that betel embellishes and perfumes the mouth, softens the voice, renders one more attractive, improves and brings luck in adventures. It cures coughs and other sicknesses.

The *Skanda Purāna* describes various kinds of betel. The preparation of betel is considered a fine art. According to Varāhamihira, the ingredients of betel are cardamom, catechu (katthā), lime (chuna) and betel nut (supāri), to which other ingredients may be added.

Some texts consider that the hair, beard, and body hair should be shaved at full moon, leaving only a lock on the top of the head. There are different opinions with regard to keeping one's hair and beard or not. Traditionally, all hair should be eliminated, but some people believe that keeping hair and beard prolongs life.

7 Two main meals should be taken each day, in the morning and in the evening before nightfall.

The morning is divided into three periods according to one's occupation. One eats in the fourth period, after bathing. Eating again in the afternoon, during the fifth period, is not recommended by masters. It is advised to take a meal at the end of the day, but not if one has eaten in the afternoon. It is said, "If one's digestion has not finished, whatever one eats here and there is not assimilated. However, men who do not eat in the evening become weak."

8 After meals, quiet amusements are necessary, such as teaching mynah birds and parrots to talk, watching partridges, cocks, or rams fighting, and playing all kinds of games, subsequently conversing with the manager [pītha-

marda], one's comrade in pleasure [vita], and the facetious
secretary, before having one's siesta.

*After the midday meal, and after chatting with the parrots and
mynahs, to whom he teaches puns and how to complete quotations, he
takes a siesta, as is the custom in summer. After this he discusses with
his pīthamarda and the others about his appointments and disputes. A
siesta at the time indicated is a duty during the summer, since it
strengthens the body and is necessary for it.*

The food of the ancient Hindus is described in various works. For
refined people, it was of four kinds: food to be chewed, to be licked, to
be sucked, and to be drunk. An ordinary diet included wheat, rice, rye,
chick-peas, lentils, butter (ghee), and meat, with which the dishes were
prepared. Before the meal, salt biscuits were eaten, and afterward sweet
dishes.

After a meal, a gentleman would talk with his parrots and mynahs.
In ancient India, parrots and mynahs were companions whether inside
the harem or the hermitage in the forest. Townspeople as well as hermits had friendly relationships with these birds. Parrots and mynahs
were faithful friends, sharing joys and sorrows. At that time, people
were very close to these birds, whether in the chamber of love and the
harem or the terrible fields of battle or the ashrams of the ascetics.
Birds were companions for games, but also messengers for secret enterprises. Kings employed them widely, and they were attributed with
great intelligence. They carried ardent messages between lovers and,
during war, secret instructions. In the entrance hall of the house, cocks
and quails (kukkuta) were kept, whose fights were an after-dinner amusement. Parrots and mynahs were kept in cages in the bedroom where the
gentleman rested during daytime. He would amuse himself with their
chatter. Teaching parrots and mynahs to talk, as well as cock fights and
ram fights, belong to the sixty-four arts of pleasure of Vātsyāyana.

**9 The reception hall [goshthi] is located next to the living
quarters.**

*In the evening, at nightfall, receptions are organized with music,
dancing, singing, and instruments. When the guests are gathered, the
master of the house, splendidly dressed, enters the reception hall, located
on one side of the entrance courtyard.*

10 In the evening, having listened to music, he returns with some friends to his dwelling where, with wine and incense, he awaits the arrival of the women invited for the night.

11 He has them called, or goes to collect them himself.

12 In the company of his friends, he then greets the women who have come, with pleasant words and affectionate behavior.

13 If the woman's clothes are wet from the rain, during a sudden shower, he himself changes her clothes and gets his friends to help, for their service both day and night.

At dusk, numerous people gather for receptions, including singers, dancers, and the players of instruments.

Vātsyāyana recommends that the gentleman should go to the reception room elegantly dressed. Elegance is a matter of the quality of clothes and jewels. Bharata gives some indications in his *Nātya Shāstra*. An elegant man wears four kinds of clothes made of vegetable silk (kshauma), cotton (kārpāsa), natural silk (kaushya), or wool (rangava). Vegetable silk is made from hemp fiber and can also be made from bark.

After this, the gentleman puts on his jewels. Varāhamihira describes thirteen kinds of precious stone and nine kinds of golden jewels. The stones are: diamond (vajra), pearl (muktā), ruby (padmarāga), emerald (marakata), sapphire (indranīla), lapis-lazuli (vaidurya), topaz (pushparāga), a black stone, whetstone (kurketana), amber (pulaka), garnet (rudhirāksha), amethyst (bhīshma), crystal (sphatika), opal (pravāla).

To make up the jewels, the various kinds of jeweler were: the goldsmith (jāmbūnada), the maker of gold vessels (shātakaumbha), the chaser (hataka), the cutter (venava), the refiner of gold for jewelry (shringī), the polisher of mother of pearl (shuktija), the glazer (jātarūpa), the assembler (rasaviddha), the shaper (akaraudgata).

Jewels are of four kinds:

Āvedhya, for which the flesh is pierced: earrings, diamond in the nose.

Nibandhanīya, attached with bands: attached to the arm (angada), headband for the hair (venī), crown (shikhādridhikā), belt (shroni sūtra), diadem (chūdāmani).

Prakshepya, slipped on: ring (urmikā), nailguards (kataka), bracelets (valaya), anklets (manjīra).

Āropya, worn around the neck: necklaces (hara), necklace of twenty-seven pearls (nakshatramālikā).

Once he is dressed and has put on his jewels, the gentleman adorns himself with garlands of flowers, which are of different kinds. There are narrow rows of jasmine, like a pearl necklace, heavy garlands made of great bunches, tight necklaces, wide necklaces, flexible necklaces, rigid necklaces. After putting on a garland, he puts on some scent. The perfumes in fashion were musk (kastūrī), saffron (kunkuma), sandalwood (chandana), camphor (karpūra), aloes (aguru), kulaka, lemon (dantashatha), lavender (patavāsa), betel leaf (tāmbūla), anjana (*Hardwickia binata*), bull's gall (gorochana). These ingredients were used to scent beauty products, such as lacquers, oils, black for eyelids and eyebrows, and products for the hair and clothes. According to the season, the time, and the circumstances of his encounters, the gentleman was thus able to check the smell of sweat on his brow and in other parts of his body. He would adorn himself with durva herb (*Cynodon dactylon*), red ashoka flowers, arm ornaments and other silver ornaments known as cucumber, shell (shankha), palm leaf (tāladala) or lotus fiber. Thus scented and wearing ear ornaments and bracelets, he entered the reception hall.

Gatherings at a rich gentleman's house included seven kinds of guests: scholars (vidvāna), poets (kavi), singers (gāyaka), entertainers (masakharī), specialists in ancient history (itihāsa), specialists in legendary epics (purāna).

The same selection of participants is given in the Buddhist texts and in the lyric poems (kāvya).

According to Vātsyāyana, there were bad and good receptions. The first comprised games and drinking bouts, while the second were cultural, at which one spoke of literature and played innocent games.

Cultured gentlemen organized various kinds of reception (goshthi). Those concerning poetry (pada), the theater (kāvya), and ballads (jalpa) took place in the center of studies.

The reception hall was the scene of singing (gīta) and dancing (nritya) entertainments and concerts of instrumental music (vadya) and in particular the vīnā.

Bana speaks of the gatherings of heros that took place in time of war, during which heroic tales were told.

Gatherings for music take place in the evening, at a time when the citizen feels sensitive and romantic.

After the concert, the citizen returns to his dwelling, where his chosen woman awaits him in a comfortably arranged bedroom. This is the chamber of love, where he clasps and embraces his wife or his paramours. On the door is depicted the god of love and two pretty girls, both sides of which are lighted with luck-bearing lamps. The frescos show the god of love under an ashoka tree, holding his flower-decorated bow. Beside the bed, which is covered with a white drape, stands on one side a gilded spittoon and on the other an ivory-encrusted statue bearing a silver vase with drinking water. Round mirrors are fixed to the walls of the chamber of love, so that the beloved can be seen from all angles.

14 Receptions were organized for seasonal festivities or events [ghatā], for concerts or entertainments, for drinking parties [samapānakam], witticisms [samasyākridā], or for strolls in the garden [udyana].

Events mostly include pilgrimages to visit sanctuaries where people gather and, related to these, receptions taking place among the various social groups, at which theatrical entertainments are prevalent. In the afternoon gatherings take place for amusement and for drinking, at which are found those that drink and those that do not. Such gatherings mainly take place in the gardens, whether they are organized in one's own home or at another person's.

For the feast of the god of love, people wear orange clothes and stroll around with crowns of flowers on their head, playing musical instruments. On such days, the young people go and throw scented water over the prostitutes, who reply with abuse. They throw so much red powder that the day is darkened. The main liquors consumed include prasannā, arishtha, maireya, and mead (madhu).

15 Every fortnight or every month, on the proper days, it is a duty to gather at the sanctuary of the goddess Sarasvatī.

The proper days depend on the phases of the moon. The fourth day is dedicated to Ganapati, the fifth to Sarasvati, patron of dancing and music, the eighth to Shiva. The townspeople come to an agreement to organize dance spectacles at one or another's house, each fifth day of the lunar calendar, in order to worship the goddess.

16 The musicians, who have come from elsewhere, have to be auditioned and, on the day before, they must receive their proper fee. Then, according to the admiration they manage to inspire, they either give a performance or are sent away. One must do the same with artists, either known or who have presented themselves.

17 Artists from outside, who come unexpectedly to take part in the performance during the festivities, must be welcomed and honored. This is the rule of their corporation [ganadharma].

At gatherings in honor of the goddess, if a stranger arrives, who is not one of the guests, he must be welcomed with the same consideration as the guests and must be helped if he is in difficulty. This forms part of the duty of the faithful. Women enthusiastically take part in these festivals.

18 Whatever the divinity worshiped, strangers must be welcomed according to the possibilities and the festival rules.

19 When a reception takes place in the house of a courtesan or in the house of a gentleman, the company of friends or comrades must be chosen for their common culture, intelligence, fortune, age, and character. This makes for pleasant conversation with the courtesans.

20 When gatherings take place to discuss matters of literature and art.

21 Talented celebrities are honored and uninvited artists welcomed respectfully.

22 People go to each others' houses to drink.

Drinking parties take place at a fixed date every month or every fortnight in the house of someone or other.

23 There, the guests make the prostitutes drink, and themselves drink mead, wine, intoxicating liquors, while eating all kinds of salted fruits, salads, spicy foods, etc.

The principal drinks are made with honey [mead], molasses [rum], or alcohol distilled from maireya. Molasses alcohol is mixed with cardamom [mesha], aloes [shringī], cinnamon [tvach], and catechu [katthā].

Maireya liquor is mixed with long pepper [pippali], black pepper [maricha], and other ingredients, such as triphala [the three myrobalans]. Foam is removed from mead distilled with kapittha [wood apple] leaves. When the wine [surā] has fermented and been filtered, it is mixed with molasses. There are three kinds of liquors [surā], based on molasses [gandī], wheat [paishtī], or honey [mādhavi]. The word surā *is thus a general term, since it covers different kinds of drink.*

Three kinds of appetizer—salted and with hot pepper, salads [harita], spicy dishes [katuka]—are served separately on shigru leaves [Molioga oleifera] with cardamoms.

The courtesans are invited to drink and eat the appetizers. To start with there is no sign of drunkenness. Restrained by local convention, the signs of excitation are not apparent, but will appear later on.

24 In the same way, people drink together during country outings.

Wine was made with grape juice (angur or dākha), also called kāpishāyana or hārahūrakā. Persons of taste (rasika) regularly drink distilled liquors, mixed with dried grapes, palāsha (*Butea frondosa*), choh, māraka (black pepper), medashringī (aloes), karanjā (*Pongamia glabra*), kshīravriksha (gulara—*Ficus religiosa*), and mālaka (*Raphanus sativus*). In summer, a powder was prepared, mixing fermented sugar to which had been added a little lodhā peel (*Symplocos racemosa*) and a paste made of mahoa (wild fig), kalinga rye, turmeric, daruhaladi (*Berberis asiatica*), lotus (kamala), saunpha (mustard), chichinda (*Trichosanthes anguina*—snake gourd), sataparna (*Desmodium gigantescum*), and aka flowers (*Calotropis gigantea*), of which a handful would be thrown into the wine to flavor it. Sometimes, to improve its taste, five palas of rāva (fermented sugar) would be added.

To prepare maireya liquor, ginger peel (medashringī) was steeped and added together with molasses, long pepper (pippalī), and black pepper (kāli mircha), while sometimes triphala (myrobalan) was used instead of long pepper.

Four sorts of liquor were prepared with mango juice. The first, sahakāra surā, was mixed with wine; the second, rasottarā, with honey and molasses; the third, bījottara, was based on seeds; while the fourth, sambhārikī, was distilled.

Distilled liquors were made with pāthā (*Stephania hernandifolia*), lodhā (*Symplocos racemosa*), gajapīpala (*Scindapsus officinalis*), cardamom, triphala (three myrobalans), mūlahathi, milk tree, kesara (saffron), daruhaladi (*Berberis asiatica*), haldi (turmeric), mircha (pepper), pīpala (sacred fig).

The recipe for distilled liquor (āsava) is:

100 palas of kanthā juice (kapittha, *Feronia elephantum*)

100 palas of rāva (fermented sugar)

1 prastha of shahad (honey)

Added ingredients include: 1 karsha each of dālachini (cinnamon), chīta (*Plumbago zeylonica*), vāyavidanga (*Embelia ribes*), gajapīpala (*Scindapsus officinalis*), while for flavoring, two karshas of areca nuts (supāri), mūlahathi, motha (*Cyperus rotundus*), and lodha (*Symplocos racemosa*).

The measurements are:

1 prastha = 32 pala (1500 gr)

1 pala = 4 karsha (48 gr)

1 karsha = 16 mārsha (12 gr)

1 mārsha = 8 ratti (0.8 gr)

1 ratti = 8 chavāla

1 chavāla = ⅛th of ratti.

While drinking these beverages, all kinds of small salty things were served or brought, as well as acidulated vegetables and sweetmeats, which are called appetizers (apadamstrā). At receptions organized for drinking, the presence of courtesans was the rule. The master of the house filled their cups, or else they served themselves. On walks, girls were also present, and liquors would be drunk. Drinks were considered to give strength, courage, audaciousness, and spirit, and stimulated the gentlemen's eroticism. Care was taken not to put into the drinks anything harmful to the health of either body or mind.

25 *The country party [udyānayātrā]*

Early in the morning, after dressing and putting on one's jewels, one would mount on horseback and, taking servants and accompanied by whores, leave for the country, not too far—so as to be able to return in the evening. Having arrived at the spot, the time was spent watching cockfights, playing dice, watching the dancing, and doing exercises. Then, in the evening, one would return home, bringing bunches of flowers and green branches as a souvenir of the pleasures of the party in the country.

How were parties in the country spent?

Wearing elegant traveling clothes, they mount on horseback for a pleasure ride. The prostitutes precede them, or follow on horseback, as well as the servants who come to do their work.

Every fortnight or every month, the weather permitting, one goes out for the day. The custom of walks in the country is good for the health. When such walks take place in a garden, the time is pleasantly spent in games, cockfights, sports, or in watching the dancing. The prostitutes take part in the exercises.

In the afternoon, after a siesta, and having put on again one's elegant clothes, one remounts together with the prostitutes and servants and, as a souvenir of the pleasures of the countryside, takes back flowers and sprays, returning home with flowers behind the ears and garlands of leaves.

26 During the summer, one goes where there is plenty of water, for water games.

The organization is similar to that necessary for country walks, but the accessories are different. The games consist of throwing water at each other, which can only be done during the hot season. With a group of friends, the citizen would go to a reservoir or pond that was free from crocodiles or other aquatic animals. Reservoirs were built to store water during the summer, since otherwise water games would not be possible.

"The gentleman wears clothes as thin as a snake's skin and, scented with sandalwood and pātala flowers (*Stereospermum suavolens*), goes to a shelter close to the river, where there are pools in which the girls play, plugging their ears with steeped shirīsha flowers (*Albizia*). The water colored by sandalwood and musk reflects the lively colors of the clothes, the drops flung by the jets of water look like diamonds in the sky. The peacocks, mistaking the sound of drums for the noise of a storm, rush away" (*Prāchīna Bharata Kalā Vilāsa*).

27 For the feast of the genies [Yaksharātrī], people stay awake, in the moonlight, as they also do at the spring festival.

The night of the genies is a night of rejoicing. It takes place at the first full moon of the month of Ashvin. People stay awake and play dice. At the spring festival, which is the feast of the god of love [madana], people sing, dance, and play instruments.

The Yaksharātrī is nowadays called Divali. On that day, it is customary to worship the Yaksha, the genies, and play dice.

The spring festival belongs to the god of love. It is the day on which crowds walk around bearing images of Eros. The night is spent singing and dancing. According to the *Bhavishya Purāna*, on the thirteenth day of the spring moon, one should worship the images of the god of love and his mistress Rati (desire). In the afternoon, a festive meal is offered to the musicians and in the evening, the celebrations include music, dancing, mimes, etc.

The *Varshakriyā Kaumudī* quotes a passage from the *Shaiva Āgama* saying that for the feast of the god of love, one should, from morning to afternoon, dance, sing, and use obscene language, throwing mud and colored dye.

28 **During parties in the country, one amuses oneself by opening mangoes, eating cakes and lotus stalks, gathering fresh leaves, imitating the cry of the lion by using bamboos filled with water, making puns, gathering the red cotton plant flowers, battling with kadamba fruits [*Anthocephalus cadamba*], praising one's respective country, playing games from different regions.**

During walks, the citizen's social games consist of gathering fruits and flowers; eating mangoes and lotus stalks, which are found near the ponds; imitating the roaring of the lion with a bamboo, by blowing into the water; battling with flowers; and imitating the countrymen's way of speaking.

29 **When one is alone, one should find one's own ways of amusing oneself.**

If one is alone because other citizens are absent or do not show up, one should celebrate festivals like Yaksharātrī by amusing oneself with the servants.

30 **Later on, we shall describe the proper behavior of well-bred people with courtesans, with their mistresses, and with their friends.**

31   When a cultivated gentleman lacks money and all he
has left is a wooden bed, some soap, and oil for his body,
he should go to the gatherings and festivals of prosperous
people and assure his livelihood by giving lessons to prostitutes. By thus becoming their teacher, he acquires the
position of pīthamarda [steward and dancing master].

*No longer having the means of subsistence, having only his own
body, with neither wife nor children, he strays without resources through
the land and must earn his living in the service of others, seeking a
place to establish himself. In his own town, where he was respected, he
had studied with his teachers the sixty-four arts and the five techniques
and can therefore teach them to others.*

*He attends the receptions given by citizens and, by teaching pros-
titutes the arts, he is appreciated for his teaching and earns his living
as their pīthamarda [secretary-steward].*

According to the *Nātya Shāstra,* "Dancing and music are more
pleasing to the gods than rites and prayers. He who assiduously attends
dancing performances and takes part in them attains the same result as
those who make ritual sacrifices or practice charity."

Music, dancing, and the theater are not considered as mere amusements in India, but as a means of teaching and of achieving the four
aims of life. This is why the festivals and spectacles are organized in
such a way that all social classes can take part.

32   An intelligent and well-born man, expert in the arts,
who has dissipated his wealth and broken off with his family, but is esteemed in the houses of the courtesans and in
fashionable circles and lives at their expense is known as a
gigolo [vita].

*Having squandered his fortune on pleasure during his youth, he
now finds himself destitute, although he comes of a good family. He is
of the place and not from outside. If he has a wife, he may not leave
the country due to this bond. For a living, he works as a pīthamarda,
a man of all work, but, due to his qualities and his education, he is still
a man of the world. He is intelligent and cultivated and attends receptions as a sponger. For other resources, he stays with the courtesans,
living at their expense, despite the ill-will of their menfolk. Since he
lives parasitically on them, he is called a gigolo [vita]. According to the*

meaning of the word, a vita is someone who, to earn his living, makes love professionally and in public.

Due to his knowledge of good manners, inherited from his family, he practices the profession of a man of all work (pīthamarda) and in exchange, is nourished by the courtesans to whom he gives lessons in deportment.

33 If he does not know the tricks, he is a plaything, an object of amusement, but if he inspires confidence, he becomes a companion and amusing confidant [vidūshaka], while continuing sometimes to play the clown [vaihāsika].

A stranger, without any means of subsistence, ruined, possessing nothing but his own body, wandering, scared of everything, with nothing remaining of his former fortune, is a laughingstock. If he becomes a man of trust, however, he is welcomed by the courtesans and received in fashionable society [goshthi], since he makes people laugh. When he has gained a certain respectability among the courtesans and in fashionable society, he plays the role of confidant [vidūshaka]. At first an object of amusement to the courtesans and fashionable world, he knows how to make people laugh and is treated as an entertainer [vaihāsika].

34 Employed as a secretary [mantrī], he busies himself with the appointments and breaches, between courtesans and citizens.

He is considered a second-class citizen [upanāgaraka]. His qualities are to understand the right time and place for meetings or breaches.

35 He utilizes beggar-women, shaven-headed nuns expert in the arts, women of irregular life, or old whores, to arrange appointments.

Vātsyāyana makes it appear that riches and social position are connected. For him, the citizen means the rich bourgeois class. As a character represented in works for the theater, the confidant (vidūshaka) is generally a Brahman. Indeed, Brahmans can be found practicing the profession of merchants, but also of man of all work (pīthamarda), gigolo (vita), and confidant (vidūshaka).

36   If one lives in a village, one must surround oneself with people of one's own milieu, intelligent, willing to be amused, active, well mannered, and respecting the castes. Receptions must be organized, since people amuse themselves when they are together. In business, one must treat one's employees with kindness, even when faced with their failings. Such is the behavior of the well-brought-up man. His dependents must be respectful but, during festivals and journeys, as also in business, one must be courteous and aid each other reciprocally.

37   At gatherings, an educated man should not speak solely in Sanskrit or solely in the language of the people.

38   A prudent man will not attend meetings where there are enemies, spies, or criminals.

39   The wise predict a sure success for a man of wit with moderate behavior, who plays only reasonable games.

When attending gatherings, a person should conform to the customs of the people, going only where the atmosphere is amusing and agreeable. Only thus will he manage to acquire fame.

End of the Fourth Chapter
The Conduct of the Well-bred Townsman
of the First Part entitled General Remarks

Chapter Five

REFLECTIONS ON INTERMEDIARIES WHO ASSIST THE LOVER IN HIS ENTERPRISES

[Nāyakaśahāya Dūtakarma]

In order to arrange a marriage, an intermediary is needed for the preliminaries. Through their contacts, they ascertain that both boy and girl lead a civilized life, after which the matter can be considered. The intermediary may be a man or a woman, and is chosen either by the boy or by the girl. The business is concluded, or it is deemed preferable to abandon it, only after numerous exchanges of view.

1 Sexuality must be satisfied, in the first place, within the caste. This is true for all four castes. By marrying one's son to a virgin, as prescribed, one acquires a good reputation and general esteem.

The sacred books recommend marrying within the social group [kshatra], Brahman with Brahman, Shūdra with Shūdra, and assuring that the wife is a virgin, in the interest of the offspring, so that they can be considered legitimate. A twice-born must have sons belong-

74

ing to his social and cultural milieu. Even when there is no mutual attraction between man and woman, the word love is employed, although in this case it is a matter of social convention. The role of the intermediary is to assure the continuity of the family line of descendents, which is a man's essential duty. This is why marriage within the caste and the begetting of a son are essential, after which, one is free.

2 Sexual relations are forbidden with women of lower or superior caste, or with married women of one's own caste. This is not the case, however, of relations with prostitutes or widows, provided that it is only for pleasure.

Sexual relations are neither recommended nor forbidden with widows alone or remarried, deflowered widows, women repudiated for barrenness, if they are consenting parties, or with prostitutes or other women of that kind. Although one should avoid possessing a woman of another caste, if it occurs, one must not let it be known. It is not forbidden to possess a Shūdra girl if it is only for pleasure, but not to beget children on her. Since children born of parents of different castes are bastards [aurasa], they should be avoided. Not begetting children on widows or prostitutes is a sign of wisdom and a double advantage.

Polluted women are of two kinds: those who have relations before marriage and those who do it after marriage. The word nāraka [infernal] is used to describe the mixing of races. The mixing of races lowers the level of the best classes and gradually leads to the end of a civilization. This is why intercaste marriage is forbidden.

3 Three kinds of women are suitable for love affairs: the young girl, the widow [or second-hand woman], and the prostitute.

Girls are of two kinds, according to whether they are sought for procreation or for pleasure. The best of unions is with a young girl of one's own caste. Relations with a young girl of a lower caste are not recommended, especially if she has already been deflowered. If she is taken when still a virgin, she tends to claim the status of wife. Her virginity should be verified in all cases.

For Vātsyāyana, the best partner is a young girl, then a widow or woman who has already been used, and lastly, a prostitute. It appears that in Vātsyāyana's day, girls were free to choose, which is why they are presented as an object of desire. Marriage took place only after a period of betrothal.

"Within me has mounted the desire to marry a boy of my caste and sleep with him. He will be my husband and I shall be his wife. Our lives will be united like the two wheels of a chariot" (*Rig Veda* 10.10.7).

Given the freedom girls enjoyed, they sometimes let themselves be led into an adventure. Vātsyāyana calls such girls "second-hand" (punarbhū). Roving like bees, the boys happen upon them. This is why he describes them as famished boys and easy girls. The latter are second-hand, but so are the former, and if they love each other, they may even marry.

Vātsyāyana makes a distinction between courtesans (ganikā) and prostitutes (veshyā). Courtesans are women exceptional for their beauty, their manners, and their knowledge. They have a place in society. Even kings treat them with respect. Many courtesans have become famous as poets and artists. The sons of townsmen go to them to perfect their education. Buddhist texts are full of their praise, and they have an important role in the Tantras, since they are the instruments of the secret rites. The whole world acknowledges their usefulness and the necessity for them. Various kinds of beloved (nāyikā) are mentioned in the literature, as follows:

> Svakiyā, she who belongs to you
> Parakiyā, she who is subject to another
> Sāmānyā, she who is common to several
> Padminī, lotus, the full-blown woman
> Chitrinī, the whimsical
> Shankhinī, the fairy
> Hastinī, vigorous and sensual
> Jñāna yauvanā, the intellectual girl
> Madhyamā, a young woman (already developed)
> Praudhā, the mature woman (of thirty years)
> Mugdhā, silly and naive
> Navalā anangā mugdhā, silly young hussy
> Lajjāpriyā mugdhā, silly and modest
> Aruda yauvanā mugdhā, silly adolescent
> Pragalbhavachanā madhyā, middle-aged authoritarian
> Prādurbhūtamanobhāvā madhyā, knowing what she wants,
>   middle-aged

Suratavichitrā madhyā, perverse middle-aged woman
Samastarasakovidā praudhā, mature and experienced in everything
Vichitravibhramā praudhā, mature and bizarre
Ākramitā praudhā, mature and aggressive
Lubdhāpatti praudhā, mature, having known misfortune
Dhīrā, energetic
Dhīrādhīrā, superenergetic
Svadhīnapatikā, dominating
Utkanthitā, melancholic
Kalāhāntaritā, quarrelsome
Khanditā, rebellious
Proshitapatikā, whose husband is abroad
Svayamdūtikā, acting as her own intermediary
Samasyābandhu, linked to a close female friend
Lakshitā, the subject of remarks
Kulatā, nymphomaniac
Muditā, merry
Anushayānā, anxious
Anūdhā, shy virgin
Laghumānavatī, slightly arrogant
Madhyamānavatī, moderately arrogant
Gurumānavatī, very arrogant
Anyasambhogaduhkhinī, sullied by other sexual relations
Garvitā, vain
Rūpagarvitā, proud of her appearance
Premagarvitā, proud of her love
Kāmagarvitā, proud of her erotic skills
Uttamā, superior
Madhyamā, average
Divyā, attractive
Divyādivyā, superattractive
Adivyā, without charm
Kriyāvidagdhā, deft in action
Vachanavidagdhā, clever in speech
Kanishthā, very small.

Reflecting on those that belong to another, he says:

4   Because she belongs to another, a consenting married woman [pākshikī] forms a fourth category according to Gonikāputra.

Because she is a mother, or for quite another reason, her attachments are elsewhere.

5   However, if she agrees, she is then considered as an independent woman.

6   Since her virtue has already been ruined by many others, relations with her, even if she is of high caste, are similar to those with a prostitute and are not condemned by ethics. The same is valid for remarried women.

The purifying offering, after sleeping with a Brahman woman, is a woolen blanket; with a woman of the warrior caste, a bow; with a woman of the merchant caste, clothes; and with a worker-caste woman, a kid.

7   No scruples are needed with women who have already been used by someone else.

8   If the woman who loves me has a rich and powerful husband who is in touch with my enemy, she will arrange for her husband to injure him.

Her husband has the means to damage the fortune and social position of my enemy. Out of affection for me, she will influence her husband so that henceforth he will try to injure the enemy that wishes to harm me and bring about his ruin.

9   She will also repair the bridge between myself and one of my former friends, who has become hostile.

He left me for some reason and now seeks to harm me. She does her best to influence her husband to make him become intimate with my former friend and cause him to change his attitude, finding again the kindly feelings he previously had toward me.

10   Once my relations with her are well established, she will aid me in any matter of friendship or enmity, or other difficult problems.

When her attachment for me becomes true friendship, she will manage to help our friends through her husband. It is known that, for a friend, a man is ready to give his life and protect him with his body against the blows of the enemy. In other words, we shall overcome hostile people and difficult circumstances.

11   Once she has fallen in love with me, she may murder her husband and, having taken possession of his goods, we shall live together in luxury.

United by the affection born of their relations, they league together to kill her husband, attacking him treacherously with a stick. Having accomplished this, they seize his goods. Either she or I kill the rest of the family. We can then benefit from everything we have been able to seize and live on the proceeds of what we have thus realized, without anything appearing illegal.

12   There is nothing wrong in having a love affair with a woman out of interest. If I am penniless, without any means of livelihood, and, thanks to this woman, I can become rich easily, I will make love to her.

Whatever one does to assure one's survival is never a fault, although there are other points of view about this. It is possible to envisage making love for the purpose of obtaining material goods, if I find myself without possessions, without money, without the means of livelihood, and the chances of earning my living are remote and I am unable to feed my family. By sleeping with her, I can obtain considerable advantages. I must therefore establish an amorous relationship with her. A brief adventure would be of no use. She will give me money without difficulty if the relationship lasts. Thus my family problems will be solved.

According to the lawgiver Manu, "when one has an old mother, an aged father, a virtuous wife, and a child of tender years, one should not hesitate to commit one hundred reprehensible deeds in order to feed them."

13   However, if she knows of my problems and is violently in love with me and I show indifference to her, she will accuse me of the worst crimes and will ruin my reputation.

She passionately desires me and has my welfare at heart, but is very possessive. If, either by chance or in some other way, she finds that I neglect her, she will consider it a serious offense. Knowing my secrets, she will accuse me publicly of the worst crimes and try to ruin me. Treating me as a rake, she will have me exiled by the king.

It is therefore better to remain her lover.

14 Even if it is not true, she will accuse me of crimes of which it will be difficult for me to clear myself and will bring about my ruin.

15 Lastly, she will make her husband, who is under her thumb, angry with me, creating enmity and conflict.

16 Allying with my enemies, or else revealing to her husband that I led her astray, he will be revenged by seducing my own wife.

I am therefore forced to remain her lover.

17 We may also, with the aid of the servants and of his enemies, manage to drive her husband out of the house, at the king's order.

18 If a girl I desire is a dependent of hers, it is by establishing relations with her that I shall obtain the girl.

19 Without sleeping with her, I shall never manage to obtain the young girl, difficult to approach, rich and beautiful, whom I would like to marry.

20 In another case, if her husband is in touch with my enemy, it is through my relations with her that I can arrange to have him poisoned. These are some of the reasons for seducing other men's wives.

21 However, unless one has serious reasons for doing so, it is better to avoid taking the risk of seducing other men's wives for mere amorous dalliance.

Thus end the reasons for sleeping with other men's wives.

According to Gonikāputra, four kinds of women are suitable as mistresses (nāyikā). It is not advisable to contemplate the matter from a moral or social point of view. From the moral point of view, to seduce other men's wives is a sin. However, Gonikāputra does not envisage things from the point of view of ethics or virtue. He is only interested in strategy (nīti). The texts on strategy (*Nīti Shāstra*) say, "Under all circumstances, one must consider one's own interest." An intelligent man has to achieve his aims by whatever means. Each individual must utilize the means that best serve his interests.

Gonikāputra was not merely a specialist in sexual behavior, but also in the art of governing. Vātsyāyana, in many places in his work, takes up the arguments of Gonikāputra, who is an unrivaled authority on matters of society and behavior. Although his theories concerning the wives of others are intelligent, logical, and well argued, they do not, however, constitute a rule of behavior. According to him, each must seek for the best possible success in society and, to do so, use every means available. The normal ambitions of a man are to obtain a wife, money, and social standing, the means for achieving which Gonikāputra sees in the seduction of other men's wives.

There is a great gulf between theory and practice. In our behavior, we must consider two aspects, one which is individual, and the other social. Not everything described in the *Kāma Sūtra* is to be put into practice. Theory is general, while practice varies according to circumstance. After Gonikāputra, Vātsyāyana takes into account the opinions of Nārāyana, Suvarnanābha, Ghotakamukha, and Gonardīya.

22 Apart from the four categories of women mentioned above, Nārāyana mentions as a fifth category the wives of the families of ministers or sovereigns, or others of the same milieu, as well as widows occupying an important position.

23 According to Suvarnanābha, a sixth kind of woman is the nun [pravrajitā], the itinerant ascetic.

Here he refers to a widow who has become a religious, belonging to the family of the king, a minister, or an influential family, whose circle she frequents, who has been married young and has accomplished her duties as mistress of the house.

24 According to Ghotakamukha, the daughter of a prostitute or a still-virgin maidservant constitute a seventh category.

The daughter of a courtesan, even if still a virgin, untouched by man, is all the same unmarriable. A woman in the master's service, even if married, may also be a woman of culture and know how to write.

25   For Gonardīya, a young girl of good family, just out of childhood, who can only be seduced at the price of much effort, makes an eighth category.

26   According to Vātsyāyana, since they do not play a different role, these different kinds of mistress belong to the previous four categories.

27   To these must be added the third nature [tritīya prakriti], the inverts or homosexuals who have particular practices and constitute a fifth category of sexual partners.

Inverts form a third sexual category. Not being manly, they behave like women. They take pleasure in practising buccal coition. They are considered as a fifth category of partner, due to their appearance and behavior, although from the point of view of pleasure games, they differ from prostitutes.

It is because they practice buccal coition that inverts form a fifth category. Homosexuals are sometimes confused with eunuchs and impotent men. An impotent (napunsaka) man is one who, although having a sexual organ, has no virility and therefore cannot copulate. Some are so from birth, others by accident. There are two kinds of eunuch, according to whether or not they have a visible organ. They were much used in harems. Boys of the third sex behave like women. Although he mentions inverts as a third nature and recognizes the place that is due to them, Vātsyāyana, in later chapters, does not however consider them as a fifth kind of partner.

28   Types of lover:

The first type of lover, whose role is known by all, is in some way official. Another sort of lover is one whose relationship remains secret. According to the importance or the deficiencies of their aptitudes and defects, lovers are considered as being superior, average, or inferior.

An official lover is like a husband. The others generally have some reason to conceal themselves. They will be described further on.

29   Thirteen kinds of women should be avoided:

Lepers, madwomen, women thrown out of their caste, those who are incapable of keeping a secret, unchaste women, those who are too old, those whose skin is too white or too black, and those who smell bad, as well as kinswomen, those with whom one has friendship, those who have taken monastic vows, as well as the women of one's family, the wives of one's friends, of Brahmans, and of persons belonging to the royal family.

30 According to the Bābhravyas, when it is certain that a woman has had relations with five men, there are no longer any prohibitions.

Although married, if she sleeps with five men besides her husband, she is a profligate, or public woman. One or two lovers are not considered sufficient in this case, only more than five, according to Parāshara's treatise on ethics. The Bābhravyas explain that Draupadī had relations with Yudhishthira and her other four husbands. The story thus shows that a woman can be faithful to several husbands.

31 But, according to Gonikāputra, one should also avoid having relations with the wife of a friend, a female friend, the wife of an officiant priest [shrotriya], or a woman of the royal family.

In saying that there is no objection to frequenting a woman who has had relations with five men, reference is made to a married woman who is known to be profligate and whose vulva has been penetrated by other men. However, in the case of her being the wife of a friend, or a woman with whom a friendship already exists, if she is the wife of an officiating priest, someone belonging to the royal family, or of an aged master, even if she has already been corrupted, one should not unite with her either publicly or secretly.

32 *Friends*

A bosom friend [snehamitra] may be someone with whom one has played in the sand as a child, someone to whom one has done a service, whose qualities, behavior, and nature are similar to yours, a comrade of schooldays from whom nothing is hidden, someone who has shared the pleasures of adolescence.

33 One may give one's friendship to a person who has the following qualities: whose family is attached to yours by traditional ties of affection and kinship, with whom one never has quarrels or disagreements, whose nature and behavior are not changeable, with whom there is mutual trust, who is constant and disinterested, who does not frequent bad company, and who knows how to keep secrets.

34 According to Vātsyāyana, besides these, townspeople may form friendly relations with all those who might serve as intermediaries or messengers, such as laundrymen, barbers, gardeners, perfumers, goldsmiths, beggars, cowherds, betelsellers, jewelers, managers [pīthamarda], gigolos [vita], and jesters [vidūshaka]. One should also be friendly with their wives.

Laundrymen and other suppliers who have access to the house may serve the hero's interests, especially the perfumer who comes to sell his wares. The goldsmith also enters the harem, and no one reproaches the mendicant monk who comes begging his food. Women can penetrate houses where men are not allowed. Women must therefore be trusted.

35 The role of the intermediary [dūta] is suited to a man who is well known and esteemed by both parties, particularly by the woman who must trust him.

36 The qualities of an intermediary are: skill in making contacts, tact in conversation, lack of prejudice, the ability to seize the slightest sign. He must know how to recognize when the woman is most vulnerable and, if there is any risk, he must be prompt in deciding and always find the right trick to attain his ends.

37 In this connection, a quotation: "The enterprising townsman, assisted by his friends, who is enough of a psychologist and knows how to take advantage of time and place, manages to possess the most difficult woman."

Vātsyāyana does not at this point appear to consider employing female intermediaries. He thinks that women are more effective in creating disputes rather than ties. It is male messengers who are most effective, under any circumstances. In his Artha Shāstra, *Kautilya describes the role of the intermediary in much greater detail.*

An essential quality in the go-between is his swiftness in seizing the slightest opportunity, without making any mistakes. The perfect lover is described, not as being immoral, without scruples, and scheming, but, on the contrary, as a man of good family, intelligent, sociable, artistic, and well mannered.

Here ends the Fifth Chapter
Reflections on Intermediaries
and the First Part entitled General Remarks
of the Kāma Sūtra *by Vātsyāyana*

Part Two
Amorous Advances
[*Samprayoga*]

Chapter One

STIMULATION
OF EROTIC DESIRE
[Rata avasthāpana]

*In order to seduce a woman, it is necessary to know erotic technique.
The penis should not be introduced without preparation. To achieve
one's ends, preliminaries are indispensable, the methods of which will
be indicated. For erotic success, the peculiarities of both parties must be
known before commencing to embrace. Skill is required to cause excitation, taking into account the dimensions of the sexual organ, the
duration of the act, and the degree of emotional lability.*

There are different types of man and woman according to the size
of their organs, their moment of sexual enjoyment, and the violence of
their sexual impulse (kāma samvega).

*Having determined the right moment and state of mind for in-
troducing the penis, its size must be considered before starting action.*

1 According to the size of his sexual organ, a man is called
a hare [shasha], bull [vrisha], or stallion [ashva]. The
woman, according to type, is called doe [mrigī], mare
[vādavā], or cow-elephant [hastinī].

2 Those that are matched form three balanced pairs.

89

3 On the other hand, unequal relations number six.

*In cases where the man is superior, there are two forms: superior
and ultrasuperior coition. Similarly, there are two forms of inferior
and ultrainferior coition, the rest being equal. Although it is possible
to unite organs of superior or inferior size, relations between equals are
preferable, the worst being the coupling of extremes. Those between
intermediates are neither good nor bad.*

4 Relations on equal terms are preferable to those between superior and inferior organs. There are thus nine
sorts of sexual relations according to size.

*The stallion and the mare can have an acceptable union. The bull
with the doe is bearable up to a certain point. But the cow-elephant
with the bull and the mare with the hare are not recommended.*

A successful sexual relation must be preceded by preliminaries.
This is the reason why this part is entitled "Amorous Advances"
(Samprayoga). Since the sexual organs are the instruments of copulation, Vātsyāyana commences by indicating their dimensions. It is because of the size of their organ that men are called hare, bull, or
stallion and the women doe, mare, or cow-elephant. This classification
does not merely refer to the physical aspect, but also implies a certain
kind of temperament. It may be asked why, since he does not speak
of the other parts of the body, he gives a detailed explanation of the
shape and size of the sexual organs. The reason is that we are dealing
with erotic science, which is largely based on the said organs. The
Taittirīya Upanishad, speaking of sexuality in terms of prajā—the begotten, prajana—procreation, and prajāti—the begetter, refers to categories that are similar to those of the *Kāma Sūtra*. Knowledge of the
various parts of the body is itself part knowledge of the divine plan,
and its study leads to knowledge of god (brahmavid), through perception of the divine plan in the human sphere.

According to the *Atharva Veda*, the man who realizes that his
body is the image of the heavenly city (brahma nāgarī) that floats in
eternity perceives the creator through the divine work, or in other
words, in corporeal faculties, such as vision, life, procreation. The man
who realizes that he only resides in the divine city that is his body, is
called purusha (city-dweller). Until old age, he will keep his sight and
his other senses, as well as the breath of life. Ayodhyā (the invincible)

is the name of that city of the gods, with nine centers (chakra) and nine gates, over which reigns the light of intelligence and where, in a gilded sheath (hiranyamaya kosha), lies paradise (svarga), made of bliss and enjoyment. This gilded sheath, the image of paradise, is fixed to the soul at three points and in three regions, in which dwells the divine principle (brahma deva), or intelligence. As a result, he who knows the secrets of the body and the conduct suited to the heavenly city becomes invincible (ayodhyā) and attains all his desires.

The body is the product of the male seed and the female seed, coming from the father and the mother, from whom the child inherits his appearance, his tendencies, and his weaknesses. This body that is transmitted by heredity lasts eternally, and for this reason is known as the immortal city (amarāvatī). It must be kept with care. The description of the size, length, depth of the penis and the vagina concerns not only pleasure, but also the product of their union. The fetus is the product of semen, and represents the physical achievement of the substance of a living being. Through him is manifest the invisible, inconceivable, indescribable presence of the soul, and its power.

If we consider only the pleasure of the union, copulation is limited to sighs, pleasure, and ejaculation. What is most important in the sexual act, however, are the transmittable characteristics, the shape of the body and the size of the organs. Vātsyāyana contemplates three types of man: the hare, whose organ is six fingers long, the bull, whose organ is eight fingers, and the stallion whose organ is twelve fingers. As far as women are concerned [the doe, the mare, and the cow-elephant], it is a question of the width and depth of their vagina. Those whose sizes match are termed equal.

The stallion man has elongated ears, head, and lips, a thin body, thick hair, long fingers, a luminous look, heavy thighs. He is fast and has beautiful nails.

The hare man has small feet, figure, buttocks, hands, and ears, a gentle voice, beautiful and well-spaced teeth, a lively body. Always with a smile, his face is round and his nails hard.

The bull has a thick neck, an impressive bearing, red palms, an assured air, clear skin, a nice round stomach. He is always lucky.

The doe woman has beautiful hair, a thin body, golden skin; her organ is as cold as the ray of the moon. She has strong teeth, a low voice, abundant hair, and a lymphatic temperament. She eats little, her face is narrow, her sexual secretions are scented. She never cries out.

The mare has wide, strong nostrils, is slightly knock-kneed, has thick thighs, and her sexual organ is always hot. She has tender fat arms on which drops of sweat appear; her body is of a clear color, her sexual secretions smell of meat, her limbs are regular, her belly small. She is of bilious temperament.

The cow elephant is tall. She has a massive body, often has long teeth, and her skin is reddish in color. Her constitution is dominated by the element of air. Her body is strong and harmonious. She is now cold, now hot, speaks much, is changeable, her menses smell like elephant's sweat.

In his *Ratirahasya*, Koka describes four kinds of female partners, whom he calls padmini (lotus), chitrini (whimsical), shankhini (fairy) and hastini (cow-elephant).

The lotus woman (padmini) has tender limbs like lotus stems; her sexual secretions smell of lotus. She has the eyes of a startled doe; the edges of her eyes are red. She hesitates, out of modesty, to expose her beautiful breasts. Her nose resembles a sesame flower. She is virtuous and respectful by nature. Her face is white like a jasmine flower. Her sanctuary of Eros seems like a full-blown lotus. Her body is thin and light and she walks delicately like a goose. Her words are mixed with sighs, like a goose, her figure is slight, her belly divided into three parts. She eats little, is modest and wise, but proud. She loves beautiful clothes and flowers.

The bearing of chitrini (the whimsical) is graceful. She is of average height and her figure is slight. She has opulent buttocks and thighs, and thick lips. Her sexual secretions smell of honey. Her neck is marked with three lines, and her voice is like that of a partridge. Her sanctuary of Eros is rounded and soft inside. She is skilled in artistic techniques, has little hair on her body, and abundant sexual secretion. She appears agitated, loves caresses, kisses, and other external forms of lovemaking. She likes unusual and colorful clothes and jewels. She eats little and has a sweet tooth.

Shankhini, the fairy, is tall, with a well-fleshed body. Her fingers are long. When she is angry, tiny veins shine on her body. She loves red flowers and clothes. Cupid's den is covered with thick hair. Her buttocks are elongated, her sexual secretions smell like ashes. When making love, she likes to dig in her nails. She is of bilious temperament, spiteful and scandalmongering.

The cow-elephant has an ugly bearing and not very graceful body. She is tall. Her features, fingers, thighs, and buttocks are massive, her hair yellowish. Her body is strong. She has a cruel nature. Her sexual secretions smell like an elephant in rut. She likes sharp, sour food and cold dishes. Her lips are very thick, her vagina is very deep. She stammers and eats standing.

Vātsyāyana and Koka's descriptions of men's and women's characteristics are given with a view to promoting properly matched sexual relations. Whatever the moral or social point of view, whether it is a question of marriage or individual amusement, the main point is always the union of man and woman. So long as sexual relations between them do not take place, even if they are married from a religious or spiritual point of view, or if there are considerations of a social or political nature, or simply affectionate relations, these considerations are of no importance.

Before a marriage, the astrologers compare horoscopes in which eight points must be taken into account: racial compatibility (caste), compatibility of character, the state of the heavens at birth, sexual type (hare, etc.), the planets and their conjunctions, social standing, state of health according to the Āyur Veda, character.

When sexual relations take place:

5   Feeble temperaments [mandavega] are those that during amorous advances show little ardor, whose semen does not flow abundantly, and who do not support being bitten, scratched, etc.

He desires action, yet if he obtains no result after a while, he gives up. There is thus a contrast between cause and effect. The cause is his erotic desire, which is why he makes amorous advances, but the result is the absence of any erection. Failure may be relative, middling, or total during relations with the woman he loves, even if he is mentally excited. The sperm ejaculated is not abundant. Furthermore, he cannot stand the girl's attempts to bite or scratch. A feeble temperament is shown by lack of desire or inability to sustain an erection.

6   On the other hand, there are also middling [madhyama] and passionate [chanda] temperaments, and the same goes also for women.

7   Here too, as for size, there are nine sorts of coition [rata].

8   Similarly, as far as the duration of the act is concerned, there are rapid, average, and slow men.

When their sexual drive is similar, a couple is well matched. If their speed is not the same, enjoyment is not perfect.

If there is a difference in the capacity for enjoyment between man and woman, there can be no true satisfaction in love. This is why the organs must be matched and the moments of enjoyment and ejaculation correspond. Otherwise, copulation is animal. However, many authors doubt that it is possible for the woman to reach orgasm at the same time as the man.

9   As far as women are concerned, opinions vary.

10   Since, according to Auddālaki Shvetaketu, her sexuality is less strong than the man's.

Because she has no ejaculation of sperm. Then why does she unite with the man?

11   Only friction with the man's penis calms the itching of her vulva.

With the prospect of sexual relations, an itch appears which can only be calmed by copulation. The itch, arising from desire, may be subtle, feeble, average, or strong. Its intensity is the effect of the god of love. This is why she seeks a man and is only calmed by sustained action. Otherwise it becomes intolerable. But she can also satisfy herself with an instrument of some kind.

12   Although she can bring herself to sexual enjoyment, she prefers another form of satisfaction.

Although she can satisfy herself, she needs other forms of pleasure. Having calmed her itch with the aid of a small stick or an earpick, her desire grows for other sensations such as kisses. With other sensual pleasures in mind, she seeks the means for them and, in particular, feels the lack of the fertilizing emission of sperm. Finding herself in a continual state of excitement, she desires to enjoy a man.

By practices such as kisses, caresses, bites, and blows, which stimulate her erotic desire, she experiences true sensual pleasure that she can only achieve in union with a man.

How can one know whether a woman does or does not experience sexual enjoyment similar to a man's?

13   Neither man nor woman can know the pleasure experienced by the other. One cannot perceive a man's feelings. How could one describe his sexual enjoyment?

A man's feelings, by their very nature, are beyond the range of the senses. How could he know the feelings of a woman, which words cannot describe? A woman enamored of a man gives him pleasure by her behavior, but even if she questions him about it, she will not be able to know the nature of his feelings, nor know whether his enjoyment is different to hers, since it cannot be expressed in words. Auddālaki expresses a doubt as to whether her experience is different to a man's. According to him:

14   "How can one know therefore whether a woman feels a pleasure similar to a man's? A man's excitement ceases once he has ejaculated. A woman's need is not satisfied at that point, since woman's nature is not like a man's."

A man calms down when he has come, when he has taken his pleasure. He no longer desires the woman, even if he loves her. Women are not the same. If she came like a man, she would be willing to separate from the instrument in order to rest, but it is not so. Even if the man does not want to go on, she wants him to stay inside her. Sometimes, if the opportunity arises, she will continue with another. "If there is no wood, fire does not spread in the water. Among human beings, death makes no distinction between man or woman." The woman's desire does not calm down after she has been satisfied like that of a man after ejaculation.

15   One thing certain is that a man whose activity lasts long pleases women, while on the other hand they complain of men who reach orgasm rapidly.

Satisfied tranquility is not to be found among women after an erotic experience with a man who reaches orgasm quickly. Women love and are pleased by men who ejaculate after long copulation. A man whose ardor is rapid, who ejaculates quickly, detaches himself after experiencing his pleasure. Men who have a habit of finishing quickly are not well looked upon. It is on this that women's attachment or contempt depends, and on this basis they decide which deserve to be used or not. The wife of a man who has difficulty in making her reach orgasm becomes hostile to him. Thus it is that, from a certain point of view, a woman's love or indifference is connected with the man's possibility of making her reach orgasm. Women appreciate the virility of a man who performs the longest copulatory act. It is almost impossible for a woman to desire to sleep with someone who ejaculates quickly. Love's delight is only possible if she reaches orgasm at the same time as the man of whom she is enamored.

This is why the man who pleases women is the one who gives them complete pleasure, and not the contrary.

> **16 Yet it is not so. Once her itch has been calmed, she wants the act to continue for a long time. Duration is thus an essential element.**

The penetration of the penis does not give rise to a feeling of love, even though it is sufficient to calm the excitement that rapid action suffices to eliminate. If women desire long—and even prolonged—action, it is not to reach an ejaculation, which they do not have, or to calm their itch. It cannot be stated that ejaculation or being freed from an itch is the reason for their attachment. With a man who ejaculates quickly, they can in no way manage to experience pleasure. The woman therefore does not behave like a man.

A woman's desire does not stop when she has reached orgasm. She experiences a continual enjoyment. Her need for a man continues even when the itching of her clitoris has been calmed, which is why her need for signs of affection is independent of her desire for enjoyment.

A verse of Auddālaki Shvetaketu expresses his point of view:

> **17 "In coupling, the friction of the man's member calms the woman's excitement. But it is in signs of affection [abhimāna], kissing and caressing, that she finds her pleasure."**

From another source:

> **18 According to the sons of Babhru, a young woman gets a taste for the thing if the duration of the act is prolonged. If the man repeats his performance, it is the best way to achieve it. If, for lack of duration, she does not experience enjoyment, she is unable to conceive.**

Procreation depends on both. From the moment she is penetrated by the instrument [yantra], a woman needs uninterrupted continuity. She wants to be possessed by the man. She shrinks at the contact, like a cracked vase losing its water. When the man has achieved his pleasure, the woman only reaches hers if [the act] continues, but in the meantime, the man has reached the end of his pleasure and pours out his semen.

According to size and according to different durations of the act, there are differences in orgasm. For procreation, a simultaneous orgasm must be reached. It has been said elsewhere that a woman only conceives if she is fully satisfied during the procreative act. According to Charaka, the author of the great medical treatise, "Having vigorously spurted out his sperm, his member subsiding, the man, proud of himself, is no longer interested. Once his semen has been seized by the vagina, his virile member is satisfied and the man has a feeling of achievement."

He does not scatter his seed to get rid of it, as the woman does with her menses. Inflamed by desire, the man and woman establish body contact. Like a fire stimulated by a poker, the sperm excites the menstrua. Who at that moment can imagine the result, know whether the semen is used to impregnate the woman? However, it happens that, on contact with a man, the woman is impregnated, since that is the goal of copulation.

According to the Sushruta [medical treatise], sperm is produced with a view to procreation. Amorous desire is the outcome of the generating substance, which seeks the opportunity to encounter an ovum. The spermal substance is produced by the spinal cord.

The disciples of Babhru say that a man achieves sexual enjoyment at the moment of ejaculation, after which he has finished. When the woman begins to experience pleasure, however, her pleasure continues without interruption. It is a well-known fact that if she has no desire to reach orgasm and experiences no pleasure, fecundation does not take place.

19   Not having been proved, these two opinions must be examined.

In the case of rapid enjoyment, there is only the feeling of copulation. The excited man achieves his purpose. However, if she is unsatisfied and he does not recommence action, a problem arises. Even to calm the tickling of the clitoris, a certain time is needed. When this excitement appears, rapid action does nothing to calm it. During penetration, the titillation does not last long. The desire to conceive not having been satisfied, a continuation of the union is therefore desired. Rapid action is pleasant for the man, but a lengthy duration puts the woman into a good humor. From the man's point of view, it is also quite satisfactory, since both experience the same pleasure.

The questions raised by the sons of Babhru and Auddālaki will be solved later. This is why:

> 20 The woman develops a taste for it by means of continual stimulation. At the start, she is moderately interested, and is not ready to put up with much. Then, gradually, developing a taste for the union, she no longer defends her body. In the end, if he wishes to rest, she will not allow him to do so.

The question is, if the woman experiences pleasure throughout the act, what is the reason for which, at the outset, when the excited man is growing agitated, the woman stays calm, without any impulse, refusing to be scratched, bitten, or massaged, when in the end it is she who wants the man to continue in action? In reality, it is a mistake to believe that a woman experiences pleasure from the start to the finish.

At the beginning of coition, she is moderately interested, and does not wish to be bitten, scratched, etc.; she is not ready to put up with it. But little by little, gradually, during the union her indifference changes. With no consideration for her body, she is ready to put up with everything. Then, at the end, when he desires to free himself, it is she who, after one performance, wants another.

> 21 When the potter starts his wheel moving, the speed, initially slow, increases little by little, then slows down and stops. It appears that it is the same in exciting a woman from the beginning to the end.
>
> 22 According to the text of the Bābhravyas, man experiences pleasure up to ejaculation, while the woman's pleasure is continuous. When he has ejected his semen, he seeks rest, whereas she wishes to continue.
>
> 23 Vātsyāyana's opinion is that a woman, like the man,

experiences the same sexual enjoyment from start to finish.

24 How is it possible for two beings belonging to the same species and practicing the same act not to feel the same pleasure?

25 Differences exist only in advances and in secondary actions [caresses, kisses, etc.].

26 Vātsyāyana does not believe that there is any difference in the pleasure itself. Difference of sex is a fact of birth. It is generally admitted that the man is active and the woman passive. The man's action is therefore different to the woman's. The man thinks that he is enjoying the woman, while the woman thinks that the man is enjoying her. There is thus a difference in attitude and experience, but not in enjoyment.

Difference in behavior is innate: it is a question of nature. Man and woman have an identical structure. The organ [meha] of the one is open, while the other's is erect. If one of these organs seizes, the other is seized. There is a difference in action and, consequently, in behavior. There is only a difference in behavior and in emotive aspects. He enjoys the girl selfishly, but the desire for caresses arises in both of them. They are only different in the action they agree upon during the act. Which confirms the author's thesis.

27 A difference in behavior does not imply a difference in result. The difference in behavior is the result of the characteristics of him who acts and the characteristics of her who submits to the act, but there is no difference in the effect.

Once more, the objection can be raised that if there is a difference of behavior and action between man and woman, why should there not be any difference in the pleasure of coition? The answer is that there cannot be. Although there is a difference in their organs, there is no reason why the goal of the union, which is enjoyment, should be different, since both man and woman belong to the same species.

28 When two actors do a job together, the job accomplished is one. Each pursues his own goal, which is, however, connected with that of the other. When a man and

woman unite for the same purpose, which is enjoyment, it would appear mistaken to say that the pleasure they both receive from the union could be of a different nature.

29   This is not so. It is clear that the couple pursue a common goal, like rams fighting, like two halves of a fruit, like a wrestling match.

There is no difference in the actor, even if there is a difference of role. As far as behavioral differences are concerned, they are established in advance at birth, but for both, the obtaining of pleasure must be similar.

The reality of different kinds of couples must be considered, such as rams fighting, the two halves of a fruit, a pair of wrestlers. The rams, fruits, and wrestlers seek the same goal. It may be said that with the rams, fruits, and wrestlers, there is no sexual difference, but between man and woman there is no difference in nature since both are human beings. Sexual difference is a part of their nature. The result is that the experience of pleasure must be the same for both.

30   Because they belong to the same species [jāti], man and woman seek the same pleasure in sexual relations. This is why desire must first be stimulated by preliminary attentions.

The woman has to be excited with kisses, caresses, kneading, and other exterior play in such a way as to arouse her desire before the man's. After which, to satisfy his own desire, the man can copulate rapidly.

31   Similarity having been demonstrated, there are nine forms of the sexual act according to the moment, desire, and the size of the organs.

32   In order to describe the sensual delight [ānanda] of pleasure [rati], the words rasa [taste], rati [pleasure], prīti [love], bhāva [sensation], vega [ardor], and samāpti [conclusion] are employed. And for the sexual act, sambhoga or surata [copulation], samprayoga [amorous advances], rata [coition], raha [being alone together], shayana [to sleep], and mohana [to seduce].

33   According to organ size, moment, and mood, there are nine forms of balanced sexual relations. Going outside the

norm, these possibilities are so numerous that it is impossible to count them.

34 According to Vātsyāyana, one should copulate after reflecting on the contradictory arguments concerning these different forms of sexual relations.

Unequal relations should be shunned in favor of equal relations, and should not be risked without thought regarding size, moment and mood, and how to proceed with the union. One must be aware of inequalities and ascertain whether the relation is practicable or not.
According to the Bābhravyas:
When the male organ slides into the other, the best result is when both mood and moment are shared. If the organ causes an injury on penetrating, the act must be interrupted. If moment and mood are not shared, the relation is of no interest. Relations between corresponding types are the best. Unequal relations make for bad copulation. In all intermediate cases, the relation is better if it is from strong to feeble. The very strong should always choose the moment; hares too should seek the right moment. The cow-elephant has to be touched everywhere, especially her vulva. With a mare, a ram will need a lot of time. Due to the difference in size, he will need to make a considerable effort. The power of force is not always sufficient. A stallion, even when excited, needs a lot of time. The man with an inadequate duration and size must do the best he can.

35 On starting the act, the man's ardor is so strong that he seeks to conclude as quickly as possible, but later on, it is otherwise. In reaching sexual enjoyment, the woman's behavior is exactly the opposite.

From the beginning of the act until ejaculation, the man's ardor is so strong that he tries to reach his conclusion immediately. If, however, he performs copulation a second time, the man takes a long time to ejaculate. This suits the woman's nature. During the first intercourse, her feeble erotic fire gradually lights and lasts very little. The second time, it lasts longer. Therein lies the difference between male and female sexuality.

36 All agree on the point that in sexual intercourse, the man reaches orgasm more quickly than the woman.

By nature, woman is submissive, but even if she is not, she quickly learns the art of kissing, caressing, and using her hands to attract affection. Only her passivity is natural, the rest is artifice. She seems passionate when she feels very little passion. Man too is often tender by nature, the rest is invented. That is the opinion of the ancient masters, to which all agree.

37   However submissive or reticent the woman may be by nature, she is quick at learning the games of love, the specialists explain.

External acts, kisses, and caresses make a gentle woman rapidly discover the pleasure of love and she finally becomes enterprising. It is the same for a woman who is not very cooperative to begin with. Man is also tender by nature. All the rest is fabricated. On this subject, the whole world agrees, if one thinks about it.

The authors of treatises on eroticism consider that, due to the sweetness of her nature, a woman is more rapidly stimulated than the man. The fires of desire are rapidly lighted by kisses and caresses. This contradicts the opinions given previously.

38   What has been said up to now concerning sexual relations has been said briefly, being intended for intelligent men. We will now explain in greater detail for people who are hard of understanding.

According to Auddālaki Shvetaketu:
"The woman feels an itch in her sexual organ that is partly calmed during sexual intercourse, but continues after the man's ejaculation, since the woman's desire is not assuaged."

According to the Bābhravyas, there is a great difference between the sexual enjoyment of the man and of the woman. At the outset of intercourse, the woman experiences violent pleasure, while the man experiences pleasure at the moment of ejaculation. The woman's pleasure can be compared to the action of the potter's wheel, slow to start with, then fast in the middle, and slow at the end, but with a continuous movement.

According to Vātsyāyana, amorous attraction (prīti) is of four kinds: born of habit, of the imagination, of memory, or of interest. Man is the active element (kartā), and woman the passive support (ādhāra). In copulation, the man plays the dominant role, but the woman has to cooperate. If the woman stays indifferent or frigid, neither of the two will really experience pleasure. When the man's member penetrates the woman, they are gradually stirred up by the friction. The man's desire stops when he has ejaculated, and, if the woman has also reached orgasm at that moment, their intercourse is a success. For success, preparations are required. This is why Vātsyāyana takes organ size into account for successful copulation. The man and the woman have to be excited before starting action. When both man and woman are greatly inflamed, the itching of the vulva and the nerves of the sexual region being involved, the pleasure is much more intense.

It should also be noted that the first encounter may be a failure, if loveplay is not known. The man must be more careful than the woman in the act of copulation, since he does not know how to restrain himself, while the woman is always hesitant. The responsibility lies with both.

In his *Nāgarasarvasva*, Padmashrī explains how to prepare for sexual intercourse. In order to stimulate her partner, the woman should alternately hide and expose her body. She should approach the man, stimulating him and resisting. If he takes her hand, she should show reluctance. If he seizes it, she should appear astonished, startled like a doe, and hide her sex, then gradually let herself go. Any place that he seeks to touch, look at, scratch, or bite, she should hide, then suddenly let herself go eagerly. While he is caressing, biting her, and so on, she should sigh and protest and then abandon herself to it.

The question of knowing on what basis the man and woman are attracted to each other remains open. Attraction and enjoyment are mental phenomena.

39 Those who know the mechanics [tantra] of relations say that attraction [prīti] is born in four ways: from practice [abhyāsa], from imagination [vichāra = abhimāna], from substitution [sampratyapāda], or from the object [vishaya].

40 *Love born from practice [abhyāsa]*

All activities of the senses, starting with speech, require continuous practice in order to manifest themselves. Love is born of long practice, like the love of hunting for the hunter.

In saying, "starting with speech," allusion is made to dancing, singing, playing instruments, drawing, sculpture, etc.

41 *Imaginary or intellectual love [abhimāniki]*

A person with no previous experience of a form of action can develop an attraction born of imagination (samkalpa), which is termed imaginary [abhimāniki].

One may desire something without having any experience of the act, like a hunter without experience who develops a passion for hunting. It is different for someone who is used to it. If one has no experience of the thing, of how it is performed, as with other physical activities, one's interest for it is imaginary. Imaginary love, which is a kind of affective condition, is termed pure mental invention.

Imaginary love without any experience is a mental condition, and is distinct from the love of real objects. Why is it contemplated in this treatise?

Sexual fantasies.

42 This is a matter of activities such as buccal coition for inverts or for women, or else kisses, caresses, etc.

It has to do with acts that inverts and women do with their mouths instead of the vagina. By practicing them, a love for the physical act gradually develops. It is the same, although they belong to another order, for kisses and caresses, as well as scratches, bites, blows, etc., which, even among those who have no experience of them, exist at the level of fantasies. In such a case, they are often sought by a form of intellectual eroticism connected with a desire that is not of a physical nature. It is an experience tied to the feeling of touch. Pain inflicted on the body, which cannot be called love, represents a purely mental satisfaction, and is not of a physical nature.

43 *Substitute love [sampratyaya]*

In the absence of someone, one becomes attached to another. This kind of tie is called substitute attachment.

In the absence of somebody, or of a former love, a man or woman can mentally transfer their feelings to another person, attributing to the new object the qualities of the other. Since this kind of attachment is born of an attribution, the authors of the Kāma Shāstra call it substitute love.

When the features of an unknown person evoke those of a loved one, it is a substitute attraction.

44 *Mercenary love [viṣhayātmika]*
Whether manifested openly or implicitly, love based on the desire for material goods, in which gain is primordial, is of another nature.

Love for objects of the senses is common to all. But love born of the desire for objects of the senses is another matter.

45 Having examined from a theoretical point of view the various forms of affective ties described in the texts, each man must act as he prefers.

The temperament and state of mind of both man and woman must be taken into account, so that a mutual affection can develop.

End of the First Chapter
Stimulation of Erotic Desire
of the Second Part entitled Amorous Advances

Chapter Two

EMBRACES
[Ālingana]

There are sixty-four elements in loveplay prior to copulation.

1   It is claimed that the preliminaries to sexual intercourse involve sixty-four elements, probably because they were originally described in sixty-four chapters.

We repeat this figure because in the opinion of the masters of old, the ancient treatises had sixty-four chapters.

2   According to certain authors, it is the body of erotic treatises that is divided into sixty-four parts.

Why did the authors of old speak of sixty-four forms of amorous preliminaries? Knowing the meaning of words, such authors must have had a reason for using this figure. It could have to do with a particular aspect of this science, or the body of theories.
Is it a local opinion, or a part of the science itself?

3 The arts number sixty-four, and are considered as forming part of the practice of love. As a body, they are mentioned as the "sixty-four."

The *Rig Veda*, comprising ten chapters, is mentioned as "the ten." Such an interpretation could also be valid in this case. The disciples of Babhru, who came from Panchāla country, used this number out of respect.

Why did the people of Panchāla use this figure, if not for the same reason that one speaks of "the ten" in the case of the Rig Veda? *This is particularly the case here, in this chapter of preliminary practices, which comprise ten elements: caresses, kisses, bites, scratches, sighs, blows, stretching out against one another, inversion of roles [purushāyitam], buccal coition, and intercourse with boys [narāyitam].*

The great sages of Panchāla divided the Rig Veda *into sixty-four parts. The Bābhravyas, according to the tradition of Panchāla, speak of sixty-four parts of the* Rig Veda, *and of the same number of erotic practices. These various authors were natives of Panchāla, and it is out of respect for erotic science that they compare it with the* Rig Veda.

The Bābhravyas try to consider embraces as something sacred, though there is nothing virtuous about them, and explain why they should be honored, remarking that they are practiced by cultivated people as well as by the humble and by the courtesans' corporation. Who does not worship a young girl [nandini]?

The Bābhravyas also mention the different kinds of embrace suited to married people and those practiced by men without ties.

5 Division into eight categories would not appear to be acceptable. Blows, cries, sodomy [purushopasripta], bizarre tastes [chitra rata] belong to other categories. Here we are dealing with penetration [pravesha]. For Vātsyāyana, it is merely a manner of speaking, as when one speaks of "a seven-leafed tree," or offerings with five ingredients.

6 Before copulation [samāgama], in order to arouse the penis with desire, the following four kinds of caress [ālingana] are practiced: contact [sprishtaka], bruising [viddhaka], baring [uddhrishtaka], and squeezing [pīditaka].

7 These four actions are known as external or preparatory acts.

Each of these caresses is defined below.

8   *Contact [sprishtaka]*
It is termed contact when the boy and girl are face to face,
body pressing against body, uniting the areas involved.
Although in contact, there is no question of penetration.

9   *Bruising [viddhaka]*
In an isolated spot, finding her seated or standing, he seizes
her breasts. Since the boy hurts her by catching hold of
her, it is called bruising.

*The girl does not refuse the advances of the enterprising boy and
does not go away. She allows him to continue, but there is no question
of sleeping together, since they are not yet lovers. Even in an isolated
spot, she is reluctant to uncover her breasts. What can he do in order
to knead them? Having drawn close, he finds some pretext to place his
hands on her breasts. If she resists, the boy puts his arms around her
and, uncovering his own sex, presses it against her from behind. Then,
freeing her from his embrace, he kneads her breasts until she experiences a certain pleasure, sliding his penis between them and bruising
them.*

10   These two practices may be performed by lovers who
only just know each other.

If they are not excited and do not speak, it will not work.

11   *Baring [uddhrishtaka]*
In the darkness, if people are present, or otherwise in an
isolated place, they stroll slowly, showing their bodies to
each other, not just for an instant, but for some time.

*The boy shows his body, the girl only the area involved. They
caress each other and are both excited. Or else, he only exposes himself,
while she remains covered.*

12   *Squeezing [piditaka]*
Leaning against a wall or pillar, he presses his erect organ
against her.

13   These two last contacts are practiced by lovers who
have not yet passed on to the act.

14 Four kinds of embrace are employed in preliminary loveplay: encircling like a liana [latāveshtitaka], climbing the tree [vrikshādhirudhaka], rice and sesame [tilatandulaka], and milk and water [kshirajalaka].

15 *Encircling like a liana*
Encircling her lover like a liana around a sāl tree [*Shorea robusta*], she bends her face toward him for a kiss and then withdraws with a small sigh. Assured and showing off her beauty, she seems to entwine around him like a liana.

16 *Climbing the tree*
Resting one of her feet on the man's and with the other attacking his thigh, she embraces him with her arm across his back. Her other arm clings to his shoulder and neck. With a slight sigh, she makes an effort to climb onto him to kiss him, just as if she were climbing a tree.

17 These two embraces are done initially.

Before passing on to the act.

18 *Rice and sesame*
Both lying with arms and legs entwined, they rub against each other and become deeply entangled.

If the man is on the right, he places his left leg between the woman's thighs and his left arm on her right side. The woman clasps him. Arms and legs are entangled like rice with sesame, whence the name.

19 *Milk and water*
Blinded by desire, unable to wait, they press against each other with the same passion, face to face, whether seated or lying down.

This is possible when the woman is sitting on the man's lap, facing him, encircling his waist with her legs, breast to breast, or else when they are both stretched out on a bed.

20 These two embraces are done in moments of passion [rāga].

21 Such are the preliminary embraces described by the Bābhravyas.

22 Suvarnanābha indicates a further four kinds of embrace concerning a part of the body.

23 *Embracing the thighs [uru upagūhana]*
Squeezing one or both thighs of the other party as hard as possible in the grip of one's own is called embracing the thighs.

24 *Embracing the sexual area [jaghana upagūhana]*
Thrusting his groin firmly against the girl's pubis, he seizes her by the hair and stays crouched over her in order to scratch, bite, and strike her.

Lying on his side, either he rests his best limb [varānga] on her as on a brood mare, or else lying on top of her, the part of his body below the navel resting on the woman's pubis, he presses his instrument against her without penetrating her. At that moment, the women's sex opens out, overexcited, particularly if she has a large organ. He seizes her by the hair and, if she wishes, scratches and bites her, lying on top of her for a long time.

25 *Embrace of the breasts ([stanālingana]*
Inserting her breasts between the boy's thighs and resting there with all their weight, is known as the embrace of the breasts.

Either seated or lying, she lowers the top part of her body and pushes her breasts strongly between the boy's thighs. Feeling their mass between his thighs, he experiences pleasure at the contact.

26 *Joining brows [lalātikā]*
Face to face, gazing into each other's eyes, their brows join, the one against the other.

27 *Sundry caresses [samsparsha]*
Some deem that caresses should be counted among embraces.

So long as one feels pleasure at the contact.

28 But, according to Vātsyāyana, since they take place at other times, have another scope, and are an ordinary ac-

tion, caresses do not belong to erotic play properly so-called.

For him, caressing is not enjoyment but fatigue. Not being a means of enjoyment, it cannot be termed an embrace.

Caresses are mostly practiced by men and submitted to by women. They are thus not common to both. The sixty-four arts, singing, etc., are also erotic stimulants, as well as pulling hair, slapping, and kissing, which will be dealt with as variants.

29 Asking questions, whether hearing or talking about embraces, immediately excites sexual ardor in men.

And they will experience pleasure if they put the same into practice.

30 Other kinds of stimulating contact exist, which are not described in the texts. They are perfectly honorable and may be practiced by those that like them.

All kinds of practices are encountered in various countries, serving to arouse amorous excitement. One should not hesitate to try them, according to circumstances and place.

31 The subject of this treatise does not concern men who lack a sexual temperament. The texts and methods indicated for an erotic nature are not for them.

Vātsyāyana has described the sixty-four arts considered to be the best introduction for love.

In his *Nāgarasarvasva*, Padmashrī mentions sixteen feminine states of mind (bhāva) during the preliminaries of love. A woman can be tender, restive, contemptuous, excited, perplexed, mocking, relaxed, seductive, importunate, disagreeable, vain, bored, complaining, incapable, anxious, or charming.

These sixteen states of mind appear when a woman is in love. It is in understanding them that the man must practice the embraces, kisses, etc., that are the prelude to copulation (maithuna). If he does not perceive the woman's emotional state and, when he is burning with desire, begins his effusions without worrying about the woman's reaction, a man will always meet with failure. Neither he nor the woman will experience true satisfaction.

When the first experience takes place at a tender age, and the god of love agitates the heart most deeply, love's troubles are manifested in signs, marks, and indications: this is known as amorous feeling (bhāva).

In the *Ujjvala Nīlamani*, agitation and the desire to seduce (hāva) and gestures of affection (hela) are a young girl's charms. Beauty, courage, bloom, radiance, perspicuity, gentleness, and wiles are the qualities that make women attractive, to which are added ten attitudes or states of mind (svabhāva), which are as follows:

Feeling (bhāva)
> When one is seized by the taste for love (shringara rasa) and desire (rati) awakes, the first confusion the god of love sows in the heart is called amorous feeling (bhāva). The implementation of the feelings established in one's consciousness is called experience (Anubhāva).

Affection (helā)
> When a woman embraces a man forcefully, drawing him toward her, begins to twine around him, and lays her trembling thighs on those of the stretched-out man, showing that her state of mind is disposed toward erotic activities, this is called affection.

Refusal (vicchitti)
> When a woman is angry with her lover, throws away her ornaments, and spurns his love, this is refusal.

Contempt (bibboka)
> Even if her lover brings gifts that please her, she rejects them with contempt.

Excitement (kilakinchita)
> Seeing her lover return from a journey, the woman is full of joy and weeps without shedding tears, or even starts laughing.

Perplexity (vibhrama)
> When the woman sometimes smiles, sometimes loses her temper, throws away the flowers she asked for, then picks them up again, goes to sleep at a girlfriend's house while her lover is looking for her, or walks about here and there.

Amusement (līlā)
> Imitating all her lover's words and making faces.

Flirtation (vilāsa)
Approaching her lover, then going away, getting angry when he calls, then smiling at him, turning away with a grimace when her lover calls, pointing the finger of scorn at him, pacing up and down.

Seduction (hāva)
Fluttering her eyelashes, making her eyes dance, laughing, talking, and interrupting herself, feeling a deep love for her lover and behaving accordingly.

Inopportunity (vikshepa)
When her lover is not in the mood, approaching him and showing all the signs connected with desire.

Boredom (mottāyita)
When, while talking, the woman yawns on several occasions or stretches herself.

Moaning (kuttamiti)
The woman feigns pain.

Stupidity (mugdhatā)
When difficulties in sexual life are due to ignorance.

Anxiety (tapana)
When her lover is late in arriving, contesting her friends and weeping.

Charm (lalita)
Moving her lashes, eyes, hands, and feet artfully is called lalita bhāva. Such behavior is frequent in women, with the aim of exciting the man.

A man must not let himself be led by his desire, but take into account the woman's mood. In the presence of such behavior as described, a woman's state of mind can be easily understood and met. In order to understand these states of mind, it is necessary to interpret the slightest signs. Padmashrī explains that, for a man possessing every quality and expert in the sixty-four arts, a woman will drop her unmannerly husband without subtlety, like a garland of faded flowers.

According to Padmashrī, however expert a man may be in arts and science, however famous and important, if he is scorned by women in the art of love, he is a dead man.

In his *Nāgarasarvasva*, Bhikshu Padmashrī describes the symbols (sanketa) used to communicate in secret language (vakrabhāshā).

Thus, the man is called "the fruit," the woman "the flower," the family "root." If he is a Brahman, he is called "pomegranate," if a Kshatriya "gourd," if a Vaishya "banana," and if a Shūdra "mango." A prince is called a "half-moon," the king "cloud"; a girl with no family is known as a "black flower"; someone who criticizes everything is called an "arrow." A young man is called "midday," a child "raw," an old man "cooked." A Brahman woman is called "flower of the pool," the king's daughter "chameli flower," a courtesan's daughter "jasmine flower," a girl of low caste "water lily," a merchant's daughter "pink lotus," a minister's daughter "blue lotus." The lover is known as a "bee," his beloved as a "mango shoot." To call, the word "ankusha" (elephant goad) is used; to stop, the word "wall." Chandra, the moon, means a "nocturnal meeting"; Sūrya, the sun, "during the day." Early in the morning is "shellfish," during the morning "conch." "Lotus" means midday, "great lotus" the afternoon, "passion" late in the afternoon, "tranquility" (rāma) the evening, "rest" (virāma) the beginning of the night, "renewal" midnight, "dawn" the night's end. When the boy lurks around the house and the messenger encounters him and says, "Why does the bee (the boy) stay on the wall, even if the moon is hidden; the mango shoot, like a lotus flower, will blossom at the renewal," he understands that he can meet his girlfriend during the third watch of the night.

Besides spoken language, there is also a language of the parts of the body (anga sanketa). If one takes care while asking a question or saying something, one can also use body language. Touching the ear means "silence."

Touching the hair indicates erotic desire. Touching the breast with both hands signifies "love." To ask the time or circumstance, place the middle finger on the little finger; when the time arrives, join both hands (anjali) and, to call, lift joined hands.

To indicate directions, the thumb signifies east, the little finger south, the middle finger west, and the index north. From the base of the little finger to the line beneath the thumb, there are three lines for each finger, making fifteen lines, which represent the days of a fortnight, from the first day of the moon to full moon. For the clear half, use the left hand, and for the dark half, the right.

Small symbolic packets (potali sanketa)

To indicate love, they contain betel nut and catechu together with scented ingredients; for passionate love, cardamom, nutmeg, and cloves; to indicate the end of a love affair, a piece of coral; after a long relationship, two pieces of coral; in love's fever, a bamboo object; for an immediate love call, a bunch of grapes. A cotton fruit means, "I am all yours." Cumin means, "I give you my life"; bilva (wood apple) means "attention"; turmeric (haldi) means, "nothing to fear." Small packets containing a little ball of wax, marked with the nails of all five fingers, bound with a red thread, are used as a message in the games of the god of love. The wax indicates attraction (anurāga), the red thread a love relationship, the nail marks represent the wounds inflicted by the god of love.

There are also clothing signs (vastra sanketa). To indicate the state of one whose body has been lacerated by the arrows of the god of love, clothes of good quality are worn, but torn. To show violent love, one must wear yellow- or orange-colored clothes, and torn clothes in the case of separation. For refound love, resewn clothes are worn; for a single love, a single garment; for two loves, a garment of two pieces.

There are also five kinds of symbolic betel (tāmbūla), made up into little packets: the first is without points or seal (shalākā); the second in the shape of a hook (ankusha); the third is triangular; the fourth rectangular or square. To indicate strong affection, an open betel should be used, the inside being filled with care; the hook-shaped betel is used for quarrels. To indicate the wounds of love (madanavyathā), an arrow shape is used. To sleep together, a rectangular betel is given, while the square shape indicates that one is not free.

If one is not in love, the betel is prepared without nutmeg (supāri); but to indicate sincere feelings, betel with cardamom is offered.

As a sign of breaking off, tie the betel with black thread and present it upside down.

To ask for a meeting, put a betel in your mouth and touch your mouth with another betel tied with red thread, which is to be offered.

To indicate that you are leaving, break the betel in two and tie it with black thread.

To indicate the moment of death, tie the betel with red thread.

In cases of intense passion, cut the betel nut into small pieces, place saffron (kesara) inside, and smear sandalwood on the outside.

The meaning of flower garlands (pushpa mālā)

To indicate passion, use red flowers; orange flowers are used for separation. For absence or disaffection, the garland is tied with knots of black ribbon.

The authors of erotic treatises compare woman to the opal (chandrakānta). Just as the opal, touched by the fresh rays of the moon, becomes damp, so the woman becomes moist (dravita) on contact with a man. An intelligent man must take great care in enjoying a woman: a man in love must not behave like an animal. Even if he is under pressure, he must retain his human discernment. The scope of the works of the *Kāma Shāstra* is to prevent a man in love from behaving like a beast. He must reach the moment of action after studying the signs, contacts (kisses, caresses, etc.), and behavior of the woman from both physical and psychological points of view.

Bhikshu Padmashrī explains that the lover who wishes to possess or seduce another man's wife must be very careful. According to the signs, he must understand whether or not the woman is accessible. Padmashrī goes on to explain that, apart from the fact that seducing other men's wives is a sin, one must know in advance whether the woman with whom the man wants to make love has already been led astray or not, and moreover, whether the woman is easy or reached only with difficulty. Knowing that she cannot be reached even with a great effort, it is pointless to run after her. If, on seeing a man, a woman lets her arms drop, hides her eyes, thrusts out her belly, arranges herself so that her breasts can be seen in some way, then one knows that she can be easily had; and also, if she has a child with her, she caresses and kisses it; if she several times muddles and rearranges her hair. If in bending and straightening out, she allows her body to be seen. If she arranges her clothes, makes up her eyes, polishes her nails. If she coughs, spits, or yawns on several occasions. If she becomes attentive when she hears the voice of the man she desires; if she stretches, stops her ears, speaks and looks while laughing.

Not much effort is needed to seduce a woman whose husband is sick, without resources, cruel, or deformed, or else a woman whose husband lives abroad or is very inconstant. Highly modest or virtuous women, or those who fear public opinion, must be considered beyond reach. The favors of those who suffer or are not interested in money can never be attained. Padmashrī considers that adolescents and very young women are a good catch (patya). In his view:

an adolescent (bālā) is a girl of sixteen;

a young woman (tarunī) is from sixteen to thirty;

a mature woman (praudhā) is from thirty to fifty;

and an old woman (buddhā) is over fifty.

In summer and autumn, intercourse with a young girl (bālā) is beneficial; in spring and winter, a taruni; in spring and the rainy season, the praudhā.

The author of the *Rati Rahasya* explains that, before making love with a girl, the lover should know how to make her moist (dravita). Just as the moon grows and wanes in sixteen crescents, just so, during the clear fortnight and the dark fortnight, the influence of the god of love grows and wanes in the woman's special parts. During the clear fortnight, starting from the very first day (pratipaksha), the god of love installs himself successively on the toe, the foot, the thigh, the navel, the breast, the armpit, the neck, the cheek, the lips, the eyes, the eyebrows, and the forehead; then from the first day of the dark fortnight, he descends from the head to the feet. This is why, according to the days indicated, the astute man seizes the woman's hair, kisses her brow and eyes, bites her lips, kneads her breasts, and pats her torso and belly to awaken the god of love. The fifteen places mentioned corresponding to the digits (kalā) of the moon are those where the god of love dwells more particularly. For this reason, before enjoying her, it is essential to kiss and embrace these places. Embraces make a woman moist and then, with a joyful heart, she is ready to pass on to the act itself.

The five arrows of Eros are represented by the letters A, I, U, E, and O. Five parts of the woman's body are the targets of these arrows. The target of arrow A is the heart; the target of I is the breast; the third, U, is aimed at the eyes; the fourth, E, at the forehead; and the fifth, O, at her vagina. The man must clasp the woman, taking these zones into account, since her desire is then aroused.

According to the *Sushruta*, the treatise on medicine, a man's semen comes from his whole body, like the juice of the sugar cane, butter in milk, oil in the sesame seed, which come forth when the cane is cut, the milk churned, the seed crushed. When a man thinks of a woman, sees, hears, and caresses her, he feels pleasure. The semen then leaves the various parts of the body to gather in his testicles, whence, during copulation, it penetrates the woman's belly and the fetus is formed.

Sperm is the essence of the living being, through which the invisble, inconceivable, indescribable soul materializes and is made manifest. The seed contained in the sperm is the support of the soul, and should not be put to bad use. This is why the sages have defined the activities that precede and follow that of procreation.

According to Bhikshu Padmashrī, twenty-four differently placed nerves arouse the desire for copulation. One is located in the woman's vagina, hidden by the parasol of Eros, which must be gently massaged with a finger. If the girl is young, this must be done with a finger. With a mature woman, the neck of the uterus should be caressed with the fingers or with the penis. Of the other nerves that stimulate eroticism, two are found in the mouth; two in the eyes; one in the neck; one at the base of the index finger. By pressing these spots, sexual desire is rapidly aroused. In the same way, by driving one's nails into the ears, the thighs, beneath the shoulder blades, or into the brow, desire is aroused.

Six great nerves called satī, asatī, subhagā, durbhagā, putrī, and duhitrinī, which are located in the vagina, provoke violent desire. Putrī and duhitrinī are to the right, at the very bottom. Satī is to the left, and asatī to the right. At the entrance, subhagā and durbhagā are to the right and left respectively. If satī is pressed, asatī flares up; if asatī is pressed, satī is contented. By stimulating subhagā, the woman has good luck, while by stimulating durbhagā, she has troubles. She becomes red, weak, and ages prematurely. By stimulating putrī, a woman stays young. With duhitrinī she bears sons, while with putrī, daughters. If both centers are activated at the same time, the child will be homosexual. Abortion is caused by massaging satī heavily. By caressing the woman's sides, asatī is stimulated. In kissing her posterior (adhara), subhagā is stimulated; in caressing her waist, durbhagā; in kissing her mouth, putrī. By caressing her buttocks, duhitrinī becomes restive and eroticism is kindled.

These particulars about embraces are mentioned by Charaka in Ayurveda medicine.

Thus, prior to the ritual of coition, Kāma, the god of love, must be invoked, and having installed him in every part of the body, copulation may be performed.

End of the Second Chapter
Embraces
of the Second Part entitled Amorous Advances

Chapter Three

PETTING AND CARESSES

[Ālingana]

Kissing is as much a part of lovemaking as blows, scratching, and biting, but one must know when and how to do it.

1 There are no special moments in which kissing, scratching, and biting should be employed, since they are constantly used in amorous relations and preliminaries. Slaps and sighs are also a part of sexual practice.

When seized by passion, no particular order has to be followed. These practices usually take place prior to the penetration of the instrument. They are recommended for provoking or arousing excitement before the male and female are united by the instrument. The blows that stimulate desire are also employed beforehand, as well as the sighs that they cause. With kisses, scratching, and biting, there is no before and after, since in erotic excitement there is no order or reason. These practices are generally used to stimulate excitation. Moreover, blows and sighs also continue during copulation. That is one opinion: its opposite is also given.

119

2   Passion knows no rules, nor place, nor time, Vātsyāyana
declares.

*People bursting with ardor know no rules, but less active persons
are sometimes perplexed.*

3   During the preliminaries, they should not be overindulged
in, and once confidence has been established, they should
be used prudently. Even when excitation is evident, great
care should be taken, especially if they are combined the
better to inflame desire.

*These five practices [kisses, scratches, bites, blows, and sighs] should
not be violent. While pursuing one's goal, self-control is necessary and
the various practices should be tried one at a time, not together, either
a kiss or a scratch, a kiss or a bite, a kiss or a few blows. If one strikes
a blow, caress the hair twice the right way and then twenty times the
wrong way.*

*To begin with, desire is weak. When interest is relative, one does
not put up with much, and it is best to control oneself. Later on, as
desire for intercourse increases, the body is no longer fearful. The thighs
can then be stroked, then whatever part one wants, and one finds
twenty ways of doing things that can be suggested to increase desire, so
that intercourse is not tasteless, and establishes a lasting relationship
between the two. Kissing and the other activities must be practiced in
succession. The order to be followed is determined by increasing confidence. One thing must be done after the other: it is not possible to do
everything at once.*

4   Kisses can be placed on the brow, the cheeks, the throat,
the eyes, a boy's chest, a woman's breast, the lower lip,
inside the mouth.

Kisses in other places are not recommended by the authors of old.
In the mouth means sucking the tongue. At the same time, one
also embraces the thighs, the armpits, the groin, the navel. When passion is aroused, there is no part of the body that cannot be embraced.
Vātsyāyana says that it is not possible to count all the parts of the body
where men place their lips.

The inhabitants of the Lāta country also embrace the thighs, the armpits, and the vulva. According to the intensity of desire and local custom, different parts are embraced.

According to Vātsyāyana, while kisses play a role in causing excitation, they are better when accompanied by scratches and bites. When feeling amorous, one should start with kisses and continue with scratches and bites. It is a mistake to believe that during the first moments there are no rules. As long as one keeps one's senses, one is aware of what one is doing. Later on, all control is lost. Under the word rāga, Vātsyāyana studies the erotic practices of the whole world. He calls rāga the fifth degree of desire (rati). During the preliminaries, when desire is gradually increasing, he calls it love (prema).

Just as the sun's heat makes butter melt, so, when love melts reason (chitta), affection (sneha) is formed. With increasing affection comes consideration (māna). When consideration grows, confidence appears (pranaya), and when confidence is full, rāga (passion) develops. When passion reaches its highest level, it is known as anurāga (infatuation).

Vātsyāyana considers it normal to lose self-control when in a state of passion, and that there are no longer any rules about kisses, and so on. In a state of passion, man and woman suck one another like lumps of sugar. They find pleasure, whether in embracing or in scratching and biting. A sugarloaf is sweet at whatever point it is cut. In approaching the spouse, or at the start when lovers unite, great precautions are necessary. The seed of desire, born of mutual attraction, must develop. To make it grow and flourish, much delicacy is needed. It must be watered with the ambrosia of kisses and caresses.

Once desire has grown and become strong, taking on the aspect of passion, the moment has come for kisses, scratches, and bites. Once passion has developed, there is no further need to worry about using them. It is no longer the concern of the man alone, since the woman too, once the prey of passion, is ready to respond to all the man's attacks. Her amorous desire (vāsanā) is so activated that, losing all respectability, shame, and shyness, she herself embraces the man with force, responding to his kisses with her own, and to his scratches and bites with her own scratches and bites.

Vātsyāyana draws attention to the fact that if, at the start of activity, the man, carried away by his excitation, begins to embrace, scratch, and bite, attacking the girl's tender body, she will not experience pleasure but, on the contrary, will develop a feeling of repulsion toward the man, a hostility that will be established forever in her mind. Women are not only fragile in their limbs, but also in their feelings and mind. Considering her like a flower, she must be treated in such a way that she will not close up, but will diffuse her scent. If she is squeezed and embraced brutally, fear, doubt, rage, and contempt will develop in her mind and will stay with her for the rest of her life. She must be treated with an understanding of her state of mind and fragility. It is important to realize on what part of her body she prefers to be embraced, at what moment she likes to be bitten or scratched. During the first three days, the man must be very careful, since it is during this time that she can take a permanent aversion to him. At this time, with patience and sweetness, the man must drive away the woman's natural apprehensions, and be careful of her ethical problems and modesty. Women prefer to make love in the dark. If the young man prefers a light in order to look at her, scratch and bite her, a virtuous girl will see the man's efforts as the work of a devil and will continue to do so: she will consider the man as something inhuman.

Happiness both given and received is mutual enjoyment. For this shared happiness and pleasure, a man is willing to give himself entirely. For a man as for a woman, the total gift of self is a source of wonderful happiness and luck. Sexual intercourse is not merely a pleasure of the senses: more important is the sacrifice of oneself, the gift of self. To understand the mystery of sexual intercourse, to know and make use of what is fitting is the essential difference between man and beast.

Love and pleasure are the two main mental aspects of sexuality. Love creates the impulse and feeling, but amorous desire follows its own path. Many believe that a couple has no need to learn erotic arts, and that nature will teach them everything. Those who believe that, on reaching middle age, become unhappy and desperate. Their life in common no longer has any savor and mutual hostility develops. Often, they lose their trust in each other. Vātsyāyana explains how, in order to guard against such a change, the preliminaries of copulation can be used, kisses and caresses that awake desire and, when amorous stimulation (kāma samvega) has reached its peak, continuing immediately with kisses, scratchings, and so on.

As places to kiss, Vātsyāyana indicates the brow, the hair, the cheeks, the eyes, the chest, the breasts, the lower lip, and the tongue, but he also adds that the people of the Lāta country kiss the thighs, the joints, the armpits, and the sex (pedu). The possibilities of kissing vary according to the country. It is the custom of the people of Nishada that one should embrace at night, never during the day. King Nala, when his beloved Damayanti was unsatisfied, said craftily to one of her companions, "Tell your friend to forgive the shortcomings of this wretch that I am, since the kisses I practice at night are forbidden to me during the day." Vātsyāyana also indicates how the people of Lāta embrace, and in his *Naishadiya Charitra*, Shrī Harsha makes his hero Nala say, "Well beloved, the clothes that cover your body have an immense fortune: they are like a lucky man who embraces your buttocks, your sex, and your breasts."

Bhikshu Padmashrī too, acknowledges that, according to place and character, women like kisses on certain parts. They take their pleasure according to their nature, and so it is necessary to fall in with their habits. If one kisses contrary to custom and local sentiment, it is an amusement which no longer has any meaning and becomes distressing, like the air from a fan to someone who is cold.

5 The people of Lāta country [Gujarāt] also lick the labia of the vagina [nābhimūla], the crotch [urusandhi], the underside of the arms and the pubis [pedu].

Nābhimūla: the root "navel" really means varānga [the best of members, i.e., the sex].

6 Vātsyāyana's opinion is that in the heat of passion, and following local custom, people lick these parts and places, which does not, however, imply that everyone should do the same.

Kissing the thigh joints and other parts, as practiced in Lāta country, are not practiced elsewhere.

These parts are considered indecent by well-thinking people. The places reached by lowering the head are considered kisses because the face takes part in them. They are performed the one lying on the other, in an inverted position, which many people consider degrading.

Here follow the three kinds of kisses.

7 Kisses given to girls are of three kinds: nominal [nimittaka], vibrant [sphuritaka], and rubbing [ghattitaka].

8   *Nominal [nimittaka]*

Seizing her head with his hands, he applies his mouth forcefully on hers, but without violence.

Out of delicacy, he does not seek to seize her lower lip: this is termed a nominal kiss because it is limited to lip contact. In the hope of inciting the woman to suck his lip, the man places his mouth on hers, but she does not open her lips.

9   *Vibrant [sphuritaka]*

He seeks to insert his lip into her mouth, but does not attempt to seize her mouth. Since her lips tremble, however, she does not allow him to seize her lower lip.

When the lover presses his lip to the woman's mouth, the latter shyly tries to press their lips together. Because her lower lip trembles slightly, out of shyness her upper lip remains closed. This sort of kiss is called sphuritaka [vibrant].

10   *Rubbing [ghattitaka]*

Holding him loosely, she closes her eyes and covers his eyes with her hands. She then rubs her lover's lips with her tongue.

After having begun to feel the pleasure of their relation, she seizes her lover's lip, which he has inserted into her mouth. Feeling shy, however, she closes her eyes and, placing her hands over the boy's eyes, she rubs her lover's lip with her tongue. This sort of kiss is called ghattitaka [rubbed].

11   There are a further four kinds of kiss: equal [sama], crosswise [tiryaka], reverse [udbhranta], and pressed [pīditaka].

Equal [sama]; face to face, the man and woman make contact with their lips.
Crosswise [tiryaka]; turning the head slightly, the lips are caught by making them round.

Reverse [udbhranta]; being seated behind, catch the head and cheeks and turning them toward one, sucking the lips.

Pressed [pīditaka]; when the lips are closely pressed together in any of the three previous kisses.

12 *The fifth hold [panchama grahana]*

A fifth kind of kiss is performed pressing the lips very closely, bringing the fingertips together and pressing the cheeks, then pressing the lips together without letting the teeth touch.

With the nails, press both cheeks, seizing the woman's lips with the mouth, in such a way that the teeth do not touch. This is what is known as pīditaka, pressing closely. Such are the five kinds of kisses.

Vātsyāyana proposes three kinds of kiss suitable for very young girls (kanyā). According to the *Dharma Shāstra*, kanyā means a seven-year-old girl, which does not seem very practicable in this context. The author of the *Kāma Sūtra* probably wishes to indicate the sexual use of girls who have attained sexual maturity by perching them on a stool. They are attractive, but have not had relations with men. The word kanyā—very young girl—must mean a young unmarried girl. The *Mahābhārata* defines the word as meaning a desirable unmarried girl.

The order indicated for these kisses is envisaged from a psychological point of view. If, during their first relations, the boy wants to force the girl to suck his lip and press her lips on his, she will allow it to be done, but will not respond to his desire. This is what Vātsyāyana calls nimittaka, nominal. The girl desires the kiss, but is shy and dares not respond. Later on, she will be the one who takes the initiative. The boy will then consider that he has been successful.

When she makes love a second time, the girl is less shy. She presses her lips to his and rounds her mouth in order to suck his lower lip, but her upper lip remains immobile. This is the kiss that Vātsyāyana calls "vibrant" (sphuritaka), because one of her lips trembles.

To begin with, the girl is paralyzed with fear, modesty, and hesitation. Doubt is subsequently replaced by pleasure. The desire for enjoyment and copulation develops. The boy no longer needs to make an effort to get kisses, it is she who seizes his lips. In speaking of the third kiss, Vātsyāyana explains that although the girl no longer hesitates or is upset, due to her remaining modesty, she closes her eyes. She remains still undecided between her desire and her hesitation.

13 *The kissing game*
A game is established.

Only kisses on the mouth are intended, not anywhere else. Passion is stirred up by a kissing competition. It is a game, since there is a winner and a loser.

14 The first to seize the other's lip is the winner. As in a game, it is necessary to take the other by surprise. Since there is a winner, a quarrel is inevitable, which is also a stimulant.

15 If she loses, she cries a little and wrings her hands, she sighs, threatens him, bites him and then, turning round, she draws him to her forcefully, ill-treats and insults him. If he wins again, she ill-treats him doubly.

16 *The trick [kapataдyūta]*
Taking advantage of the self-satisfied hero's inattention, the heroine catches his lip with her teeth and immobilizes him. If he protests, she threatens him, shakes him, dances about joyfully waving her arms and telling him some home truths.

She loudly boasts of her victory. If her lover gets cross, she challenges him, her eyes dancing and arms waving until he shows his strength. Thus finishes the affectionate conflict of the war of kisses.

17 The ways of scratching with the nails, biting with the teeth, and striking, which are also games of combat, will be described below.

18 The lovers make use of them because they are both in a moment of acute excitation.

And may their sexual games long endure.

19 *Kissing the upper lip*
While the woman is sucking the lower lip of the boy, the

latter seizes her upper lip with his lips. This is called kissing the upper lip.

Two ways of kissing are described for the couple:

20   In the first, called the box, both lips are seized between the teeth and are sucked. This is called shutting the box [samputaka], and can be practiced by either boy or girl.

So long as the boy does not wear a moustache.

21   *Tongue combat [jihvāyuḍḍha]*
Having performed the closing of the box, rubbing the tongue lengthily over the other's teeth and palate is called the combat of tongues.

22   It is thus that mouth wrestling and teeth conflict should be understood.

23   *Special kisses [chumbanavishesha]*
Besides the ones already described, there are a further four kinds of kisses called: equal [sama], pressed [pīdita], devouring [ashchita], delicate [mridu]. They consist of embracing particular parts of the body, and are known as special kisses.

These kisses are performed otherwise than face to face.
Sama [equal], is done on the brow or elsewhere, on the thigh-joint, the armpits, the pubis, neither too hard nor too soft.
Pīdita [pressed], on the cheeks, the armpits, the sexual region.
Ashchita [devouring], on the brow, the chin, and the body up to the armpits.
Mridu [delicate], lightly touching the eyes.
Such are the special kisses.

Sama, seated or lying next to each other, kissing or nibbling the thighs, chest, armpits. Pīdita, seizing the breasts, cheeks, buttocks, navel and pressing and kneading them. Ashchita, tickling and kissing lightly below the breasts and the armpits. Mridu, lightly touching the neck, breasts, buttocks, and back. These are the four kinds of kisses.

Vātsyāyana explains how to introduce an element of competition into kissing: of the boy or the girl, who will be the first to seize the other's lips? The aim of these games is to fire passion, establishing physical intimacy between the boy and girl which will lead to coition. It is not so in every case, however. If the boy and girl are very ardent, they have no time to lose before getting to copulation.

According to the *Ujjvala Nīlamani* of Rūpagosvāmī, "a sexual relationship without preliminaries is incomplete. Desire, affection, love create a lasting state of mind, through which the boy and girl, stimulated by caresses and kisses, abandon themselves wholeheartedly to the act of love."

24   *The inflamer*

Seeing the mouth of her sleeping lover, she kisses him in order to reach her own ends. This is the inflamer kiss [rāgadīpana].

In order to arouse his desire, she embraces him and wakes him with a kiss, so that he immediately understands her intentions. This kind of kiss is called the inflamer.

25   *The encouragement*

When the boy seems distracted or in a bad mood, or for some other reason looks elsewhere; if he seems to be asleep or falls asleep, the kiss of encouragement [chalita] should be used.

If he is distracted by music or reading, or if, out of vanity, he is looking for a quarrel, or stays offended after a quarrel; if he looks elsewhere or seems sleepy or falls asleep, in order to shake his indifference or whatever, he needs a kiss of encouragement.

When the boy seems indifferent to the girl, quarrels with her, or shows interest in other girls, or falls asleep, in order to attract his attention, appease the quarrel, wake him from sleep, the girl must embrace him, which is known as the kiss of encouragement [chalita].

26   *The awakening [pratibodhika]*

When her lover returns home late and kisses the sleeping girl, his intention is clear. This kind of kiss is called the awakening kiss [pratibodhika].

27 When the girl has thus been awakened by her lover, she should put his love to the test by feigning to sleep when he arrives.

28 When he sees his girl's shadow in a mirror, on a wall, or in the water, the lover should kiss the shadow to show his feelings.

29 A young man [bāla] who kisses a portrait painted by an artist, also kisses a reflection.

He takes the portrait and clasps it to him, or else, placing an image of clay or wood in front of him, he kisses the imaginary resemblance that he attributes to the object of his love. With tender words he kisses the illusory presence or image. Thanks to this fiction, he claims the right to kiss it, then, seized by excitation, he touches it with a heightened sensuality and it is evident from his reaction that he feels erotic satisfaction.

His emotional state can be seen when he seizes, kisses, and clasps to himself the portrait or image.

30 At nighttime, during entertainment or family meetings, he approaches her intentionally, he kisses her hands or fingers, or, throwing himself to the ground, her toenails.

31 Although she does not want to, due to sleepiness, she is affected, attracted by the look of the boy, who rests his head on her thigh and kisses it, arousing in her the desire for amorous games.

Somewhat affected by the boy's contact, and noting his appearance, even if she does not wish to be kissed, she is charmed by the boy's look and, feigning sleepiness, lets him rest his head on her thigh and kiss it, and suck her toes, moved because he is at her feet. She does not reproach him for his behavior, since she is charmed to see him at her feet, desirous of an amorous encounter, for the contact of their two bodies and to exchange a few words. Taken by the same feeling, they give themselves over to simulated kisses [chāyā] if other forms of contact are impossible under the circumstances.

If the girl whose foot the boy is squeezing is attracted by or enamoured of him, to show her feelings, she will let him lay his face on her thigh, suck her big toe. She will, however, pretend to be asleep, so that those present believe that it is due to the effect of sleep that she allows the boy to lay his face on her thigh.

It is necessary to know the right time for preliminary play.

32 Each of the two lovers must respond action with action, blow with blow, for each activity the same activity, for each kiss a return kiss.

For any practice or aggression, the same practice or aggression should be inflicted by way of example. With blows and kisses, the same coin should be repaid. For indecent acts, however, kisses practiced by animals should not be repaid in kind, nor similar ways of copulating. At the same time, if he makes use of uncommon practices, he should be repaid in the same coin.

Before making love, in order to stimulate desire, the woman should behave just as the man. Whatever the man practices on the woman should also be practiced on him by her. The woman should kiss just as the man does. Whatever the circumstances, open or secret kisses cause both man and woman wonderful pleasure. When lovers kiss, their purpose is to draw close to each other, to develop love and mutual trust. Kisses, quarrels, blows, scratches, and bites arouse amorous ador and pleasure.

Lips play an important role and are one of the most sensitive areas of the body. Caused by contact, an electric current passes through the lips. When a boy and girl experience such a shock at their first kiss, they become mad with desire and want only to go aside somewhere to copulate. In their kisses, they find love's oneness, a feeling so strong that they can no longer see each other's faults. Young people kissing become radiant. The kiss is the gateway to bliss and amorous experience. The kiss provokes erotic ardor, agitates the heart, and is an incitation to the natural gift of self.

The kiss is a tradition to be met with everywhere: its instruments are lips and teeth. Women like being bitten, since bites cause rapid excitation. Kissing with the teeth is an art that must be practiced gently, and is particularly efficacious when the tips of the breasts and the buttocks are nibbled.

Kisses are described by numerous authors.

According to Bhikshu Padmashrī, if one simultaneously strokes the clitoris and squeezes the breasts, the kiss is known as vipīdita (insistent). Kissing with the teeth on the brow and the lip, while turning the head, is called "the vagabond." Kissing while lifting the head and embracing the eyes and brow is the "joyful" kiss. Kissing the navel, the cheeks, and breasts, and kissing while turning back the lip, is the "vibrant" kiss. Kissing with both lips together on the heart, the leg, or thigh, is the "satisfied" kiss. Kissing while turning the head, on the cheeks, the neck, and the chest is the "twisted" kiss. A kiss with tightened lips first on the cheeks, then all over the body, is called a "bowed" kiss.

End of the Third Chapter
Petting and Caresses
of the Second Part entitled Amorous Advances

Chapter Four

THE ART OF SCRATCHING
[*Nakharadanajāti*]

After kissing, the usage of scratching and biting is described.

1 The nails are used for scratching and scraping in order to increase excitation.

2 The nails are used for scratching and scraping in the heat of passion, or, by contrast, to show vigor when enthusiasm is lacking, or on the evening of an amorous encounter, on returning from a journey, or prior to a departure. This practice is also a sign of anger, joy, or intoxication, but it cannot be practiced in every circumstance.

It is a mark of affection, to recall passion by keeping the souvenir during an absence. It is also the visible sign of anger, joy, or drunkenness in a young man.

3 Biting with the teeth, like scratching with the nails, is a sign of possession.

Both have the same effect of increasing excitation and showing domination.

4 The marks left by nail imprints are of eight kinds:

1 the knife stroke [achchuritaka]
2 the half-moon [ardhachandra]
3 the circle [mandala]
4 the dash [rekha]
5 the tiger's claw [vyāghranakha]
6 the peacock's claw [mayurapadaka]
7 the hare's jump [shashaplutaka]
8 the lotus leaf [utpalapattraka]

5 The best parts to scratch are the cheeks, the breasts, the neck, the back, the thighs, and the crotch.

6 According to Suvarnanābha,
"In the heat of union, people are not aware of the parts of the body that they can scratch and those they should avoid."

7 The nails of the left hand should be long and pointed. Some people cut them into two or three points. They are then known as nails of aggression.

This cannot be done with the right hand, which is used for too many other purposes. They are cut into three points, like a raven's claw, thus allowing them to lacerate a wide area. Less violent people cut their nails into half-moon shape.

8 Fingernails have eight qualities: the cross-lines are of the same color as the nails themselves; they are all of the same length, shiny, clean, without broken edges, strong, smooth, nice to look at.

9 The inhabitants of Gauda [North Bengal] consider long nails to be an ornament of the hands. Such nails are an attraction for the girls of the region.

10 The southern peoples' nails are small, resistant, well suited for practicing any kind of scratching, and can easily be inserted anywhere.

11 The people of Mahārāshtra keep the nails of both hands short and aggressive.

Different kinds of scratches are used to mark the various parts of the partner's body.

12   Seven areas of the body are suitable for scratching. First scratch the breasts and lower lip with a light hand and a continuous stroke. A light touch causes gooseflesh. When the pressure applied is stronger, it is termed the knife stroke [achchuritaka].

With moderate force, slide all five nails to the spot chosen, which has been prepared by pulling the skin gently and pinching it fairly hard. It is a matter of practice. It should be done very lightly, so that it does not make any wound, but only a mark. A mere touch suffices to cause gooseflesh. The thumbnail can be used instead of all the nails together, if it has sufficient effect. Grating may have the same effect as a scratch, even if no cut is made. A girl should be able to show her scratch marks on her chin and her bottom, even if she does not expose any other nail marks. It should be done especially on the breasts.

Joining the fingers of one hand, lightly touch the cheeks, breasts, and lower lip, in such a way as to cause gooseflesh. Then make a mark with the thumb, reinforced by the other fingers. This scratch is called the knife stroke, and can be practiced on various parts of the body, according to the occasion.

13   When a girl is receptive, agitates her limbs, scratches her head, removes her blackheads out of nervousness, it is a sign that the time is ripe to mark her cruelly.

14   *The half-moon*

The semicircular mark left by the nail on the neck or below the breasts is called the half-moon. Very cruel when done with the little finger, it is more permanent when done with the middle one.

15   *The circle*

Two half-moon marks made by nails face to face are known as the circle.

16   The parts of the body suited for marking with the circle are the lower belly, the crotch, and the buttocks.

17   *The dash*

A straight line may be traced with the nails on any part of the body, but it must be short.

18 *The tiger's claw*

A line curving inwards, traced near the breasts or on the face is called the tiger's claw.

19 *The peacock's claw*

When the nipple is seized by all five nails and pulled outwards, the nail marks around the breasts are known as the peacock's claw.

20 *The hare's jump*

If the woman enjoys the peacock's claw, the mark left by pulling the tip of the nipple harder with the nails is called the hare's jump.

21 *The lotus leaf*

On the side of the breasts or on the buttocks, a mark looking like a lotus leaf is known as such.

22 When a man leaves on a journey, in order to remind his mistress of him, he traces three or four lines on her breasts or thighs with his nails.

23 Apart from the above, he may also mark her in other ways.

24 Since imagination knows no limits, variations are innumerable when practiced with astuteness. Nail scratching being so widely used as an erotic stimulant when practiced properly, how could the authors of the *Kāma Shāstra* enumerate all its varieties?

When a man is excited, he takes pleasure in scratching, but at that moment he does not think about the art of scratching and the different signs that his nails may leave.

25 Passion feeds on varied practices. Variety fosters mutual attraction. The courtesan is interesting to an erotic man due to her particular talents, an interest which is mutual. In treatises on the arts of war, the texts speak of the need for a diversity of weapons. What should we say in our own case, asks Vātsyāyana.

In order to renew excitation after having been satisfied, unusual practices are required, whence the taste for fancy dress, bizarre practices, different positions, which cause a mutual interest. Variety is required to satisfy the need for change. From a strictly erotic point of view, however, are these particularities really necessary?

When they take an unusual position, the courtesan and her lover, whoever he may be, are depersonalized. For the courtesan, her lover, whatever his appearance, is the very god of love. If they wish to play in a special way, they come to an agreement between themselves, seeking, however, to avoid any degrading act. It is thus that the most bizarre forms of amorous relations come into being. The same problems are met with in archery, fencing, or any other applied science. The treatises teach both theory and practice. In archery, it is a matter of piercing with an arrow, and quantities of different arrows are aimed at this target. Why should one question the various ways of reaching one's goal set out in the Kāma Sūtra? Where is the difference?

On this subject, Vātsyāyana considers that, in a state of amorous excitation, a desire is aroused for the most varied and strangest acts. The man and woman derive satisfaction from the most curious forms of intercourse. People used to sophisticated sexual relations utilize women who are specialized in the art of pleasure. Men who are expert at the art of loving are sought after by the courtesans, themselves expert in the art of enjoyment.

Just as in the art of war, defined by the *Dhanur Veda*, skill in managing arms is indispensable, so in the art of love, skill in technique and adaptability to all circumstances are also essential.

26 One must not leave nail or tooth marks on other men's women. They can only be marked with the nails in their secret parts, as a souvenir and to increase their excitation.

27 On seeing nail marks on her secret parts [guptānga], a girl feels affection awake for a lover, whether new or old.

28 If there are no nail marks to recall the lover's presence, it means that passion has long since disappeared and love has been overcome.

Nail marks serve to recall the beauty, youth, and qualities of the object of passion.

If there are no longer nail marks on the girl's body to remind her of her lover's beauty, youth, and qualities, love has long since passed away and ended.

29 When a man sees, even from afar, nail marks on a girl's breasts, he feels interest and desire for her, even without knowing her.

30 Similarly, it often happens that when a woman sees nail marks on the various parts of a man's body, her spirit awakens and takes her to him.

31 No acts can be compared to scratching and biting for increasing amorous excitation and driving to action.

This is true for both men and women.

Vātsyāyana indicates eight main ways of scratching, as well as the best moments and places and the methods for doing it. Scratching is an art (kalā) and, as with all arts, it must be studied and practiced, which is the scope of this chapter.

It is important to note what Vātsyāyana says: while making love, man appreciates a certain fantasy in the various acts, because it excites him. Sensual women appreciate a man who is expert in erotic fantasy, and desire to sleep with him.

For Vātsyāyana, nail marks are also souvenirs of sexual relations. On seeing these marks on her secret parts, a girl who believed she had broken off her relationship finds renewed desire for the boy who marked her so. Scars from nails and teeth awaken memories of youth. If such marks no longer exist, it means that the amorous relationship has been over for a long time and that love is dead. Scratch marks are not only a souvenir, but bring to life the lover's youth, beauty, qualities, and performance in love. Nothing can be compared to scratches and bites to increase erotic excitation.

From the point of view of sexuality and psychology, acts such as scratching and biting form part of the art of living. This does not only mean mankind, since the very same acts can be observed in the male-female relations of all species. The purpose of these acts is to arouse the desire to couple. When, with a view to copulation, excitation increases, scratches and bites are useful to ensure its success.

The places recommended by Vātsyāyana for bites and scratches are those that erotic science considers as centers of stimulation. The body's erogenous zones are the best suited for caresses, kisses, scratches, and other erotic activities prior to copulation. All the places indicated by Vātsyāyana are generally acknowledged to be centers of sensual excitation and play an important role from the erotic point of view.

In order to increase passion and experience full satisfaction, it is essential to know the art of scratching and other practices. The lover's prime virtue (dharma) during preliminary practices is to arouse the woman by titillating her limbs so that she reaches maximum excitation. It was with this practical aim in mind that Vātsyāyana wrote this chapter on scratching. However, just as in the case of copulation, Vātsyāyana divides people into categories such as hare, hind, etc. In practicing scratching, the categories must also be differentiated from a physical and psychological point of view, although the general structure of all individuals is similar, their sensitivity differs, as well as the choice of the point of attack. The finding of these points of attack is easy according to the pleasure felt in touching or scratching them. According to medical science, some areas of women's skin are connected with the ovaries. Under certain circumstances or sudden excitation, a contact will produce not only a stimulation, but a true orgasm. A negative reaction to pressure in these areas can cause fainting. This is why, to protect the woman's mental and physical health, she must be scratched and bitten in places that stimulate her sexually.

End of the Fourth Chapter
The Art of Scratching
of the Second Part entitled Amorous Advances

Chapter Five

BITING

[*Dashana Cheda*]

A description of biting follows that on scratching with the nails. As far as the ways of biting are concerned, as for embraces, local custom should be consulted. One should not be led by a state of excitation into performing acts that are considered unfitting. The subject comprises two aspects: the areas of the body to which pain may be caused, and the areas to be avoided.

1   As for kisses, all parts of the body are suitable for biting, except for the upper lip, the tongue, and the eyes.

There remain the forehead, the lower lip, the neck, the cheeks, the chest, the breasts; then, the sides, the crotch, the armpits, and the sex, parts that are not acceptable to everybody. It is unnecessary, therefore, to list all the places to be bitten that are the same as those to be embraced, and in which the teeth leave their mark, since they have already been described in dealing with kisses.

2   Teeth quality includes evenness, with an attractive shine,

139

colored with betel, of the right size, close set, and sharp.

3   Defects include irregularity, badly aligned, decayed, too small or too large, uneven, or overlapping.

4   There are ten kinds of bite, known as: discreet [gūdhaka], impressed [ucchunaka], pointed [bindu], necklace of dots [bindu-mālā], coral jewel [pravālamani], necklace of gems [manimālā], scattered clouds [khandābhraka], the chewing of the wild boar [varāha-charvita].

5   For the discreet bite, the teeth gently press the lower lip, so as to leave red marks that do not last.

6   The impressed bite is similar, but the lip is bitten hard.

7   The discreet, impressed, and pointed bites are made on the lower lip.

These are light bites on the lower lip.

8   The impressed, pointed, and coral jewel bites are made on the cheeks.

9   Kiss marks on the ear, as well as scratch and bite marks on the cheeks are considered ornamental.

10   The coral jewel is when the same spot is squeezed several times between the top teeth and the lower lip.

11   Coral jewel marks in a line are called necklaces of gems.

12   The pointed bite is the mark left when a small piece of skin is seized between the teeth and pulled.

13   Numerous pointed marks made in the same area are known as the necklace of dots.

14   The two necklaces are made on the neck, the sides, or close to the sex.

Because the skin is more tender there.

15   The necklace of dots can also be made on the forehead and the thighs.

16   A circle of irregular small tooth marks beneath the breasts is called the scattered cloud.

17   A wide area of bites close to one another beneath the

breasts forming a red center is known as the nibbling of the wild boar.

18 The two latter bites are made in a state of great excitation [chanda vega].

This closes the description of the bites, followed by the habit of placing one's mark on things.

19 It is a frequent custom to mark with one's teeth and nails the leaves she uses to put rouge on her face, the flowers she wears at her ears, the betel leaves that she will chew, and the palm leaves on which love letters are written.

As regards peculiar local customs:

20 One may treat women according to local conventions, or according to one's own customs.

There are five kinds of behavior to be adopted or rejected according to one's own tastes and local custom. In one's own country, even if one has particular tastes, no problem arises. With regard to kisses, and so on, one can always follow the customs of one's own country. Women have no objection to this since they do the same.

21 In Madhyadesha, the population is mainly Aryan, and the women are very careful of their purity. They do not care for kisses or injuries from nails or teeth.

According to Bhrigu, Madhyadesha stretches from the Himalayas to the Vindhya mountains, while for Vasishtha it is the Ganges plain. The women of this area are very puritanical.

22 The same occurs among the women of Bāhlika [Balkh] and Avanti.

Balkh is north of Gandhara [Afghanistan], while Avanti is the country of Ujjaina.

23 They are, however, attracted by unusual loveplay [chitrarata].

24 The women of Mālavā and Abhīra are much given to embraces, kisses, nail scratching, biting, and blows, but not to injuries. They are very fond of sucking the penis.

25 Those who live in the region of the Indus and the Sutlej rivers are very fond of fellatio [auparishtaka].

26 The women of Aurāntaka, Sahyādri, and Lata [Surat, Baroda] are very erotic and sigh gently.

27 To satisfy the women of Koshala and those belonging to the regions where matriarchy is practiced [strīrājya], violent practices [kharavega] and brutal sexual behavior are needed. Dildos [apadravya] are much employed.

28 The women of Andhra are gentle by nature and sensual. They are shameless, and their tastes are not very decent.

But they are delicate and are not fond of blows. They like to dominate men, and know no limit.
They are very independent.

29 The women of Mahārāshtra are skilled in the sixty-four arts, but their language is obscene, coarse, and hard. They are very impetuous in bed.

30 The women of the great city [Pātaliputra] act in the same way, but practice the arts in private.

31 Due to friction during possession, Dravidian women have slight losses of blood.

Due to friction, the instrument's going back and forth when it penetrates during possession, even when great precautions are taken.

32 The women from the north of Vāna country [Konkarna] have a moderate temperament. They bear everything—embraces, kisses, blows, scratches, and bites—but they hide their sex, and the sight of their partner's sex makes them laugh. They loathe men who behave vulgarly, or in an obscene or brutal manner.

33 The women of Gauda [South Bengal] speak softly, are affectionate, and have delicate limbs.

34 According to Suvarnanābha, it is more important to

follow one's nature than local custom as far as kisses, embraces, scratches, and bites are concerned.

35 However, local custom must be attended to as regard the times for making love. Furthermore, the garments, behavior, and amusements of the place must be adopted.

This is why it should not be thought that the habits and behavior described in this book are valid everywhere.

In some cases, behavior that would be considered normal in one country is condemned in another. For this reason, it is better not to worry about it and to follow one's inclinations.

36 Stimulating entwinings are performed to start with, unusual practices follow.

Embraces, kisses, scratches and bites, blows and sighs: these six external actions are practiced one after the other for the purposes of arousal. Of these, sighs are born of pleasure caused by pain, while blows are classed as manual contact. Bites are heavy contact. Scratches also count as aggression, while kisses are gentle contacts. Next in order come special practices, including blows. All these practices, if lightly performed, arouse desire and provoke sighs when they take place in those parts of the body that are not very accessible.

It is thus that, reflecting on local convention and one's own tastes, one should practice those cutting attacks that are useful for lasting affection. They are of two kinds: those that leave permanent marks and those that are merely transitory.

37 The more a man increases the violence of his blows, the more the girl receiving them should repay in kind. If they become very violent, the victim should double her own.

38 She should respond to aggression, a bindu for a bindu, a necklace of bindus with a necklace of bindus, and repay also the wild boar's bite, attacking the boy, as if she were in anger.

39 Lifting his head by the hair, she glues her lips to his, and forcing him to lie down, she bites his whole body like a madwoman.

She seizes him by the hair with one hand, and with the other takes him by the chin to lift him. She bites him wherever he had bitten her and rejoices at his efforts to free himself.

She embraces him with such force that their bodies become a single body, then she covers him with bites.

40   Sitting on her lover's chest, she raises his face with one hand and with the other encircling his neck, she marks him with the necklace of gems [manimālā] around his neck and neighboring areas.

41   During the day, when the boy shows various persons the marks his mistress made, the latter, without a glance, should start laughing.

42   Then, turning her head away, or accusing her lover, she should show everyone the wounds he has left on her body.

43   Whether they continue having sexual relations, or live chastely together, true love never decreases, even after one hundred years.

End of the Fifth Chapter
Biting
of the Second Part entitled Amorous Advances

Chapter Six

ON COPULATION
[*Sambhoga kriyā*]

AND SPECIAL TASTES
[*Vichitra rata*]

Methods of Penetration
[*Sanveshana vidhi*]

While taking into account local mores, personal inclinations, entwinings, and other means of excitation, the various methods of penetration [sanveshana] envisaged in this chapter are divided into two parts according to posture and special acts.

1   At the moment of the act, a hind woman must open her organ [jaghana] to be penetrated by a big caliber [uccharata]

when the penis is erect for penetration. A large organ, such as that of the horse man, cannot penetrate unless her aperture is stretched.

Similarly, when a bull man penetrates a hind woman, she must open her thighs, since the relationship is unequal.

2   On the other hand, the elephant woman contracts her sex to receive a small caliber.

She opens her thighs in order to be penetrated, then contracts like a mouth being pursed. In order to receive a bull size, she contracts since her aperture is too wide, but she disdains small sizes, such as the hare.

3   When they are of the same category, penetration is easy.

The woman need not open or contract her organ.

4   As far as the mare woman is concerned,

when she is used by a horse, who is of superior caliber, she has to dilate, while contracting for a hare. With a bull, whose size matches hers, penetration is effortless. It is the same for the hind or the cow-elephant.
The rule is to "open her thighs for larger sizes and tighten her thighs for smaller sizes." Coition is equal for matching sizes.

5   She seizes the boy's sex with her vulva.

Lying down, the woman's sex can take the man in three ways: by contracting, dilating, or normally.

6   If the boy is of very small caliber, dildos [apadravya] may be used.

These artificial instruments are used by bull and hare men to satisfy mare and elephant women. For matching coition, an instrument of the same size is employed. When the man is of larger size, the use of dildos is unnecessary.
If the man's organ is too small and cannot satisfy the woman's desire for enjoyment, an artificial organ is utilized to satisfy her.
He then pushes the object back and forth between her thighs.

7   The hind woman can control the width of her vulva in three ways: blossoming [utphallaka], expanding [vijrimbhitaka], and Queen of Heaven [Indrānika].

Matching copulation methods have popular but not theoretical names. In practice, sleeping together can be done either in peasant or city-dweller fashion, and there are two ways of penetrating the girl: on the side, or lying down on top of her, to which a third can be added: pitcherwise, from behind.

In peasant fashion, the girl [pramadā] sits on her lover's lap and opens her thighs. For the city-dweller fashion, the woman sits on the boy's knees and encircles him with her legs. In the third case, she is penetrated while bent in three.

8 The blossoming is realized by lowering the woman's head and raising her vagina.

The raised vagina is thus higher than the woman's inclined head. In order to widen it, although it does it by itself, the hands should be placed one over the other, from behind, on the woman's buttocks, putting her legs on the hips on both sides: the raised vagina spreads and opens.

9 Thus the way is open.

In order to let the boy's instrument penetrate her, she raises her waist. The boy gradually withdraws until he is only halfway in, then suddenly thrusts. The skin of the boy's sex is turned back and physicians say that the foreskin may be hurt.

Sometimes, he places a pillow under the small of her back.

10 The woman having raised her thighs, the boy takes the lower part of her body sideways and penetrates. This is known as the expanding position.

Lying down, she lifts her thighs and feet, placing herself sideways. In order to penetrate her, the boy must also place himself sideways on.

The woman opens her thighs and raises them very high to open her sex properly, while the boy, putting his sex in sideways, penetrates her. This is the expanding position.

11 Encircling the woman's sides with his thighs, his knees at her side, he widens her. This position, which requires practice, is known as the Queen of Heaven.

He opens the woman's sex forcefully with his hands to the maximum extent. This position is so named because it was invented by the spouse of Indra, the King of Heaven.

The man opens the woman's thighs with both his hands.

12 Small sizes should practice copulation lying face to
face, in the box posture.

*The Queen of Heaven position is suitable if the man is of very
large size, whether a bull or even a horse, in a state of sexual frenzy
or even of great excitation, since then the larger sizes manage to penetrate. The blossoming and expanding positions of the mare are best for
the bull. This position is also recommended for the horse.*

If the man and woman are of very different sizes, as for example,
a hind woman with a horse man, the Queen of Heaven position allows
them both to reach orgasm.

13 To receive smaller sizes, the box position [samputaka]
is always recommended.

14 As in the case of a very small organ with an elephant
woman.

*In the case of a hare who is unable to insert, the box position is
guaranteed to allow them to find pleasure. Even the mare, in the box
position, manages to receive a hare.*

If an elephant woman has a hare partner, she will be able to satisfy
him in the box position.

To bring small or very small organs to orgasm.

15 Four kinds of penetration are recommended: the box
[samputaka], great pressure [pīditaka], envelopment
[veshtitaka], the mare [vādavāka].

16 The box [samputaka]

The box is when both lie face to face.

17 It is of two kinds: side by side, or one on top of the
other.

*When the man and woman lie face to face on their sides for
coition, it is known as the lateral box [parshva samputa]. When the
woman is lying down and the man, stretched on top of her, possesses
her, it is called the closed box [uttana samputa]. It is the most widespread position and the easiest, since it presents no difficulty for the
penetration of the instrument.*

For the lateral box, the boy presses his body to the hip of the stretched-out woman. When both lie extended hip to hip, the instrument penetrates her, but sometimes injures her.

Vātsyāyana gives another description of the box: the woman folds her knees against her breasts, while the man faces her in a doubled-up position and presses his hips against hers. This is known as frontal box. Since the thighs are doubled back, the vulva cannot be contracted and the position is thus not suitable for small sizes with a cow-elephant, but is appropriate for matching sizes. The lateral position is very popular.

18 In sleeping, the man must lie to the right of the woman: she should always be on the man's left.

In sleeping, the woman's right side is in contact with the man's left side in order not to cause difficulties if one seeks her while asleep. The contrary should be practiced, however, in copulating with a cow-elephant, since it is proper that preliminary contacts with the intimate parts should be done with the left hand.

19 Strong pressure [pīditaka]

In the box position, the instrument is made to penetrate violently between the thighs.

Whether the box position is on top or sideways, when the instrument is in place, it is made to slide inside. If the girl resists, she should be violated. To enforce the box, press strongly while covering her like a lid.

While in the box position during coition, both man and woman press their legs hard against each other.

20 Envelopment [veshtitaka]

For envelopment, she crosses her thighs in view of being penetrated by the instrument in the box position.

In order to let the instrument penetrate in the upper box position [flat], she covers one leg with the other, placing the left over the right or the right over the left and covering it completely. This is known as envelopment.

To contract her vulva as far as possible, the woman crosses one leg over the other.

21   The mare [vādavāka]
Like the mare who seizes the instrument without moving, the same name is given to a similar performance.

Without moving, she seizes the man's sex in the opening of her vulva, just as the mare does. This method, which is very vulgar, requires a certain experience. Trying to do it directly, suddenly, is never successful.
Rubbing her sexual organ against the horse's, the mare seizes the latter. Similarly, the woman rubs her sex on the man's and catches it without any embrace or kiss. This position is known as the mare. It requires a certain practice and is mainly utilized by whores.

22   According to the disciples of Babhru, this form of penetration is particularly widespread in Andhra country.

Here ends the description of the positions of copulation [sambhoga-āsana] given by the Bābhravyas.

23   We will now go on to the opinions of Suvarnanābha
24   Bent [bhagnaka]
For the position known as bhagnaka, both thighs are raised in the air.

The girl raises her thighs, which she clasps with her arms. The boy, too, lifting his knees, grips her and fucks her.

25   Gaping [jrimbhitaka]

She raises both her legs and places them on the boy's shoulders. It is the knee-joint that rests on the shoulder.

26   High pressure [utpīditaka]
"High pressure" is performed with both legs bent back.

The girl folds both her legs, which the boy presses against his chest. The boy puts his arms around the girl's neck and presses his chest against her retracted legs. Both their chests are compressed, which is why it is called "high pressure."

Lying on her back, the woman folds her legs beneath the chest of her partner, who is lying on top of her. The latter, crushing her with his chest, possesses her. This is known as high pressure.

27 Half-pressure [ardhapīdita]

If only one leg is folded, it is called half-pressure.

The woman, lying on her back, stretches one of her legs out and folds back the other. He, resting his chest on her folded leg, possesses her. She then does the same thing changing legs.

28 The broken flute [venudaritaka]

One leg resting on the boy's shoulder is then removed, and subsequently replaced on his shoulder several times.

The left foot placed on the boy's shoulder is then abruptly taken off and lowered. She then replaces a foot on his right shoulder and relaxes the left leg. This is known as breaking the flute.

Lying down, the woman places one of her feet on the shoulder of the boy who is lying on top of her. Then lowering the first foot, she places her other foot on his other shoulder. If she is being possessed at that moment, it is called the broken flute.

29 Impalement [shūlāchitaka]

The woman places one foot on the boy's head and extending the other, allows herself to be penetrated. This position, known as impalement, requires practice.

She then places her other foot on his head and, stretching the first leg, gives him enjoyment alternately. Sometimes, she places her foot only on his shoulder.

30 The crab [kārkataka]

Like a crab folding its claws, the woman, lying down, folds her bended legs over her vulnerable part, the boy pressing his navel against her legs. Intercourse in this position is called the crab.

The girl bends her knees against her stomach while the boy penetrates her sex.

31 Tight [pīditaka]

When the girl crosses her raised legs, it is known as the tight position.

She crosses her left leg over her right, or right over left. It is called tight, because she restricts her vulva.

32 The lotus position [padmāsana]

Spreading the thighs is the lotus position.

Having opened her thighs, the girl places her right foot on her left thigh joint and her left foot on her right thigh joint. This resembles the lotus position in yoga.

33 The spin [parāvrittaka]

Embracing from behind the woman who has her back to him, he turns her round. This is the spin, which requires practice.

Having deeply penetrated from behind the girl he clasps in his arms, the boy makes her turn to face him, while remaining in position. Practice is necessary for this position, which cannot be improvised.

The seated boy penetrates deeply. Then, after a moment, he turns her around and, without separating, they find themselves the opposite way round. This is a difficult practice requiring considerable experience.

The various positions are not considered as special practices [chitra]. The methods of making love standing up, from behind, or from the side are normal throughout the world. Other positions considered to be special will now be described.

34 Making love in the water [jalasambhoga]

According to Suvarnanābha, certain positions can be practiced immersed or half-immersed in water. Many amusing positions can be practiced in this way, since they are easier.

While difficult when dry, many methods of copulation can be performed in the water, keeping one's head above the surface. The

*strangest kinds of copulation one could desire, which are difficult when
dry, can be practiced in the water. Any form of embrace that the boy
can imagine is possible, whether standing or sitting, but not lying
down. Among these special forms is impalement, which thus becomes
easy.*

According to Suvarnanābha, one can make love in the water either
standing or sitting, but not lying down. Coition in the water is much
easier than on land.

**35 According to Vātsyāyana, all this is senseless, since this
way of behaving is not envisaged by respectable persons.**

*To say that it is easier means nothing, since it is forbidden by any
author. According to Gautami, copulation in the water leads to hell,
while the Bhārgavas [disciples of Bhrigu] indicate the penances to be
performed after such an act: "When the sperm comes into contact with
water, as a penance one should fast for a month [chandrāyana]." For
this reason, one should make love when dry.*

Thus end the thirteen methods of sexual penetration [sanveshana].

Vātsyāyana condemns sexual acts in the water. Being thus opposed
to the propositions of Suvarnanābha, he claims that the whole matter
is senseless, since making love in the water is condemned by all authors
and respectable people.

**36 Unusual or special sexual practices [chitra] will now
be described.**

Certain of which are surprising [adbhuta].

37 Standing intercourse [sthitarata]

**Both are standing against each other, leaning against a wall
or column.**

*Lacking any other support, they lean on each other. In one case,
the girl leans on a column, while at other times, the boy does. In the
standing position, she can also fold her legs, supported by the boy's
hands. Lifting first one of her feet and then the other, the girl puts
them in the boy's hands, her sex open, facing him. She then squeezes
the boy's shoulders with her knees, which can easily reach them.*

38   Hanging [avalambitaka]

The boy stands leaning against a wall. The girl sits on the seat formed by his two hands. Encircling his neck with her arms, she stretches her legs along the wall, imprisoning him between her thighs. This is the hanging position.

The wall may even be a column. She puts her arms around his neck, grasping his topknot, then squeezes him between her thighs, stretching out her legs. Gradually she slides her feet along the wall, bending her waist and holding on to the boy's neck. This strange position makes them both laugh.

The boy is standing against a wall. He makes a seat with his clasped hands on which the girl sits, putting her arms around his neck and raising her legs against the wall. Spiked as if by a stake, she reaches orgasm in this position, known as the hanging position.

39   The cow [dhenuka]

The woman places herself on all fours on the ground, in the posture of the cow ready for the bull's assault. This is the position of "the cow."

The boy holds her by the waist in order to take her.
He enjoys her from behind, like a bull.

40   What is generally done between the thighs is in this case done from behind.

41   In the same fashion, one can imitate other animals, mounting the woman like an ass, playing with her like a cat, attacking like a tiger, stamping like an elephant, pawing the ground like a pig, riding horse-fashion. Thus one learns a thousand ways to copulate.

Thus, all kinds of amorous practices can be observed among the quadrupeds.
So, when inspiration is lacking, the boy can find models for his amusement.

42   Group sex [samghataka rata]

Making love with two women who like each other and have the same tastes is called group sex.

This falls under special practices. The two women lie on the same bed, and the boy makes use of them both. While he is mounting one, the other, excited, kisses him, and after pleasuring one, he brings the other to orgasm.

If the women are his, and are fond of each other, the man can devise loveplay with both of them.

43 The herd of cows [goyūthi]

When performed with several women, this kind of intercourse is called "the herd of cows."

This kind of special copulation is performed with a group of women, as a bull does with his herd of cows.

44 It is also interesting to imitate the elephants' water games, the behavior of the he-goat, etc.

One can amuse oneself with the women by imitating the water play of the elephant and cow-elephant, the bleatings of the he-goat with the nanny goat, or the behavior of a stag. In imitating these various love games, copulation is performed in the cow position.

Group sex play is usually between a man and two or more women, or else between one or two women and several men. When a group of boys gather for sexual purposes, it is also group sex. If there are two of them, more often than not it is out of a desire to sodomize each other [purushāyita]. They penetrate one another between the thighs from behind. The one has his sex in the air, while the other mounts him as a bull does with a cow-elephant.

In certain herds of cows, the boy is the only male, like the bull with his herd. The imitation of elephants' water play is considered as being one of the amusements of the herd of cows.

45 In country villages and in the Strīrājya, matriarchal country, as well as in Balkh [present-day Tajikistan], the women closed in their inner apartments often hide young men.

Highly sensual women sometimes hide several.

46 The young men hidden in this way satiate the women's desires either one by one, or as a group.

The boys split their activities as follows:

47   One of the boys holds her in his arms, while another penetrates her. One embraces her thighs, and another busies himself in the middle, vying with each other to satisfy her.

One of them holds her seated on his knees, while another takes her mouth and embraces her. One bites and scratches her, while the other penetrates her sex or licks her vulva. She is scratched, bitten, and beaten separately by one after the other, or by all together, after which they fornicate with her successively. One of the practices that satisfies a woman and calms the excitation of her hole of pleasure, the opening for the passage of liquids, or vulva, consists of one of them servicing her sex with his mouth, besides all the other games.

One of the ladies who reside in the inner apartments sits on the tender knees of one of the boys, while another attacks her with his teeth and nails, a third enjoys her, a fourth kisses her lips, and a fifth bites her breasts. Thus each of the young men continues to excite her and give her pleasure until the woman is fully satisfied.

Besides the places indicated, he mentions others.

48   This kind of group sex [goshthi parigraha = samāhita sambhoga] is especially practiced with prostitutes, but also with kings' wives.

Group sex does not only involve prostitutes and gigolos, but also other men's wives. Together with the young men, they secretly practice this high deed in the regions of the East. Whores, as well as other women, take delight in a gigolo or a young boy. Many of these group amusements are practiced by men with their wives.

The pleasures of group sex are especially sought after by whores, but sometimes even kings' wives entertain young men in order to procure this kind of amusement for themselves.

49   Sodomy [adhorata]

Inferior copulation [adhorata], meaning in the anus [pāyau] is particularly practiced by the peoples of the South. Here ends the subject of special intercourse [chitrarata].

It is termed lower because the excremental route [apāna] is below the vulva. This kind of intercourse is of two kinds, according to whether it is practiced with a man or a woman. It is special inasmuch as it is an abnormal way [vimarga] for the penis.

Oral intercourse [auparishtaka], which concerns people of the third sex, is not classed among the special forms of copulation, except sometimes when performed by a woman on a man.

Anal intercourse, which is practiced in the South, is a matter of local custom. It is considered a perversion because the penis penetrates by the bad route [vimarga].

The lowest form of copulation is in the lower opening, the anus (gudā).

Here ends the description of the astonishing [adbhuta] or bizarre ways of copulation.

50 Homosexual practices [purushopasriptaka] will be described in the chapter on role inversion [purushāyita].

Homosexual practices or reciprocal penetration among boys, for which there are innumerable opportunities, will be described in the chapter on inversions, in dealing with the third sex. Anal intercourse is of two kinds, according to whether it is practiced with men or women. For both man and woman, it is a deviation.

Here ends the description of special forms of sexuality.

51 Sexual relations can be diversified by studying the movements of domestic and wild animals, as well as insects.

Domestic animals bestir themselves from behind, wild beasts mount on top of one another, the playing of insects and birds can be seen. Their efforts, their shudderings, and the particular noises of their bodies should be studied with a view to imitating them in the company of women so as to vary the ways of making love. Either partner can utilize them.

By imitating the curious ways in which animals, wild beasts, and birds make love, women can be seduced and their affection assured.

52 Those whose sexuality follows their fantasy and local custom inspire affection, desire and esteem in women.

In this chapter, Vātsyāyana describes the acts of sexual union (sambhoga kriyā), the ways of penetration (samveshana prakāra), and unusual intercourse (chitrarata). Although dealing with the same subject, he differentiates between ordinary methods of penetration and bizarre copulation.

The first part describes normal sexual practices in civilized society, but among the types of bizarre copulation, he describes the habits of people whose behavior is entirely immoral.

What can be the purpose of the author of the *Kāma Sūtra* in describing acts that are antisocial and against nature? This question comes to the mind of every reader and of all normally behaved persons. The answer is that knowledge is not something fragmentary, but must cover a whole subject.

End of the Sixth Chapter
On Copulation and Special Tastes
of the Second Part entitled
Amorous Advances

Chapter Seven

BLOWS AND SIGHS
[*Prahanana-sītkāra prakarana*]

To facilitate penetration of the instrument during intercourse, blows
are employed. This chapter, describing the technique of blows and the
resulting groans, is divided into two parts. It might be wondered how
blows, which are usually hostile acts, can be adjuvants of pleasure.

1   Sexual relations can be conceived of as a kind of combat, and eroticism as a contest and perverse behavior
[vāmashīla].

This apparent conflict is in reality a struggle, since in order to
assert themselves and overcome each other, both man and woman violently oppose one another, bringing to light a state of mind that could
not be achieved by affection. For successful intercourse, a show of cruelty
is essential. According to a quotation from the Kirātārjuna of the poet
Bhāravi, "Aggression with nails and feet, embraces, kisses, cruel bites
are acts leading to much greater enjoyment than loving behavior."
Although love is generally acknowledged to be associated with the
quality of gentleness, cruelty has its place in sexual acts. The nature of

Eros is thus of two kinds, and according to whether its cause or its effects are contemplated, behavior differs.

Sexual games may be described as a combat, a struggle between the lovers, serving to stimulate their aggressiveness at the moment of sexual union, since eroticism is by nature conflictual and perfidious (kutila).

> 2   Good places for giving blows are on the shoulders, the head, the gap between the breasts, the back, the sexual area, the sides.

The blows exchanged are part of the pleasure of intercourse.

> 3   There are four ways of hitting: with the side of the hand, with the palm of the open hand, with the fist, with the ends of the fingers joined.

After which, we will pass on to the second subject of this chapter.

> 4   The woman groans [sītkrita] under the blows, because they hurt her. Since the blows vary greatly, sighs do too.

The kind of cry corresponds to the pain felt. As the result of the blows suffered, the groans are the sound expression of the pain felt. As described by the authors of old, groans are of many kinds as are the forms of violence.

> 5   Cries [virutāni] are of eight kinds.

Since they are produced by the places that articulate speech, the various cries are limited by what sounds can be issued. Born of sexual excitation, with or without blows, they express a state of mind which forms part of erotic aggressiveness.

> 6   They are called:
>   Himkāra (nasal "hee")
>   Stanita, roll of thunder
>   Kūjita, hissing
>   Rudita, weeping
>   Sūtkrita, sighing

Dutkrita, cry of pain
Phutkrita, violent expulsion of breath

Himkāra is a nasalized "hee," starting from the throat and mounting to the nostrils, and breaking out as a light sound.
Stanita, the sound "ha" from deep in the throat to the nose, like the rolling of thunder.
The meaning of rudita, "weeping," is clear, but it should be moving.
Sūtkrita, sighing by drawing in the breath.
The meaning of kūjita and phutkrita will be explained. These seven groans can also be silent.

Himkāra "hee," stanita a deep "ha," kūjita a slow "kou-kou," sūtkrita "sou-sou."

7   Some cries are words that have a meaning, calling for mother, pleading for release, to stop, or to continue.

For example, Ari! Mummy! Not like that! Stop! That's too much! I'm dying! Mercy!

8   When she groans under her lover's blows, the woman's cries are like those of:

the pigeon [pārāvata]
the cuckoo [parabhrita]
the turtledove [hārāta]
the parrot [shuka]
the bee [madhukara]
the nightingale [dātyuha, papiha, chātaka]
the goose [hamsa]
the duck [kārandava]
the partridge [lāva]

Cries are of all sorts, usually appearing when the woman is beaten. They also serve on other occasions.

Sighs mixed with other sounds are as attractive as a song, when the embrace is loosened. It is also a question of imagination.

9   With the girl sitting on his knees ready for love, he strikes her back with his fist.

10   Pretending that she cannot bear him, with a long breathed-out "Han" and tears, the girl gives him the same back.

11   When the instrument penetrates her as she is lying on her back, the space between the breasts should be struck with the side of the hand.

12   Begin gently, then, when she starts liking it, strike harder and harder, finally striking in other places.

When she has been put into a good mood by the blows in the heart region, strike her in the three sensitive areas, the head, pubis, and heart, which will make her violently excited.

Strike first gently, with the fist, then, if she gets to like it, strike harder until she is well aroused.

13   One must judge from the girl's sighs whether the blows given are insufficient, and if the moment has come for going ahead without restraint.

From the seven ways of moaning, it can be understood whether the light blows to the heart are insufficient. Realizing that the moment has come to strike harder, it can be gradually accelerated without hesitation.

If she does not give any audible cry indicating suffering, no rules or order need be followed any longer: she should be struck with the fist until she lets her cries be heard.

14   Excruciating [prasritaka]

Excruciating [prasritaka] is the name given to a way of striking the head with joined fingers, making her scream when she is thus assailed.

In attacking her, the fingers resemble a snake's head. If she is not satisfied by the blows given by the hand and needs a different kind of attack, since the first blows were found insufficiently stimulating, her head must be hammered with blows, as if to open her skull, first gently then harder in order to excite her finally and make her cry.

If the woman finds pleasure in the blows struck by the side of the hand, and wants more, then in order to satisfy her, the boy, joining his fingers like a serpent's head, strikes her on the head, as if to lacerate her skin.

15 Thus cries and sighs issue from the girl's mouth.

16 After reaching orgasm, she sighs and weeps.

Quite quietly.

17 The panting that accompanies the action is called "the effect of pain" [dutkrita].

18 At the moment of orgasm, she utters a sound [*phut*], which is similar to a jujube fruit falling into the water.

19 Once she has groaned, her whole body having been attacked by kisses and blows, she must do the same to him.

In turn, she must subject him to the same ill-treatment. The saying is, "to render blow for blow."

20 When, under the effect of excitation, the boy starts to ill-treat her, in order to protest and to stop him, the girl calls out "Mummy! Mummy!," weeping and sighing and continually uttering cries of pain and other protests.

The sighs, tears, and cries are a result of the suffering inflicted. She makes sounds like the cooing of pigeons. At the moment of pleasure, when she is penetrated by the penis, she stops agitating her legs. He then slaps her with the palm of his hand on her sides and the lower part of the body, after which, having sated the desire for blows, they calm down.

21 When she is struck on the breasts, her cries are like those of a partridge or a goose.

Thus ends the subject of blows and sighs.

22 Quotation: "Vigor and audacity are manly qualities. Weakness, sensuality, and dependence are female characteristics."

A man must have a strong body, be decided and audacious. These are both qualities of the ardent man [tejas], of him who likes beating. Lack of strength, the incapacity to hurt, even though the softest hands make her suffer, dependence, lack of character, the fact of desiring to be beaten by men, the wish to receive blows, all are part of women's nature.

If, without having been beaten, she begins sighing during intercourse, what she wants to receive are blows in response to her sighs.

Vigor, steadfastness, and endurance are the natural qualities of a man. Incapacity, suffering undergone, defensiveness, weakness, and fragility are the intrinsical qualities of a woman. This is why a man attacks a woman, and why she groans.

> **23   Sometimes, out of passion, custom, or temperament, the woman inverts the situation. This is only temporary, however, and nature ends by taking back its due.**

During the act, roles are sometimes inverted. Carried away by passion, local custom, or her own temperament, the woman puts aside her natural behavior and, with a man's ardor, begins slapping and beating. The boy, in turn, changes his own behavior, and starts whining and groaning. This does not last very long, however, and after a few moments, the situation reverts. He says, "What's all this?" and rediscovers his true nature to fuck her. Since intercourse against nature is not possible for lack of the instrument, they go back to the old formula, being without any means of changing it.

Sexual characteristics are not universal. Occasionally, in certain countries, at certain times or under particular circumstances, it happens that the woman, at the height of her excitation, becomes hard and fearless, dominating the boy, who then starts groaning. This kind of role changing is not very frequent, nor does it last very long.

The methods of slapping differing from the four previously mentioned will now be indicated.

> **24   Besides the four forms of aggression mentioned, four others are utilized by the peoples of the South, which are:**
>
> **the nail [kīlā] on the chest**
> **the knife [kartarī] on the head**
> **the borer [viddhā] on the cheeks**
> **the pincers [sandanshikā] on the breasts.**
>
> **These make eight in all. In the South, "nail" marks can be seen on the girls' breast. This is the custom of the country.**

The nail [kīlā]
Joining thumb and little finger, with the middle finger reinforcing the thumb from behind, one strikes from the top downwards.

The knife [kartarī]

The knife is of two kinds, with the fingers straight or bent. The straight-fingered kind is also of two sorts: with one hand it is called the great knife [bhadra-kartarī], while with hands joined it is known as the twin knife [yamala-kartarī].

Bending the fingers, with the thumb tip above joined to the index is known as the speaking knife [shabda-kartarī]. In using it, the scratching of the finger makes a slight noise. Some people call it the "blue lotus leaf" [utpalapatrikā]. In both cases, the nail of the little finger scratches the head.

The borer [viddhā]

The index, middle, and ring fingers are bent toward the middle of the thumb, as with a fist. This is called viddhā [the borer], the fingers facing the thumb graze the cheek cruelly.

The pincers [sandanshikā]

With closed fist, pinching with the thumb and index, or index and middle finger, is known as the pincers. This is usually practiced on the breasts or sides, pressing hard, pulling the flesh and bruising it.

To these four kinds of blows using the hand must be added a further four practiced by the people of the South, which, according to the experts, are the four that leave the most visible marks.

Kīlā, the nail, is characteristic of the girls of the South, who wear the mark on their breast. Kartarī, the knife, is done on the forehead, close to the hair parting. Viddhā, the borer, is especially made on the cheeks. To satisfy fantasy, custom, or passion, one tries to leave one's mark, even at the risk of wounding or disfiguring.

Throughout the South, one can see "nail" marks on the breasts of young men and women. This is one of the local customs and the people of the country act accordingly. This does not mean, however, that such practices should be transferred elsewhere.

25   Vātsyāyana's opinion is that causing suffering is not an Aryan practice and is not suitable for respectable people.

These are regarded with suspicion, both as defects and uncivilized behavior.

26   These practices are allowed in certain areas and not in others.

The customs of one country should not be exported to another.

27 One must in all cases know when to stop if there is a risk of mutilation or death.

28 Chitrasena, the king of the Chola country, struck the courtesan Chandrasenā so violently with the "nail," in the blindness of his erotic excitement, that she died.

29 In the land of Kuntala, King Shātakarni Shātavāhana caused the death of the great Queen Malayavatī by striking her with the "knife."

30 The chief of the army, Naradeva, in Pandya country, attracted by the dancer Chitralekhā and attempting to strike her cheek with the "borer," struck her eye, making her one-eyed.

31 A countless number of people are imprudent and igno-rant of the rules and, driven by passion in the ardor of their erotic practices, are unable to measure the conse-quences.

There are two kinds of erotic man [kāmī]: he who knows the rules, and he who rejects them. It is not by knowing the theoretical works that one is able to count the various methods of striking. But he who knows the rules is less imprudent than another and, even in the heat of passion, remains conscious of the consequences.

When a man blinded by passion throws himself into intercourse, he considers neither the injunctions of treatises nor possible conse-quences. This is why passion alone is responsible for unfortunate con-sequences.

32 The fantasies a man invents under the effect of erotic excitation are not imaginable even in dreams.

33 Like a speed-maddened horse, flying at a gallop and seeing neither holes nor ditches, two lovers blinded by desire and making furious love do not take account of the risks involved in their conduct.

34 This is why in his sexual behavior with a girl, an edu-cated man takes into account his own strength and the fragility of his partner. He knows how to check the vio-lence of his impulses, as well as the girl's limitations of endurance.

35 In love, not all kinds of action can be practiced at all times with all women. In amorous practices, the man's behavior should take into account the place, the country, and the moment.

At the moment of intercourse, blinded by passion, the man strikes the girl on her head, shoulders, between the breasts, on her back, her sex, her sides. Being hurt in these sensitive places, the girl starts to groan, but soon becomes the victim of her pleasure. All the boy has to do gradually is to strike her, squeeze her, and slap her with the palm of his hands.

Recapitulating the instructions of ancient authorities, Vātsyāyana explains that the man must beat the woman only after evaluating her fragility and endurance, at the same time, taking due account of the woman's ardor. When her erotic ardor is intense, instead of hurting her, the blows give her pleasure. From Vātsyāyana's point of view, blows do not belong to the customs of civilized society, but rather to louts and savages. In erotic practice, however, a man becomes so maddened and blinded that he has no discernment or conscience. He forgets in what places he risks causing a wound. As proof and example, Vātsyāyana cites cases in ancient times of women who have died or been disfigured. He gives a warning that not all the various kinds of acts can be practiced at any time or with any kind of woman. Local custom, the moment, and the woman's state of mind must all be taken into account before indulging in blows and other practices.

End of the Seventh Chapter
Blows and Sighs
of the Second Part entitled Amorous Advances

Chapter Eight

VIRILE BEHAVIOR IN WOMEN

[Puruṣhāyita]

After repeated intercourse, incapable of recommencing, weary in all his members, his passion calmed, the boy no longer desires anything but rest. The girl, behaving like a man, then takes control over the quietened boy. This is what is known as virile behavior [purushāyita]. This chapter is divided into two parts, since it includes the sodomization of boys [purushopasripta] among the various practices.

1   When the boy, wearied after his uninterrupted sexual exercises, seeks rest and is no longer dominated by passion, with his agreement, the girl descends to his anus [adhah] and, with the aid of an accessory [sāhāyya], imposes her virile behavior on him.

After repeated copulation, exhausted in all his members, the boy rests. The girl, whose excitation is not yet satiated, without asking his leave and despite his protestations, obliges him to behave like a woman and, without any modesty, behaves like a male, placing the boy beneath her. Not having the necessary, she has recourse to an accessory [sāhāyya].

When the woman behaves like a man, it is called virile behavior (purushāyita), or inverted sexuality (viparitarati). When the man has spent his strength after repeated intercourse, and the woman is not satisfied, she lies on top of the man.

2 Whatever his intentions may be, she is decided on practicing this fictitious intercourse.

If he does not agree, a struggle ensues, but she is determined on that kind of inverted intercourse known as virile behavior.
The woman manages it through her dominating will.

3 Or else with the boy's agreement.

Noting the boy's surprise and seeing that his opposition has weakened, she introduces the object and goes ahead.
Even if the boy is not tired, he allows himself to be treated like a woman in order to have a new sensation. With the girl on top of him, they find their intercourse amusing.

4 She is determined to unite him with the instrument that she is inserting into his anus, so that he gets the taste [rasa] for one pleasure [rata] after another. This is one of the ways of proceeding.

There are two ways of proceeding with the inversion of roles. In the first case, she holds firmly the instrument [yantra] to unite the boy with this fake sex [shālya] in a doubled up position. Being excited, the girl grips it in her arms and, mounting him and bestirring herself, possesses him. Seeing that he is developing a taste for a sensation of pleasure that is different from the other, she lets the instrument slide once more into its target [sandhana]. He feels a pleasure unknown before, since up to then he had not had any inclination for that kind of experience. However, he suddenly interrupts this pleasing sensation, since it is of a kind that is not acceptable for a young male [kāmina]. In such a case, despite her efforts, the girl's desire is not fulfilled.

5 The second way consists of taking him by surprise.

Pursuing her goal, her desire once more awakened, she begins again and, behaving like a man, without any beating about the bush, she spreads his buttocks apart and lets the instrument slide inside. This is the second way of doing it.

There are two forms of virile behavior, exterior and interior (bahya, abhyantara). The first form is described as follows:

> 6 Tearing the flowers from her hair, laughing until she is breathless, in order to bring their faces together, she presses hard with her breasts against the boy's chest, forcing him to lower his head several times. She copies in every detail his previous behavior with her, dominating him in turn. Laughing, she mocks him, saying insulting words to him. Then, again, if he shows modesty, wishing to rest from his labors, she mounts him [upasripta] and sodomizes him.

She does her best with this unusual behavior. She makes him lower his head with shame and presses her breasts hard against the boy's chest, not to embrace him or bite him, but with the ferocious desire to force him into behaving like a woman [strairena] in all ways. Speaking like a man, she tells him violently, "I will repay you for all the torments that you have made me suffer." Then, both behaving like women, although they would like to fight, they show the need for rest. Virile behavior is the term employed for a woman acting like a man. It is sometimes used for upasripta [to mount a man], meaning to sodomize him [upasarpet].

> 7 These practices will be explained.

The practice known as the sodomization of boys will be described. It is of two kinds, exterior or interior. The exterior kind will be described first.

> 8 Having made the boy lie down, the woman distracts his attention with her words while she unties his undergarment [nīvī]. If he protests, she embraces him to calm his apprehension.

Having decided to sodomize the boy, in order to implement her virile behavior, the woman seizes him and declares laughing that it is she who will play the man. Making him lie down, before starting her enterprise and to avoid his being embarrassed out of modesty [lajjā], she distracts his attention with her chatter in order to untie his nīvī, the knot of his undergarment. If he protests, she kisses him on the cheek until he agrees entirely and the undergarment can be easily removed.

9 When his penis is erect, she caresses him in various places.

Being excited, he allows the girl's hand to caress his sides, thighs, breast, putting him into an erotic mood. Then the boy is suddenly possessed by an object of copulation [sangatāya], which she slides without difficulty between his thighs.

10 If penetration [sangatā] is blocked to start with, she caresses the inside of his thighs.

If, to start with, the object of copulation cannot penetrate due to contact with the undergarment, which comes untied, or because he clenches his thighs out of modesty, she slides her hand into the cleft in order to widen it.

11 She behaves in the same manner with a girl. After winning the girl's trust and overcoming her modesty, she scratches and caresses the inside of her thighs, having unknotted the folds of the garment that passes between the legs.

12 Then, crushing her breasts and resting her armpits on the girl's shoulders, she puts her arms around her neck.

Making her hands slide everywhere and likewise placing her lips, despite the girl's hesitations, she strokes her beneath the arms, on her shoulders and thighs, and clasps her with her arms around her neck.

13 How the lesbian sets about it when she couples with her similar. In order to kiss her goatee [alaka], she seizes hold of the chin [pubis], slipping her finger into the slit.

A woman known for her independence, with no sexual bars, and acting as she wishes, is called svairinī [homophile]. She makes love with her own kind. She strokes her partner at the point of union, which she kisses. Once she has won the girl's trust, the svairinī practices the acts mentioned above, pitilessly, ill-treating the girl's pubis.

14 During the first intercourse, the girl is intimidated by
the other's contacts.

*At the first contact, the girl is reticent about the enterprise, out of
modesty and shyness, not completely trusting the lesbian. But, by employing the four exterior preliminaries of possession—untying the garment between her legs, touching her, stroking her, and inserting the
accessory—she inspires trust in the girl lying down and begins to kiss
her and perform other acts.*

In the event of her rejecting penetration:

15 The girl's reactions must be studied to find out at what
moment she has her orgasm during sexual intercourse.

*In this case, sexual intercourse means coupling with the instru-
ment in order to bring her to orgasm. Through external amorous
approaches, it can be determined how and to what point internal possession can go.*

16 According to Suvarnanābha, once the girl is possessed
[upasripta] by union with the instrument, the moment when
her eyes start vacillating is the moment to make her suffer.
This is the secret of young girls.

*When the girl is possessed using an accessory properly in place and
wedged into the vagina, her eyes start vacillating under the onrush of
pleasure, and the pupils of her eyes start moving. This is the right
moment to hurt her. The partner must then agitate the accessory in a
violent manner and, by making her suffer, rapidly increases her excitation. This is the secret of young girls. Since there are no visible signs,
a girl's excitation is determined by other means.*

*According to Suvarnanābha's authority, such practices are not
forbidden. Opinions differ considerably as to the possibility of enjoyment. One of the theories is that one must touch the places on which
she sets her eyes and, if she rolls her eyes back, hurt her in that place.
This is one of the ways of proceeding.*

*For many, wherever the girl turns her glance is the place to slap.
According to another opinion, she should not be hurt in the place to
which she turns her glance while bowed. The texts differ, especially as
regards the area of the hole. These different opinions should be studied.*

*The state of mind of girls who can be possessed is of three kinds:
accessible [prāpta], cooperating [pratyāsanna], hostile [sandhukshamāna].*

17 Her limbs relaxed, glances meeting, the disappearance
of all modesty, close contact, these are the characteristics
of the woman who is "accessible" for sexual intercourse.

*Relaxed limbs, and looking straight into the eyes are the sign of
the state of mind of the accessible girl.*
*The disappearance of modesty and shyness in sexual relations here
refer to copulation with the instrument.*
*Closely united means that she presses her pubis against the "male"
pubis of the virile woman. Such is the cooperative girl [pratyāsanna].*
These are the states of mind of accessible and cooperative girls.

18 *The hostile state of mind [sandhukshamāna]*

Approached for libidinous purposes by the virile woman,
she pushes her away with her hands. Perspiring and biting,
she refuses to be mounted, kicking with her feet.

*She will not let herself be possessed by the instrument. She rejects
any contact of her sex with the virile woman in the prey of her masculine desires.*

19 Before inserting the instrument, she strokes the girl's
vulva [sambādha] with her hand as would an elephant's
trunk and, when the vulva decontracts, she inserts the instrument.

*Knowing that the other shares her tendencies, excited before the
instrument is inserted and knowing that after reaching orgasm the
other will no longer desire it, she utilizes four different procedures. It
is said that, "Inside, the woman is like a lotus petal on which shines
a pearl of dew, or else her vulva may be all folds, rough as a cow's
strong tongue." In such a case, it should be stroked with the hand,
rubbing hard to make it relax. Once it is relaxed, the instrument can
be inserted. The girl is ready to be penetrated and must be rapidly
made to come to orgasm. The elephant is referred to as a comparison
for the hand, which takes the same form. It is a question of "the
position of the hand, with the ring and index fingers joined together*

*with the middle finger, known as elephant by analogy." Penetration
using the hand is similar to the use of an artificial object, and is thus
counted as one of the forms of internal sexual attack with an artificial
object.*

20   The forms of virile copulation [purushopasriptāni] are:

Normal copulation [upasriptaka]

Churning [manthana]

The rod [hulā]

The devastator [avamardhana]

The cruel [pīditaka]

The thunderbolt [nirghāta]

The wild boar's thrust [varāhaghāta]

The bull's attack [vrishāghāta]

The bird's amusement [chātakavilāsa]

The box [samputa]

Such are the forms of virile copulation.

Upasriptaka [normal copulation]
The union of phallus and vulva is always termed normal copulation.

21   Generally, union with a rectilinear object [riju] is
termed normal copulation.

*Riju means straight [praguna], and usually refers to the disen-
gaged [bared] member, while union with it refers to copulation
[upasriptaka]. The suffix ka indicates special cases [vishesha sanjñā].*
According to Vātsyāyana, only normal copulation conforms to the
rule and the other forms should not be practiced. It is the only form
that accords with decency, gentleness, and knowledge. The sexes should
unite in normal fashion.

22 *Churning [manthana]*
For churning, the phallus is held in the hand and turned
without stopping.

*Holding the phallus in the hand, it should be turned without
stopping inside the vagina, as in a churn.*

23 *The rod [hulā]*

For the rod, bend the body at the waist to practice penetration.

Bending the woman in the middle of her body, so that the inside of her vagina appears unrestricted in an upwards direction, plunge the rod in as if it were a phallus.

24 *The devastator [avamardhana]*

In the same inverse position, shaking the rod violently is known as the devastator.

With the same backward position, vagina in an upwards direction, in the arch of the buttocks, penetrate the vagina violently from top downwards.

25 *The cruel [pīditaka]*

The phallus driven in brutally is pressed forcefully in for some time. This practice is known as the cruel.

Inserting the phallus brutally right to the end [mūlam], press hard, leaving it inside the receiver as long as its intrusion is bearable.

26 *The thunderbolt [nirghāta]*

Raising the hips very high and letting them fall brutally downward is the thunderbolt.

Interrupting intercourse with the phallus and holding it firmly in place, then letting it fall abruptly back like a dart, is called the thunderbolt.

27 *The wild boar's thrust [varāhaghāta]*

Striking several times to one side is the wild boar's thrust.

On one side only, the wild boar blindly strikes several times.

28 *The bull's blow [vrishāghāta]*

Doing it now on one side, now on the other is the bull's blow.

Striking inside the vagina alternately on both sides, like a bull with his horns.

29 The bird's amusement [chātakavilāsa]
Alternately penetrating and half-penetrating, striking two, three, or four small blows, like the pecking of a bird.

30 The box [samputa]
Assuming the box position after reaching orgasm has already been described.

Since it is a natural position after pleasure, the box has already been described: "Both thighs stretched quite straight, without withdrawing the phallus, the sexual organs staying pressed hard together." This is known as the box position.

31 These acts are usually practiced by a woman with her own kind.

These forms of sexual domination are practiced between a woman and her own kind. "Usually" means it is particularly women with a sweet [mridu] and middling [madhya] temperament who are involved. The sodomization of boys is of two kinds. In its external form, the object is simply slipped between the thighs [nīvīvishleshana]. The second is internal. Sliding the object through the knots of the boy's undergarment [kakshābandha] is external sodomization [bāhyam purushāyitam]. The second form, with penetration [abhyantara], is called internal penetration [abhyantara purushāyitam].
After the sodomization of boys, we return to the forms of aggression belonging to virile behavior.

32 In virile behavior, three practices, among others, are frequently encountered. They are pinching [sandansha], the bee [bhramaraka], and swinging [prenkholita].

Forms of internal manipulation [abhyantara purushāyitam] are particularly practiced by enterprising women.

33 Pinching [sandansha]
With the lips of her vulva [vādavena = varānga aushtha]

seizing the phallus, sliding inside and keeping it tight is known as pinching.

34   The bee [bhramaraka]

Once the instrument is in place, moving it in a circular fashion is known as the bee, and requires practice.

The phallus is driven into the vagina. Lifting her body with the hands, her legs folded, make her turn on the instrument as on the axis of a potter's wheel. This requires practice.

35   To do this, raise the partner's lower abdomen [jaghana].

In order to facilitate the sliding of the instrument for the bee, the lower part of the body must be raised.

For this form of inverse coition (viparitarati) known as the bee, the thighs must be lifted.

36   The swing [prenkholita]

Swinging the ass [jaghana] in every direction, making it change position, is called the swing.

In swinging, the ass should be moved backward and forward, or else from side to side. Due to the swinging motion, it is called the swing. Making the inside part turn in a circle is churning. This kind of intercourse is practiced with a virile female partner [purushasātmyāta].

37   After which, united by the instrument, they rest face to face.

United by the instrument, they take their rest without agitating it any longer, their mutual excitation calmed, exhausted by their efforts.

38   Having rested, she recommences her virile behavior.

Here finishes virile behavior [purushāyita].
Once rested, she again makes love like a man. She recommences her virile behavior: her activity with the accessory [sahāyya] is in conformity with her nature.

In this connection, a quotation:

39 "A sensual girl, dissimulating by nature, unintelligible by her comportment [gūdhākārā], reveals her true nature when, in her excitation, she reverses roles."

Out of modesty, she dissimulates her nature, hides her impulses beneath an undecipherable appearance, dissimulating whatever could reveal her intentions. If her sexuality is inverted, she shows her desire, which she cannot hide when faced with the enterprises of one of her own kind. This is a well-known fact.

The old saw says, "A sensual girl, who out of modesty or virtue, dissimulates her nature, shows her true face when, led by passion, she practices sexual inversion."

To put matters clearly,

40   However virtuous a woman seems, or however sensual she appears, she reveals her nature in action.

It is in action, when taking the dominant role, that her entire way of behaving in sexual relations can be deduced, as well as the sexual deviations that she will also practice.

41   Women who have their period, who are about to give birth, are too narrow [hind type], who are pregnant, or are too big, should not practice the inversion of roles.

Including the sodomization of boys.

As the author of a code of behavior, Vātsyāyana has to contemplate both good aspects (shiva) and bad aspects (ashiva). After explaining the good side for each case, he indicates quite clearly what acts are contrary to ethics, antisocial, against the law, what may be practiced or must be rejected.

In this chapter, mainly dealing with questions of sexual domination and inversion, which he describes in detail, he attempts to separate the water from the milk from the point of view of an honest man. He indicates which practices are acceptable and which should be avoided. The commentary, in an enlightened examination, confirms Vātsyāyana's considerations concerning local customs, moments, and the social, physiological, and psychological aspects. He explains that, during the first contacts, a man should be prudent in his erotic approach. He should force himself to circumvent the woman's prejudices and mental obstacles before considering any physical difficulties. If at that moment, his behavior is brutal, shocking, and cruel, he will cause rejection and hostility to arise in the woman's heart, the counterblow of which will ruin the couple's future life, making it illassorted, tasteless, and distressing.

When Vātsyāyana indicates the various methods that are in accordance with ethics and custom, sources of happiness, and, on the other hand, condemns certain conduct as barbarous, immoral, of no interest, or not to be practiced, why does he then recommend that girls should study the arts of love in secret with a girlfriend or prostitute who is experienced in these arts?

It is because a knowledge of the good and study of the arts are essential. One should be able to practice and appreciate the arts, and for Vātsyāyana, this is an absolute necessity for the couple's happiness. The arts and sciences form part of sex life, for which they are a subtle necessity. Sexual intercourse is a form of yoga in which two beings blend, two hearts are united. Duality always desires unity. It is not merely a question of satisfying a marvelous and amusing desire. Vātsyāyana insists on this point, since intercourse is an act of profound significance for the spiritual life and a means of attaining liberation. Yoga and enjoyment (bhoga) are two complementary forms of action. Without pleasure, yoga leads to nothing and without yoga, true pleasure cannot be attained. True yoga leads to a complete experience of ecstasy and the true pleasureseeker (bhogi) is he who has completely mastered the art of pleasure.

The laughter, games, amusements, kisses, blows, bites, and other accessory aspects of copulation, are the means of reaching the culmination. At the moment when the peak of bliss is attained, the internal and external world vanish. The man and woman cease to be separate entities and lose themselves in the beatitude of being. All their mental powers are reabsorbed in a single central point. At that moment, no physical power, no worldly ambition can break the experience of bliss.

Vātsyāyana explains the importance of sexual yoga (maithuna yoga) and erotic positions, as well as the usefulness of blows, caresses, methods of coupling that are already envisaged in the *Vedas*. In the *Atharva Veda*, it is written,

"Young spouse! With a joyous heart prepare the happy union of the conjugal state! In giving sons to this your husband, you are as fortunate as Indrānī, the Queen of

Heaven. Happy woman! Awake with understanding, in the dawn before the rising of the sun."

"The wise men of yore united with their wives, and the latter blended their body with that of their spouse. This is why, wonderful woman! mother of sons! Unite your body with that of your spouse."

"O Supreme Being! Our protector! Stimulate the seed that I shall pour into this woman today. In order to fulfill my desire, she will spread her thighs so that my rod, inspired by desire, penetrates her vagina."

"Spouse! May the secret way between your thighs be of easy access to your husband! And may he pierce the knot of the god of the waters (Varuna), which the sun god has tied."

"Man! mount the thighs of your spouse, assist yourself with your hands, cleave to her and, full of joy, unite together, so that the sun god will grant you long life. In this marriage union, we have soiled the sheet, which we will have washed." (*Atharva Veda* 14.2.31, 32, 36, 38 and 14.1.58)

From these sacred texts, it is evident that sexual intercourse should take place at night and not during the day and that the woman should leave the bed at dawn. During the day, women are shy and modest. Daytime intercourse is contrary to custom. Furthermore, from a physiological and psychological point of view, the night is more favorable than the day for firing passion. In the second verse quoted, embraces are indicated. Embraces cause an exchange of magnetism. Fear, modesty, and hesitation are wiped away, and sexual charge increases. This is why the third verse recommends that copulation should take place with enthusiasm and gaiety. The fourth verse indicates that the way of the matrix is closed by a thin veil. In penetration, the veil is torn, which makes the woman suffer. This is why the man must act delicately. The woman must not be injured. The fifth verse describes the usual position recommended by Vātsyāyana, who declares that reverse, sideway, standing, or inverted positions should not be used, since these practices against nature may cause the birth of deformed babies. According to the fifth verse, after copulation a purificatory bath is necessary.

Vātsyāyana indicates two kinds of behavior and intercourse, beneficent and maleficent, meaning healthy or pernicious. It is better not to follow his treatise to the letter. In order to protect both the individual and society, a clean environment and honest surroundings are important. This is also expressed in *Yoga Vāsishtha* (4.3):

"The tide of desire (vāsanā) runs through good and evil. Taken together, desires are of two kinds, good and bad. If one falls into the difficulties of bad instincts, one must strive to awaken one's former good instincts. Man must endeavor to make the tide of his desires return to the right way."

"In order to flood his field, the peasant makes the water flow from another field on the same level or higher. With his hand, he prevents the water from breaking his dam and dispersing lower down."

"We must arrange for ourselves a garden in which each flower can develop freely. When all desires have been satisfied, the root of discernment is firmly planted. On the way to spiritual realization, the realization of desires is essential."

The tree of wisdom, watered by pleasure, is able to withstand storms within. Just as a peasant, to convey water from one field to another, does not carry it in his hands, but by damming the brooklets in the fields lower down, lets the water from higher up irrigate those below, so when the hand of discernment breaks through the obstacles on the road to pleasure, the satiated energy turns aside from material things.

In yoga theory, pleasure is just as essential for spiritual realization as erotic science is in the domain of material progress. Vātsyāyana explains the importance of attaining excellence in both spiritual and temporal domains.

This eighth chapter has a double scope, dealing with both the virile behavior of women and the sodomization of boys, and the various paragraphs have been divided on this basis. These two subjects play an important role in our interior equilibrium and for our behavior in life. The question is to determine the highest point a man can reach in orgasm, as well as the one at which the woman reaches her culmination, so that the woman is satiated and the man finds tranquility. The woman may practice virile behavior, comport herself like a man, and give herself up to sexual inversion when the boy is exhausted from copulation but her own passion is not assuaged. To amuse the boy, the girl mounts him and the boy submits to her as a woman. Both find satisfaction in this combination. Inverse coition creates a bond of affection and passion between lover and beloved. This kind of intercourse develops their mutual trust and is an element of bliss for them.

Sometimes, driven by a devouring passion, the woman wants to show with audacity the aggressive love she bears for the boy. In such a way, by means of sexual inversion, she can give a clear indication of her technique and her strength in the form of amorous warplay (rati yuddha). Jayadeva describes this kind of erotic struggle between Rādhā and Krishna:

> "With her sex bruised in the amorous games of the fray, at the outset of the battle, she decides to conquer her lover. She sets about mounting him, so as to confuse him. Without trembling, far from being a fragile liana, leaning firmly on his belly, their eyes gazing into each other's, she makes it clear up to what point a woman can experience male pleasure." (*Gītā Govinda* 12.63)

In order to conquer Krishna, Rādhā audaciously unleashes the conflict of inverted copulation. This required so much effort of her that her thigh movement stopped, her arm-joint was paralyzed, her heart started beating and her eyes closed. The outcome of this erotic war is brilliant. In this conflict the woman tires herself, but her passion and excitation reach their peak. When a pretty woman unleashes this conflict with audacity, her energy becomes tenfold, and madness sparkles in her eyes. Then, exhausted, she sinks onto the man's breast, somewhat humiliated, out of breath, after an enterprise that could be painted, but not described in words.

If this is the woman's behavior in sexual inversion, what then is the man's?

When the woman wants to make love like a man, it is called virile behavior. The boys whom virile women use for this purpose are known as possessed men (upasripta).

Virile behavior and sodomization are great aids in increasing lovers' erotic pleasure.

End of the Eighth Chapter
Virile Behavior in Women
of the Second Part entitled Amorous Advances

Chapter Nine

SUPERIOR COITION
OR FELLATION
[Auparishtaka]

The four previous chapters dealt with woman, ranging from the various kinds of embraces to virile behavior.

This fifth chapter, dealing with buccal coition [auparishtaka], describes the third sex [tritīya prakriti], which has two aspects.

1   People of the third sex [tritīya prakriti] are of two kinds, according to whether their appearance is masculine or feminine.

The third sex is also termed neuter [napunsaka]. Those with a feminine appearance have breasts, while those with a masculine aspect have moustaches, body hair, etc. Buccal coition as practiced by both kinds is a part of their nature.

Prostitutes belonging to the third sex are called catamites (hijrā). The first kind is described as follows:

2   Those with a feminine appearance show it by their dress, speech, laughter, behavior, gentleness, lack of courage, silliness [mugdha], patience, and modesty.

To give themselves a female appearance and imitate their behavior, they arrange their hair in female fashion and imitate their way of talking, their prattle, amusements, their dragging gait and manner of being, their flirting, sweetness, futility, their lack of courage, hesitation, silliness, their lack of intelligence and endurance, their fear of drafs and heat, their shyness and modesty.

3　They perform the act that takes place between the thighs in the mouth, which is why it is called superior coition.

This term comes down to us from ancient authors.

4　They earn their living from those that seek this form of eroticism.

5　Those who dress as women are taken for prostitutes.

Like prostitutes, they make themselves accessible to libidinous men, and experience an orgasm, or satisfaction.
The question of transvestites ends here.

6　Those who like men but dissimulate the fact maintain a manly appearance and earn their living as hairdressers or masseurs.

They too practice oral coition, but their sexual desires are dissimulated. Since they look masculine, a man does not immediately reach his goal with them. They practice the profession of masseur, and officially earn their living by massaging limbs.
Since no trust exists to start with, how do they go about getting to erotic action?

7　While massaging, he rests his body against that of the man and kneads his thighs on the side of his intimate parts [upaguha]. He draws his face closer to the man's thighs as he kneads them.

8　Continuing his investigation, he touches the sexual area at the thigh joint. Without bothering about the penis, he touches the little bag belonging to the sexual region.

9　When he manages to provoke an erection, he takes the penis in his hand, strokes it and, audaciously making fun, he starts laughing.

The boy's sex being erect when he touches the balls [jaghanabhāga] at the root of the thigh, he rubs the erect sex with his hand, like a cowherd with a cow's udder, but not immediately. Audaciously, he makes fun of the fact that the penis has become erect although he has only touched the thigh. He laughs at having reached his goal, but does not cause ejaculation [rūshya].

10 Seizing the opportunity, after clear signs of excitation, he commences action, even without being asked to.

Since the erect sex implies the man's desire, the boy seizes the opportunity. Even without any intimation to suck, he does so on his own initiative.

11 At the same time, if the man indicates his desire for this act, he first refuses, then, having protested, devotes himself to it.

If he is asked to do it, whether or not he feels an aversion for this act, he will refuse, replying, "I do not do such things." Having let it be understood that it is a woman's job, he takes it on with a show of difficulty.

12 There are eight ways of practicing this kind of contact.

These ways of practicing oral coition are given in sequence.

13 They are: casual [nimitta] placing the lips on the mast, nibbling the sides [pārshvatodashta], external pinching [bahihsandamsha], internal pinching [antahsandamsha], kissing [chumbitaka], browsing [parimrishtaka], sucking the mango [āmrachushitaka], devouring [sangara].

Then, if the desired result is not reached:

14 Having used each of these practices in turn, he shows a desire to rest.

Leaving his customer surprised and anxious for him to continue. When the boy shows his interest, what does he do then?

15 Having experienced one of these procedures, the cus-

tomer should call for the following and then, after that, the
next one.

*After the first contact [nimitta] of the lips with the mast, the man
awaits the second, the nibbling of the sides, and calls for it. When it
has been accomplished, he calls for the next, external pinching [bahih-
sandamsha] and then he requests all the others in sequence, in order
to fulfill his desire and achieve his pleasure. In coupling thus with his
customer to make him ejaculate [udānaya], the masseur himself fulfils
his own desire in this sequence of practices.*

*This kind of relation has two aspects, an external and an internal.
The external one is dealt with first.*

16 Casual [nimitta]

Clasping the penis with one hand, bringing the lips close,
while pressing, releasing, and shaking.

*Bending down if there is any resistance, taking the mast in one hand,
pressing the lips to it, rounding them over the mast, and shaking it.*

17 Nibbling the sides [pārshvatodashta]

Covering the end of the penis with one hand, pressing the
lips to the sides and nibbling slightly at the same time.
Having done this, immediately soften the bite. This is nibbling the sides.

Having bitten it, calm it down.

18 External pinching [bahihsandamsha]

Bringing his lips close to the erect penis, he presses the
mast and kisses it while sucking. This is what is known as
external pinching [bahihsandamsha].

*When the sex has been stimulated by being nibbled along the sides,
he himself, excited at the first contact with his lips, lets the end of the
penis penetrate into his mouth, pressing it and sucking and, having
bared it, he releases it. This is called the external seizure.*

19 Internal pinching [antahsandamsha]

On request, he then lets the penis penetrate further and,

pressing it between his lips, causes an ejaculation [nishthīvet]. This is called internal pinching.

This is done on request and not otherwise. When the excited customer promises to pay since he is ready to come, he lets the penis penetrate further in. Being excited himself, encircling the penis with his lips like a necklace, he causes an emission of liquid.

20 *The kiss [chumbita]*

Encircling the penis with his hand instead of his lips, he kisses it.

Seizing the penis with the hand instead of the lips, baring it and kissing it is known as the kissing hold.

21 *Browsing [parimrishtaka]*

Having done this, with the tip of the tongue, licking the mast all over and titillating the opening, is known as browsing.

In the "kissing" hold, or in others, let the tip of the tongue wander and titillate the meatus opening [vyaghana], the point of gushing forth [srotasthāna], cleaning it carefully. This is called polishing.

22 *Sucking the mango [āmrachūshitaka]*

Having bared the mast, pressing the organ hard, passionately, while half inside, and sucking while pressing, is known as sucking the mango.

With the mast thus bared, press hard on the half-entered penis and sucking while pressing, using the base of the tongue, as when sucking the juice of a mango.

23 *Devouring [sangara]*

According to the man's desire, the boy makes him come, continuing to press it up to the end. This is called devouring.

Having understood the man's desire and in order to satisfy his wish to come, he makes him ejaculate by the pressure of his tongue, until the sperm gushes out. Sangara means total ejaculation [gīrana].

24   If one wishes to, it is customary to pinch the gigolo's nipples.

According to whether the gigolo's attraction is slight, average, or strong, it is customary to pinch his nipples, although it is not becoming to clasp him in one's arms.

The object, form, result, tendencies, and ways of proceeding in oral coition have been indicated, as well as the prevalence of homophile relations in certain countries.

Here ends oral coition.

25   Buccal coition can also be practiced with corrupt women [kulatā], lesbians [svairinī], servants [paricharikā], women who carry burdens [sanvāhikā].

By corrupt women are meant those of good family who are licentious. Lesbians are independent women who frequent their own kind or others. Servants, whether they have previous experience or not, allow themselves to be taken by men. Sanvāhikā are women who do arduous work. This kind of woman can be used, and can be allowed to practice oral coition. The term does not refer exclusively to the third sex.

It is not merely a practice of inverts.

26   According to the Āchārya, the masters of learning, this practice is not recommended. It is contrary to sound morals and is not a civilized practice [asabhya]. One is defiled by the contact of the sex with the face.

This practice is forbidden by the holy books: "No penis in the mouth!" [Na mukhe meheta]. Being forbidden to Brahmans, it is therefore not a civilized practice. If the work of the vagina [jaghana] is done by the mouth of persons belonging to the family and then, in the excitation of the sexual act, the faces touch, it constitutes defilement. One says, "It is I who am the whore, not the girl."

Whether it is a woman or a boy, kissing the mouth in which one has ejaculated is shocking.

27   Vātsyāyana's opinion is that for those who like prostitutes, it is not a sin, but it is better to forego doing it with other persons.

It is not a sin for a boy who frequents prostitutes, whether or not they come from a good family. The fact of being contrary to customary morals [samaya] does not make it a sin. On the other hand, requesting one's wife to perform oral coition is a sin. Since Vasishtha the lawgiver has written "No penis in the mouth," whoever practices buccal coition with his legitimate wives [pāniorihītāyā] destroys fifteen years of celestial life of his ancestors, and it is better to forgo it, since contact with the mouth is not considered very civilized. However, mouth contact with the vulva is not forbidden by the texts, if it is a custom of the country.

The regions where these two practices can be encountered are indicated.

28 This is why contacts must be avoided with people from the Eastern area [Prāchya], who practice buccal coition.

In places where prostitutes practice the work of the vagina with their mouths, their company should be avoided, as well as any contact with their mouth. It is the women of the eastern regions who practice buccal coition.

A man who does not let himself be sucked should avoid the company of women from the eastern countries.

29 The company of the women of Ahichchatra [South Panchāla] should be avoided and, if one has intercourse with them, they should not be allowed to practice oral coition.

In the ardor of the act, without letting it be known or saying anything, they are likely to practice buccal coition, since it is the nature of the women of Ahichchatra [South Panchāla, to the north of the Ganges].

30 The people of Saketa [Ayodhya] practice it without any embarrassment.

In their relations with whores, they have no prejudice with regard to what is clean or dirty in acts performed with the mouth.

31 The people of the city [Nāgara, Pātaliputra] do not themselves practice buccal coition.

The people of Pātaliputra practice it with prostitutes, but they themselves do not perform the vulva's work with their mouth. They also avoid contacting the vulva with their mouth.

32   The Saurasenas practice everything without any hesitation.

Everything includes copulation, buccal coition, cunnilingus. They have no notion of purity. The Saurasenas live to the south of Kaushambi. The characteristics of the Saurasenas have been indicated. The people of Pātaliputra do not themselves perform any reprehensible act.

With regard to any doubts one may have about the purity of one's own wife.

33   It is said: What man, full of respect for her, considers that one can trust the virtue [shīla], cleanliness [shaucha], behavior [āchāra], good conduct [charitra], good faith [pratyaya], or word of a woman? Therefore, even if she appears guilty by her behavior, one should not desert her, even the most perfidious. This is why, according to the treatises on morals [smriti], one should consider her pure, as a matter of principle.

This is why it is said: The calf is pure when it drinks milk, the dog's mouth is pure when it seizes the game, as is also the beak of the bird that makes the fruit fall, and the mouth of a woman during the act of love.

What woman can claim to be pure and spotless in her virtue, character, cleanliness, the purity of her ointments, her behavior, in practicing the three daily rites, in conduct, in respecting the family rules, in good faith, dress, credibility, word, or pretensions? It is impossible to observe every restriction. This is why, in his own interest, a man should not judge his wife severely, even if her behavior is contrary to social and religious law, and he should not throw her out, since she is indispensable to him for realizing one of the aims of life. For this reason, from the point of view of sexual relations, the question of purity is contemplated according to social and religious criteria. According to the religious texts, we see that, apart from its muzzle, the whole cow is pure. But when the milk gushes forth, the calf's muzzle becomes pure as well as the milk coming from the udder. Similarly, the mouth of the animal that seizes the game or bites the fruit becomes pure, and the meat and the fruit are also. In the same way, during sexual relations, a woman's mouth is pure, unless she practices buccal coition. Apart from that, according to the sacred texts, all receptacles of impurity can be embraced.

In giving his own opinion, Vātsyāyana says:

34 Opinions differ on the matter of purity between the authority of the moral codes, occasional local customs, and one's own feelings. One should therefore behave according to one's inclinations.

Moralists condemn the relations of citizens of the eastern country with barbers. Their opposition is a matter of points of view. Moral codes are not revealed texts [shruti], but traditions to be consulted. This is why the phrase "according to circumstances" is used. If a woman has her menses, sexual union with her mouth is advised. If it is a question of embracing prostitutes, no problem arises. Considering alternative opinions, he says that one should conform to the local custom of the country. In such cases, local custom serves as a rule. One should follow customary behavior. One should behave according to what is agreeable or according to one's own convictions, not only according to religious texts.

Having considered buccal coition normal among women, as something which can be practiced by women, he again takes up the question of boys.

35 Sometimes, young servants, wearing bright rings in their ears, practice buccal coition with other men.

It is a question of a member of the household staff, carefully dressed, wearing glittering earrings, a young manservant, working when it pleases him, skillful in his work, pleasing to the eye. He is defined as, "beardless, who can be trusted for acts involving the mouth, wearing jewels, not disfigured by moustaches." Some of these boys, lacking enthusiasm when they get older, turn to women.

36 There are also citizens, sometimes greatly attached to each other and with complete faith in one another, who get married [parigraha] together.

Citizens with this kind of inclination, who renounce women and can do without them willingly because they love each other, get married together, bound by a deep and trusting friendship.

"Do this to me, and afterward I will do it to you." Arranging their bodies in a contrary position, they are indifferent to everything in their moments of passion. They are of two kinds, according to whether they live together openly and without complexes, or dissimulate. Women behave in the same way. Sometimes, in the secret of their inner rooms, with total trust in each other, they lick each other's vulva, just like whores.

37   This kind of activity is practiced in the same way by men on women. The manner of embracing the vulva as one embraces the mouth is not recommended.

What women do to men, men also practice on women, working with their mouth on their partner's vulva. This kind of intercourse practiced by a man is forbidden. The manner of embracing another part as one embraces the mouth is also considered a form of sexual intercourse.

Sometimes the man practices inverse coition (auparishtaka) with a woman. In such a case, he licks her vulva.

When such practices are usual between partners and represent the couple's habits, are they really a couple?

38   *The Crow*

The form of eroticism practiced on each other by the man and woman, with their bodies in an inverted position, is known as the crow.

With their bodies in an inverted position, lying face to face on their side, the man places his head on the woman's thigh and the woman does the same to unite the couple. In this position, both seize the other's sexual organ with their mouth. The boy embraces the vulva, while the girl sucks his rod. This form of buccal coition [auparishtaka] is called the crow. Like crows, the man and woman peck each other, seizing each other's sex with their mouth and experiencing pleasure. They drink each other's secretions in the heat of their passion. Kāka [crow] comes from a root meaning "laulia," an excess of ardor. It is out of an excess of desire of each for the other that they practice it.

When the man and woman lie in an inverse position, it is considered an acceptable act [sādhārana] between partners of the same social standing, and not to be recommended with persons of other castes. Acts between equals are to be preferred. As far as relations with servants are concerned, contacts with sweepers and other groups mentioned require ritual purification.

39   Virtuous, experienced, and prudent men avoid such practices, whereas prostitutes delight in road sweepers [khala], slaves, or elephant drivers.

Behavior beyond the norm is avoided by men of quality and prudence [chatura], by men experienced in life's journey. On the other hand, they please those whose natural inclinations are morally unrefined. Thus, prostitutes prefer men of low extraction, slaves or elephant drivers, to a man full of qualities, who is prudent, able to drive his way through life, liberal and generous. They prefer men of rough nature, slaves and elephant drivers, people with dirty habits, and are attracted by them because they do not draw back from unusual practices.

40   The various forms of buccal coition should be avoided by Brahmans, men of letters, ministers and other government officials, as well as by those who have become famous.

Buccal coition should not be practiced even with prostitutes. This is the case of men of letters who know the meaning of the sacred books, and all those who take part in the administration of the country, but such a prohibition is not absolute. The case of famous people, of wide esteem in the world, is different. Their glory and fame have been acquired by their acts. For them, contacts with the face are not ritual sins, but at the most a lack of decorum. In any case, the lapse is difficult to demonstrate since it is not spoken about.

If the truth is known, even the practice of kissing is not universally approved of. Religious texts contemplate it only between equals, meaning persons of the same social standing.

41   The fact of something being mentioned in the sacred books does not mean that it can be practiced. Knowledge is universal, but practice depends on the customs of each country.

Although one should act according to Scripture, this does not mean putting it into practice. The meaning of the Scriptures is too general. Embraces and so on, which are preludes to the sexual act, are instinctively practiced all the time by an erotic man [kāmina]. They are practiced in many countries and are widespread among decent people. This principle is equally valid for all other domains.

42 According to medical treatises, wine increases virile power, as does dog meat. Although this is a well-known fact, what circumspect man would eat it?

It is well known that wine and other alcoholic beverages are fortifying, but as far as dog meat is concerned, this information does not mean that one should eat it. Therefore, if something should not be done by decent people, what is the use of teaching it?

43 For some men, in some countries, in given circumstances or moments, this kind of sexual relationship is not without its own raison d'être.

Anxiety over matters such as purity or impurity have no meaning in countries like Lāta or Sindhu, where buccal coition between men or with women who make a business of it is allowed as freely as kissing on the mouth.

44 It is by taking into account the country, the period, custom, the injunctions of the sacred texts, as well as one's own tastes, that one decides whether or not to practice these kinds of sexual relations.

By taking into account local customs, the epoch, and one's own tastes, one decides whether they can be practiced with people of one's own society or with others. Although having deep respect for the texts, a man first considers his own interest to decide whether he can practice one form of intercourse or another. In this field, neither man, woman, or the third sex know any rule.
In this connection:

45 Practiced according to his fantasy and in secret, who can know who, when, how, and why he does it?

It is a matter of buccal coition, or fellation, practiced secretly in a state of mental instability, and more especially in a state of erotic excitation.

Who does it? No one else can know. How? Why? In a state of irresponsibility or otherwise. With whom? People of one's own circle or of a different social standing. For what reason does he practice this kind of sexual intercourse? Out of passion, or as a local custom. Who knows?

The practice of fellation is common among the hijrās, or male prostitutes. This practice, often considered not very refined, is not forbidden by moral texts. It is common even among civilized people, although it is not highly recommended. People with perverse inclinations are attracted by this kind of amusement.

* * * * *

Superior coition is the name given to coition in the mouth. Already mentioned in previous chapters, this act, which is often condemned, is practiced by the hijrās, or male prostitutes. According to the specialists who are our authority in this field, it is an indecent, antisocial, and uncivilized act. Although not condemned by the texts and practiced in the best society, this does not mean that it should be practiced. At the same time, there are people who, because of their evil inclinations and bad company, are subject to these undesirable tendencies and to practicing these bad habits.

These acts are clearly to be condemned and avoided. They are not something new, but of very ancient practices, transmitted by tradition, since even the sacred books mention them, though only to condemn. Buccal coition is a sexual act, is part of the erotic instinct, and represents a tradition. How can a basic work ignore it? The treatise must mention it, but also indicate any inconveniences it may have. In condemning it, the sacred text excludes it, in the interest of people's welfare. In describing the individual and society, what concerns the individual and society cannot be omitted or ignored. It is not a question of proclaiming that society is uncivilized and without refinement. This is why, while describing the practice of buccal coition, the text warns against employing it.

On this subject, Vātsyāyana, acknowledging the greater importance of men's inclinations and local customs, remarks that religious texts give no indication of what behavior should be avoided. Acts contrary to the texts, or evil practices, are not to be considered sins. Buccal coition is an act to be avoided, whatever local customs or one's own tastes may be.

When Vātsyāyana says in the third paragraph that famous people practice this kind of unusual copulation, he alludes to people who frequent transvestite prostitutes (launda). The commentator Yashodhāra makes the meaning perfectly clear by employing the word *janakhā* (transvestite-invert).

In speaking of homosexual marriage, Yashodhara, besides boys, also speaks of women, whose inclination is to lick each other's vulva. In modern terms, this is called perversion (chapatī).

End of the Ninth Chapter
Superior Coition or Fellation
of the Second Part entitled Amorous Advances

Chapter Ten

PRELUDES AND CONCLUSIONS TO THE GAMES OF LOVE

[Rata ārambha-avasānika]

Having described superior coition after the other kinds, Vātsyāyana explains how to behave before and after the sexual act. The signs of affection must be continued before and after copulation. Whatever the operational order, the performance must include embraces and other signs of affection that continue afterward, particularly in the case of an occasional fling [prakīrnakanyā], prior to copulation and also at the end, in order to create a bond.

The preliminary actions are now described.

1 Accompanied by his friends and servants, having taken a bath and being elegantly dressed, the citizen enters the chamber of love [rati-āvāsa] of his dwelling, which is carefully decorated, ornamented with flowers, and perfumed with scented smoke. He invites the woman to drink with him, and they commence drinking together.

The citizen is surrounded by his friends and servants, masseurs, carriers of betel, cupbearers, and others. The chamber of love, designed

197

for amorous games, is located outside the house. It contains a bed, and thus completes the dwelling.

Women are of two kinds, those who take care of their body and bathe in a bathroom [nepathya-graha], and those who are not very refined and should be eliminated as soon as one sees them. Once together, a little drink is necessary to enhance the mood, but not too much since drink may disturb the girl's mind. First she must be greeted with pleasant words, asking her news, and so forth, to begin with. After this, strong liquor [saraka] is taken.

2   He sits to the right of the girl, strokes her hair, and the edge of her robe, and without her knowledge undoes the part that passes between the thighs [nīvī], for libidinous purposes. He embraces her with his left arm.

He places himself on her right, holding his cup in his right hand and embracing her with his left arm. To start with, he strokes her hair and other places, then encircles her waist with his left arm, trying not to frighten her, if she is shy.

3   In order to introduce the matter, he amuses her with funny stories, making her laugh, and speaks hintingly of indecent and secret things.

At the start, very gradually he chatters. "Do you remember, my beauty, what happened here or there. You laughed so heartily!" Then, changing the subject, he goes on to speak of indecent and gross matters. Briefly he tells of hidden things, behavior that is difficult to get to know, or vulgar, little known details about people, on whose account he tells stories of which both would like to know the ending, just as in a novel [parikathā].

In order to stimulate her, he tells indecent and immoral stories, in the form of riddles, laughing and being amused the while.

4   Then comes vocal and instrumental music, whether or not accompanied by dancing. After which they talk about art, then once more, he encourages her to drink.

If she does not know how to dance, she mimes the words of the song by moving her body in a kind of sitting dance. Otherwise, they simply listen to the singing. As regards instruments, the vīnā should be played, as well as other string instruments, with an ivory plectrum. Other kinds of instruments are not suitable. In speaking of art, in order to demonstate his talent, he shows her his phallic drawings. Then, letting the matter fall, he encourages her to drink once more.

5 Once pleasure has been awakened, having scented her with flower essences and offered her betel, he sends away the others present. As previously explained, he stimulates her by his embraces and begins to undo the folds of her garment as indicated. He then begins erotic games.

Having sent the servants away, he begins his enterprise in the manner foreseen. Betel is served as a pretext for sending friends and servants away. In the manner already explained, they prepare to make love. He plucks up courage, tears off her robe, persuades her laughingly to lie down and, when she does, he slips off his own clothes and mounts her according to the various procedures for sexual possession.

6 Having finished copulating [rata], free from desire, having become modest, without intimacy, they both go separately to the toilets [āchāra bhūmi]. On returning without any embarrassment, they seat themselves comfortably, greeting each other, taking betel, and rubbing each other with sandalwood paste. He smears the girl's body with it and then makes her sit down.

Having made love as already described, their desire exhausted, they find familiarity lacking, as if they did not know each other, modest, embarrassed by one another, like strangers. Then they both go and wash, embarrassed by the sight of the virile organ. This is why they go separately to the latrines [āchāra bhūmi]. They do not go and wash themselves together in the bathroom [shaucha bhūmi]. They then return to an agreeable place, not the one in which they have copulated. Taking betel, they eat it to beautify and scent their mouths. Then, with very fine powder, they rub the body's bruises, whether external or internal. During the hot season, they utilize ointment of sandalwood or other seasonal products for the outside of the body. Then, if he wishes to, he also comes and sits down.

7   Putting his arms around her, he holds a cup in his hand and, with gentle words, invites her to drink. Then, according to the season, he offers her a light meal of sweetmeats and other preparations, which both share heartily.

Or else they remain clasped in each other's arms, one against the other, like sesame seeds.

8   Then, conversing sweetly and gently, they take a pleasant meal, a clear soup tasting of mulberries, appetizing grilled meats, drinks of ripe fruit juice, dried meat, lemons and tamarind fruits, according to the customs of the country. Then, at their ease, they drink sweet liquors, while chewing from time to time sweet or tart things.

The soup may be of two kinds, meat extract or boiled rice liquid. The meat broth implies the killing of animals. A clear and tasty broth is thus obtained. The meat extract is better than the rice broth, which is sour, since it is invigorating. The roast meat is an appetizer before drinking mango juice. Pieces of tamarind fruit in sugarcane juice, with peeled and seeded lemons, taken with small lumps of sugar to stimulate, according to the custom of the country. Eating them while drinking is a way of getting into the mood. While drinking, they pick sweet or sour tidbits from time to time.

9   Climbing to the terrace on top of the house to take advantage of the moonlight, they give themselves over to pleasant conversation. She lays her head on the boy's knees to look at the moon. He explains the figures of the constellations to her: Arundhatī the faithful, Dhruva the polestar, the garland of the seven Rishi [the Great Bear]. Thus, their games of love come to an end.

If it is too hot indoors and the moon is shining, they climb up to the terrace of the main house to sit and watch it. Whether it is hot or not, they take betel with them to eat. Their satiated eroticism having no further attraction, he continues to talk, telling her love stories. Leaning on the boy's knees, she stares at the vault of the sky, where the moon is a pleasure to the eye. He explains the figures of the constellations to her and their different components. Women are often unaware of the geography of the stars. There is the divine Arundhatī, who is hard to see. Anyone who is unable to see her will die within six months. And there is Dhruva, the unmoving polestar, which, if one can see it during the day, cancels all other defects. And there are the Seven Sages, the Great Bear, well installed in their right place. Thus he shows them to her.

He also shows her the Heavenly Ganges (the Milky Way). Then, their minds at peace, the both go and sleep in their separate apartments. *Two texts are quoted in this connection.*

10 "After making love, one's behavior should be affectionate. A solid attachment is established through friendly conversation."

Every word they say to each other after making love express the woman's gentleness and the man's love, as in the welcome given at the beginning. She is impressed by her reception, the flood of scents, the drinks, and all the other things, as well as by the soothing conversation, which are the starting point for the birth of a lasting affection.

There is a famous saying on this subject, "Embraces, kisses, small tender words, and confidences double the desire to unite together physically."

11 "Mutual affection is expressed by changes of mood, sometimes by disputes, sometimes by tender looks."

Once trust is established, a reciprocal attraction is felt by both man and woman after making love, which is shown in different attitudes. Some people remain clasped to each other, while others separate. Some seem to be seized by anger, while other throw loving glances. Sometimes they pretend to quarrel, seized by sudden anger, then, changing their behavior, they become loving and affectionate again, or else they look around them. All these attitudes increase their love in the same way as the preliminaries to intercourse.

Changes of humor stimulate desire and increase mutual attraction. One moment they turn away from each other in fury, and then the next moment they laughingly exchange loving looks.

12 The rounds and songs about faithful lovers [rāsaka] from the Lāta country, whose passion makes eyes fill with tears, have been compared to the moon's halo.

The women of Lāta country and of other regions, led by Krishna the cowherd, dance round dances while listening to the songs, their eyes turning up and dimming under the effect of love, when they see the object of their passion. They are compared to the ceaselessly moving orb of the moon, in prey to their devotion.

13   He speaks to her of the wonder of love, born at their first meeting, and of the pain felt in separating, just as the poets have described. Then, after these evocations, they embrace and exchange passionate kisses. United by their experience, their passion grows.

Love at their first meeting is sometimes born of a fleeting impression, sometimes from a simple glance. Then separation causes them savage pain. Once their love is proclaimed, they both hope to make an end to separation, a bond of mutual trust is created, which the one feels for the other. The beginning of love, whether in the adult or in adolescents, will be described in the twentieth chapter.

Thus talking about love and of their mutual attraction, while clasping and embracing each other, their contentment and passion grow.

The preludes and conclusions form part of the act of love (rata-avayava). Once stimulated, desire leads to various kinds of amorous relations. The various kinds of amorous relations are as follows:

14   Rāgavat, passionate love, born of physical attraction;

Āhāryarāga, love born from habit, the result of affection produced by long cohabitation;

Kritrimarāga, feigned love, without true feeling;

Vyavahitarāga, substitute love, through an interposed party. The man sleeps with his wife, while thinking of another woman;

Potārata, neutral sex, without feeling, practiced with servant-women or female porters;

Khalarata, degrading love, to satiate one's basest instincts, practiced with a corrupt woman or some gross individual.

Such are the various kinds of erotic attraction [rati], whether good or bad.

15 *Rāgavat, passionate love born of physical attraction*

Born in both parties at first sight, this attraction grows with the efforts made to realize it. This kind of attraction is also found on returning from a journey, or on meeting again after a quarrel.

Desire born from a first glimpse of someone's pleasant appearance, which develops with information brought through a messenger and other efforts to manage to unite, is called rāgavat, passionate love. It is the same desire felt on returning after a journey, stimulated by absence, or else when, after a quarrel, peace is made and one makes love joyously and with pleasure. This is what is known as passionate love.

16 This attachment increases until its goal has been attained.

Passionate desire fires itself and lasts until it is fulfilled.

17 *Āhāryarāga, affection born of habit*

Only an ordinary attraction exists to begin with, but little by little, it grows. This is desire born of force of habit.

To begin with only an ordinary attraction existed, a feeling of congeniality, born of a physical appearance that caused a simple desire, not the union of two hearts. Sexual attraction is consequently relative. At the outset, during their first experiences, they nevertheless feel a certain satisfaction. Later on, sexual attraction is established by routine copulation [maithuna]. They attain true erotic satisfaction. Love born of consumation also leads to true affection.

Ordinary attraction means that the lover or his mistress have a simple desire for each other, but not true erotic attraction. However, a mutual desire develops from such an ordinary attraction by practice, and creates true affection. This is what is termed love born of consumation (āhāryarāga).

18 Becoming gradually more excited by practicing the sixty-four positions, with common accord, a true passion [rāga] grows up.

The woman is aroused by the mere desire for erotic exercises.

19 *Kritrimarāga, feigned love*

Here, it is a matter of an occasional relation, while true love is for someone else. This is false desire.

Whether for good or bad reasons, it is not a case of true attraction, because the feelings of both one and the other are elsewhere. The woman is tied to another man, and the man to another woman. The enjoyment they experience in making love together is a false passion [kritrimarāga].

20 In such forms of intercourse, it is better to consult the texts.

In these two kinds of union, unlike the others, there is no spontaneous attraction. At the moment of intercourse, therefore, it is useful to consult about the methods of practicing the various forms of embrace, etc. This is why the texts are useful for information on local customs, conventions, states of mind, etc.

21 *Vyavahitarāga, substitute love*

The man whose heart is tied to another makes love with his wife while thinking of the other woman. All the marks of affection and erotic acts take place by the interposition of another party. This is substitute love [vyavahitarāga].

The state of a man who, even without other ties, or without being stimulated by another attachment, makes love without feeling is called false desire [kritrima]. Unless he does it in the hope of begetting a child, he finds no satisfaction due to lack of passion. On the other hand, if he performs with the thought of the one he loves in mind, he finds an ardor and excitation in the sexual act, which is expressed in his erotic performance. Since his performance is directed at the one he loves, it is love by substitution of the party [vyavahita]. In reality, he is uniting with the girl of his heart.

After which, occasional sexual relations are contemplated.

The first three kinds of spontaneous, habitual, or occasional sexual relations are morally acceptable and are considered pure [shuddha]. The following kinds, on the other hand, are not acceptable, since they should not be practiced by men and women of different social class. Their advantages and inconveniences are described by way of example.

22 *Potārata, neutral sex*

This refers to occasional sexual relations, due to the need for sexual satisfaction, with persons of no account, water-bearers, servant-women, inverts, etc.

This concerns waterbearers, or servants of a very lowly condition, but also wandering monks and bisexual scribes. This is neutral sex (potārata).

23 This kind of behavior is not recommended.

This kind of embrace is not respectable, or gracious. It only supplies a semblance of sexual satisfaction. In such cases, there is no need to embrace or kiss, since they are merely a convenience.

24 *Khalarata, degrading sex*

This is the case when a prostitute gives her body to a gross peasant to satisfy her perverse taste for adventure with people unlike an agreeable lover. It is the case of prostitutes, and courtesans who live on their charms, who, not being able to obtain what they desire, make use of gross individuals such as, for example, cowherds. This is degrading sexuality.

25 It is the same for a gentleman who sleeps with village girls, shepherd girls, cowgirls, etc.

For a gentleman, relations with peasants are degrading, they are merely substitutes for love. Such forms of sexual release, like neutral sex [potārata] are only possible if one disguises oneself. Of village girls, the only attractive ones are the cowgirls of the Vraja country, all the others are savages [shabara].

For a person who is skilled in the art of love, relations with cowgirls, buffalo keepers, etc., are degrading.

Only when mutual confidence (visrambha) is established, with its moments of passion, quarrels, and so on, can one practice sex without barriers.

26 *Ayantritarata, sex without barriers*

When mutual trust is well established, it is possible, with perfect agreement, to practice sex without barriers.

Mutual trust is born of long association, of a perfect adaptation of the one to the other. What the man embarks on, the woman agrees to. Sex without barriers means without restrictions, including special tastes [chitrarata], inversion of roles [purushāyitam], and other practices, which have been described in detail.

After which, loving quarrels [pranaya-kalaha] are described.

Lovers' quarrels

When sex without barriers is established, deriving from mutual trust, disagreements born of mutual affection are known as lovers' quarrels. The reasons for such quarrels are explained.

Just as sexuality without barriers is born of mutual trust, so too with lovers' quarrels.

27 As his mistress's affection increases, she can no longer bear hearing the names of his other wives, or allusions to them, or not very flattering remarks about her own family, or disagreeable words from him.

Her affection developing as her trust increases, she can no longer bear any allusion, whether light, medium, or excessive, nor that her lover should say anything disagreeable to her. This is the source of quarrels. She no longer endures the boy's faults, such as allusions to his other wives, or mentioning their qualities, or displeasing remarks about her own family, or his visits to his other women, his accepting betel from them, or making love with them, since it all implies his disaffection. As a result, she shows her exasperation.

28 So she of the beautiful eyebrows, in anger, weeping with rage, her head and body trembling, seizes the boy by his hair so as to hit him, then, throwing herself onto the ground, she tears off her necklaces and jewels.

When his other wives are mentioned, her fury is expressed in word and deed. Raising her eyebrows, the quarrel takes on the form of a succession of blazing words. In action, it becomes a fit of crying. In her affliction, she twists with pain, trembles, strikes herself, or else she seizes the boy by his hair to hit him. Tearing off her necklaces and jewels, she throws herself to the ground, but does not lie next to him.

29 What does the boy do, thus ill-treated? Lovingly, he throws himself at her feet to obtain her forgiveness and, assuaging her with loving words, he takes her in his arms and puts her back on the bed.

Never should he mock the girl lying on the ground.

30 Without replying to his words, which only increase her anger, she seizes him by the hair. Raising his face, she strikes with her feet at his arms, his face, his breast, and back, and repeats it two or three times. Then she goes as far as the door and, sitting on the theshold, weeps water-falls of tears.

Once she has hit him hard for his faults, she goes as far as the door and sits there, letting fall floods of tears.

31 Dattaka explains that, however furious she may be, she will never cross the threshold, because then she would be at fault. Drawing near, he does his best to pacify her with skillful words, seeking the right word to satisfy the lamenting one. When she has calmed down, the boy clasps the loving girl in his arms.

She remains on the threshold, neither outside, nor inside, because crossing the threshold would put her in the wrong.
Even in anger, she cannot go elsewhere. Dattaka is mentioned out of respect, since his opinion cannot be contradicted.
Approaching the girl with her eyes full of tears, tapping her foot, the boy gradually manages to put an end to her anger. Having calmed her with his skillful words, he throws himself at her feet and thus manages to give her pleasure. Then he takes her in his arms and, with affectionate words, calms her sorrow. Once she is satisfied, she shows her desire to make love.
Otherwise, if out of an excess of rage, she remains on the floor, the boy in turn gets angry and dreams of marrying a girl of a good family.

Dattaka explains that, however furious she may be with her lover, she may not cross the threshold. She hesitates at leaving the house, since the problem would be how to get in again. This is why he has to pacify her on the threshold. Even when she has calmed down, she seeks to soften her lover's heart with her moans, then, desirous of making love, she throws herself into his arms.

If she is a courtesan, who lives elsewhere, her behavior is as follows:

32 If, as a result of a quarrel, she retires to her own house, the boy goes to her seeking to persuade her.

How then does the boy manage it?

33 The lover sends his secretary [pīthamarda], a companion in debauch [vita], or his confidant [vidhūshaka] to the angry girl, in order to pacify her. Once she has calmed down, she returns with them to his house and takes her place.

If she persists in her anger, her lover sends messengers to bring her back. When they have calmed her fury, they come back with her. The lover then throws himself at her feet. Since it is forbidden for a man to throw himself at a woman's feet outside the house, she goes in with him, trampling his pride with her feet, and sits down in her lover's dwelling with the intention of making love throughout the night.

In this connection, a few quotations:

34 "In practicing the sixty-four positions described by the sons of Babhru with the best women, a man realizes his aim in life."

This is possible if he knows the sixty-four embraces. If he does not know them, even if he knows other treatises on eroticism, not only will he not be able to realize himself in this field, but he is certain to fail in the others.

If other treatises are all that he knows, he can only reach the approaches of perfection.

35 "Even if he is expert in all other kinds of knowledge, he who is ignorant of the sixty-four arts is not respected in the assembly of the wise, who are expert in the three kinds of wisdom."

Although a boy may be expert in the various sciences, if he is ignorant of the sixty-four arts, of embraces, kisses, and so on, how can he be respected in the assembly of the wise men who are expert in the means of attaining the three aims of life: ethics, material success, and eroticism?

36 "He who is expert in this subject, even if he is ignorant of the other forms of knowledge, holds pride of place in conversation at meetings of either men or women."

Since he shines in the learning that represents knowledge of erotic practices.

How can the sixty-four arts be an object of worship [pūjyatvat]?

37 Respected by cultivated people and venerated by the humble, adored in the world of prostitutes, who would not worship that which makes people happy?

This means of giving life, which is at the same time the fount of pleasure, deserves to be worshiped.

Experts in the three aims respect the sixty-four arts as a means of assuring women's faithfulness.

They are venerated by courtesans as a means of earning their living. Even those who are not very commendable, understanding their usefulness, respect them.

Who therefore would not venerate arts that are the object of veneration for all?

On this question, it is important to know the point of view not only of those who agree, but also of those who do not.

38 This art of loving so pleasing to women, whether young girls, wives, or holy women, which allows children to be begotten, has been described by sages in the sacred books.

Who would not venerate the teachings of the sages?

The sixty-four amorous practices, the source of pleasure, should be practiced by every married man, since they bring happiness and lead to success, cause motherhood, are pleasing to women, and have been described by the masters of knowledge, the achārya.

Those that know venerate these practices, especially women.

39   A man who is expert in the sixty-four arts is much appreciated by young girls, other men's wives, prostitutes, and by his own wife.

Amorous approaches are a bond in the couple's life. They are the visible or invisible cause of the opening out of the vagina (yoni), ejaculation (skhalana), and satifactory copulation (maithuna).

According to the texts:

The preludes to the act are essential; they involve touching, smelling, speaking, and looking.

In the act of love, from beginning to end, touching predominates, not only in the case of human beings, but also for insects and animals.

Among spiders, a mere contact produces violent enjoyment. Crabs are also sensitive to contact.

In their amorous games, elephants have a complete orgasm at first touch.

Cows, buffalos, deer, dogs obtain a lively orgasm by the reciprocal use of their tongue.

During the amorous preliminaries, women often resist certain contacts and their refusal must be respected, since for them touching is the first erotic experience.

Vātsyāyana attributes great importance to kissing during the preliminaries, as well as during the sexual act itself, since kissing is the best way of arousing desire in copulation. This is why it is practiced by all men and even by animals as a prelude to the act.

Between the lips and the bottom of the gums, there is a highly sensitive area, which, in a certain way, is similar to the one between the lips and interior of the vagina. At the tongue's contact, a powerful current of excitation appears in the lips and throat, strengthening sexual desire.

Each man and woman has a smell of his or her own. There is a connection between body odors and sexual excitation. At the moment of orgasm, man and woman give off a particular smell. Such smells excite and strengthen blood circulation and increase erotic ability. An erotic feeling sometimes occurs while listening or reading news of a defeat or the murder of a neighbor of one or other of the lovers, or if one sees or hears that a pretty girl of good family has given herself to an ugly person of low extraction. Faced with unexpected events of this kind, body odors are manifest more strongly. Experts say that substances that are pleasant to the taste and human smells are very similar. This is why women, in order to increase their natural odor, utilize ointments, essences, and flowers.

Scented substances may also be utilized to dissimulate or increase the odor of one's organs. Saffron, musk, amber, and sandalwood are all substances whose smell blends with that of the woman and encourages sexual excitation. This is why they are traditionally used by women. There is no doubt that body odors create an attractive atmosphere.

The sound of music, jokes, interesting stories all create a certain physical excitement. Rhythm forms part of our nature, which is why we find it pleasant and why it can be a source of excitation and enthusiasm. Singing and music are incitements to love. It is a matter of experience that music reaches the center of female sexuality.

Women find an emotional attraction in the sound of their lover's voice. Women can be hypnotized by a man's voice and be attracted by him. This is why Vātsyāyana attributes great importance to hearing.

In attraction through sight, beauty plays an essential role. It is by means of sight that lovers are attracted to each other. In the sexual life, sight is a weapon of primary importance. The poet Bihari speaks of the beauty of "clear, dark, or reddened eyes": ". . . clear, dark, or reddened, full of ambrosia or venom, each man should consider with prudence whether they are bringing him life or death." Everybody, young or old, seeks to mate and strive to carry it through. Every eye is thirsty for beauty and the desire it inspires is essential in the life of the couple.

If the birth of desire, the development of love, and even lovers' quarrels are studied from a psychological point of view, it can be perceived that both man and woman act out of egoism. According to the *Sāmkhya*, egoism is connected with the notion of self. It is in contact with things that one becomes conscious of self. Every action of the individual is based on egoism, interest, or eroticism.

"All love comes from egoistical desire." The ego is located in the very center of our faculties. It is the ego that unites the conscious and unconscious parts of our mental mechanism, which acts and perceives. According to the *Yoga Vāsishtha*, "Just as a great tree holds only by its roots, so self upholds the body. If the ego is erased, the body is destroyed, just as the tree falls if its roots are cut." The body is destroyed when the ego disappears.

Egoism (ahamkāra) directs a person's knowledge, feelings, and actions. The senses are the horses of this chariot that is our body. The mind controls the senses, as if they were horses. Both mind and intellect depend on self. The mind (manas) appears as the territory of the desires, and beyond, all the other things develop gradually.

The mental centers are where the sources of the senses are located—sight, hearing, smell—and where the various sensations are reflected.

The reflection of these sensations is the cause of our experience of the real (pratyaksha).

Vātsyāyana indicates the methods of embracing, lying together, and other actions after the act of love, which he terms the conclusion of the coition (ratāvasanika). In reality, if these things are looked at with discernment, one would rather prefer to make an end of it, and these acts thus constitute obstacles. After making love, a man's erotic power and desire are weakened. During the act itself, both man and woman feel an acute excitation, which increases their sexual power, but after reaching orgasm, they are both lacking in enthusiasm, and cool. Certain activities are useful in reawakening the ability to enjoy and strength to resist.

It is evident that the aim of these postcoital acts is not to make an end but to reawaken desire, and each desire seeks its conclusion. When desire is aroused, this excitation can awaken either favorable or hostile reactions. This kind of reaction is called feeling (bhāva) in the text of the *Kāma Shāstra*.

When this growing feeling culminates, it is termed excitation. It can be said that when feeling is awakened, ardor appears. If the feeling is connected with a memory, it can be pleasant or unpleasant. The unpleasant feeling is of conflict. Memory can engender love or rejection. Lovers' quarrels are a feature of even the best couples. Their pungency and the passions they arouse have often been described in poetry, drama, and histories of literature. Everywhere one hears stories of lovers' quarrels. Considering lovers' quarrels as characteristic of the behavior and sentiments of the couple, love quarrels are described in charming terms, full of devotion, in Vaishnava literature, the lives of the saints, Sufi texts, and on the subject of Rāma and Sītā, Krishna and Rādhā, Lakshmī and Vishnu, Prakriti and Purusha, the supreme being. Replying to Vishnu, the goddess Lakshmī praises lovers' quarrels:

"Against custom, you have spent the whole night in the chamber where I sleep. Tell me, Lord of the Gods! Is that respectable behavior, despite my desire to stay forever at your feet?"

The great poet Jayadeva, in the eighth and tenth chapters of the *Gītā Govinda*, gives a very lively and charming description of the lovers' quarrels of Rādhā and Krishna. In *Ujjvala Nīlamani*, Rūpagosvāmi describes lovers' quarrels. All the dramatic authors, Bhāsa, Kālidāsa, Harsha, etc., have illustrated lovers' quarrels in their plays and poems. The whole of Sanskrit literature is suffused with the *Kāma Sūtra*.

Here ends the Tenth Chapter
Preludes and Conclusions to the Games of Love
and the Second Part entitled Amorous Advances
of the Kāma Sūtra *by Vātsyāyana*

Part Three

Acquiring a Wife

[Kanyāsamprayukta]

Chapter One

FORMS OF MARRIAGE
[*Varana Samviḍhāna*]

A man who is trying to conquer a girl expert in the sixty-four arts does not arrange a meeting without first getting information. We will describe the preparations for organizing a meeting with a view to obtaining the girl.

There are eight forms of marriage, which are:

Brāhma, priestly
Prājāpatya, royal
Ārsha, ancestral
Daiva, astral
Gāndharva, of the heavenly musicians
Āsura, of the genies
Paishācha, of the incubus
Rākshasa, of the demons.

The first four conform to moral law. This is why the reasons for choosing are explained, as well as preferences for one kind of marriage rather than another.

1   For raising a family, the girl should be young; belong to

217

the same caste [savarnā]; without previous experience; observant of the sacred books as far as virtue and money are concerned; agreeable to the relationship; desirous of amorous relations and of having children.

She must be of the same caste as her husband, not have been intended for another in thought, word, or deed, which is what the codes call firsthand. She should, with discrimination, be respectful of the sacred books and follow their precepts.

By virtue [dharma] is meant devotion to duty and conjugal love. She should have a dowry [yautaka] and know how to look after a house, be obliging, not eat alone. She should deserve total trust.

2   One must seek a girl born of a noble family, with both father and mother alive, younger than the boy by three years at least, with a good character, rich, devoted to her family, fond of her kinsmen, having good relations with her neighbors, pubescent, obedient, pretty, well mannered, not banal, healthy in mind and body, without missing or too many teeth, nor decayed, her nails, ears, hair, eyes, and breasts without defect, without any constitutional disease.

3   According to Ghotakamukha, she should, by temperament, be interested in domestic affairs and not denigrate her own kind.

The grounds for choosing are of two kinds: from the human point of view or from the astrological point of view.

4   In order to form an opinion about her, people must be found who are connected with her father and mother and, for the purposes of this inquiry, the views of friends and persons who frequent the house should also be taken into account.

Her father and mother are questioned by friends sent by the suitor. For this purpose, kin of the suitor's family are utilized, but also occasionally friends of the boy's, so long as they have contacts with the father or mother.

The servants' views should not be overlooked.

The boy's father, mother, and other kin must strive to get information about the girl's qualities. Friends may also be used if they have some relationship with the two parties.

5 Thanks to their investigations, one is able to know of any apparent defects that could mitigate against an alliance. Qualities necessary in the investigators are that they should be of good family, enterprising, and capable of bringing their enterprise to a successful conclusion. They must take particular care to inquire into any illnesses the girl may have.

The boy's representatives will thus also learn whether she is toothless, or bald, or has other evident disfiguring defects, such as lameness, hunchback, and so on, which would make her useless. Her father will also make inquiries about the boy's family, whether he is serious-minded, does not drink, and contemplates a religious marriage. If he is satisfied, and if the girl agrees, her father, without constraining her, will decide on the marriage.

At the same time, the omens must be consulted.

6 Consulting the omens refers to the signs of destiny [daiva], omens deriving from the position of the planets, their conjunctions, influence, and meaning for the boy's future, foretelling a happy destiny for him.

The boy's representatives explain that his year of birth is favorable and an omen of peace, that the flight of crows and other birds is in the right direction and, that at the exact moment of his birth, the favorable planets were together in the same place, at dawn.

Considering the direction, moment, place, the omens, and their influence, and comparing them to his horoscope, they deduce future events, such as becoming commander in chief, or quartermaster general, or so on. Signs of good omen are considered as the basis of success. This concerns material success.

The investigators sent by the suitor, chatting like astrologers, describe the favorable signs of his birth and the position of the planets in his horoscope, announcing great material gains and the certainty of his future happiness.

7 Furthermore, they gratify the girl's mother by evoking

the misfortune that would be hers if she were to marry another.

Still under the pretext of pondering on the omens, should there be any question of marrying the girl to someone else, they describe the boy's prospects of becoming commander in chief of the army or of occupying some other important post, which are assured by the conjunction of the planets. They flatter the girl's mother, so that she will agree to the marriage.

8   It is only after having established the concordance of the signs of destiny, the moments, omens, and the position of the stars, that the girl may be given in marriage.

Destiny is the result of the good or evil actions performed in previous lives. It is called destiny because it is manifested in the planets and constellations. If the six elements do not correspond, what fool would act against the indications of destiny, after having consulted the omens according to the prescriptions of the sacred books? After watching the position of the planets on the ecliptic for the whole night, the girl's family gives her hand to the fiancé who wishes to marry her.
Having examined the compatibility of the planets and signs of the zodiac, avoiding the six and eight conjunctions, and having studied the moment and omens in the middle of the night, those who have decided to unite the boy and girl in marriage seize the moment when the conjunctions are favorable to tie the matrimonial bond.

9   Ghotakamukha says that this bond must not be established by chance, since it is not something personal, but involves the whole family and caste. If there are indications contrary to the marriage, the giving of the girl must not take place. According to Ghotakamukha's authority, it is forbidden.

It is not just the parents of the boy and girl who establish the bonds of matrimony: the agreement of the family and other kin is also necessary.

10   A girl who sleeps too much, weeps a lot, or goes out walking alone should be rejected.

If, since her earliest childhood, she has liked to stay in bed, if she has a sad humor and weeps, if she often leaves the house, he realizes that he must renounce her and, at the moment of marriage, he refuses the bond.

11 If she has a bad reputation, is secretive, breaks her word, is bald, has marks on her skin like a cow, has breasts that are too big, or yellowish hair; if she is round-shouldered, very thin, hairy, disobedient, immoral, has uterine hemorrhages [rakā], is agitated; if she has child-hood friends or a very young brother, and if her hands are always damp, she should be rejected.

One should renounce a girl who goes to friends' houses, who has brothers who are at least three years younger, who are still very small. It is said that "one should avoid a girl with young brothers aged between four and eight, because a girl who is attached to them will never settle down elsewhere."

12 In no case should one marry a girl who bears the name of a constellation, or a tree, or whose name ends with the letter "l" or "r."

13 Some opine that fortune comes when their hearts and glances are united, otherwise it would be better to renounce the marriage.

Although she is fond of her family, if her thoughts and looks express love, she will be a good wife for attaining the three aims of life, and is therefore a good choice. If such is not the case, then she is a bad choice, because she is marrying only out of obedience to her family. Without this concordance of heart and looks, one should reflect on the greater and lesser problems of life.

Examining the reasons for forming a bond with the girl's family, he says:

14 At the moment of being handed over, the girl is stand-ing sumptuously dressed, as are those who have come to fetch her, and is chatting with her longtime friends who have gathered together. For the marriage rite, she must strive to be amiable toward the people assembled and, in

the same way, during the rejoicings, show that she is satisfied with her marriage.

The girl should not appear apathetic on being handed over and must be attentive at the moment of marriage. She is surrounded by people of her own family. The previous day, she will have taken part in organizing the ceremonies, amusing herself with her friends over traveling in a palanquin, and so on, and during the marriage rite, etc., surrounded by her friends, she pretends to look at the others with astonishment.

When the girl is of an age to be married, her parents dress her in beautiful clothes. In the evening, with her friends, she amuses herself with adornments. She must be superbly dressed for the marriage rite and the rejoicing, since an object that is not carefully decorated does not attract buyers. This is why, if people do not see her in her beauty, they will not be drawn to her for the wedding.

The characteristics and conduct of the suitor will now be explained.

15 When he departs for the marriage, he must look well. Surrounded by his friends, he is welcomed by those present with respectful words.

Well dressed, having performed the ceremonies that bring good luck.

16 But the girl does not show herself to him.

Up to the moment of the handing-over, he must not see her. However, he is allowed to glimpse the girl with her jewels and luxurious garments, in one way or another.

17 Having consulted the omens, the date of the meeting is decided on, then that of the marriage ceremony.

*In the royal type of marriage [prājāpati] in which the girl is simply given by her father, the favorable moment must be determined. After examining the omens with the aid of her friends and family, the decision is taken and the moment for the marriage is established.
Beforehand, the suitor, together with a group of friends, dressed in white, goes to the altar of the funereal deities to pay his debt to his*

ancestors by offering the four offerings to the dead, prior to interrogating the omens.

18   When the suitor's party arrives, having taken a ritual bath, etc., they are told, "Everything will go well. Come back later," and they are not offered anything to eat.

The ceremony according to the royal rite of paternal gift will take place later and, on that day, the bath and other rites are not performed.

19   According to local convention or one's own desire, the Brāhma [priestly], prājāpati [royal], ārsha [ancestral], daiva [astral], or other kinds of marriage should be performed according to the rites laid down by the sacred books. Here ends the subject of marriage.

"With a joyful heart I give you my daughter, covered with jewels," is the priestly rite.

The royal rite consists of pronouncing the formula "May you together practice virtue."

For the ancestral rite, the marriage is performed with the gift of cows.

A vow is taken at the domestic altar in the astral rite.

The rites are described in the Grihya Sūtra, *or domestic rituals.*

There are twenty-three forms of marriage. The four forms of priestly, royal, ancestral, and astral marriage are the only ones that conform to the prescriptions of the holy books.

20   In this connection, it is said that one should play, marry, associate with one's equals, people of one's own circle. One should work with one's equals, not with people who are superior or inferior.

The best relationships are with people of the same religion, who have the same values. If they are different, it is more difficult to manage to have a good relationship.

21   A prudent man avoids marrying a woman of superior status, since he would lead the life of a servant.

Especially if she is rich and he poor.

22   The man who marries a woman poorer than himself behaves as a master, and the woman is like his slave. A circumspect man avoids this kind of marriage.

Such a marriage is not advised, inasmuch as habits are different as well as relations with other people.

23   When the married couple have the same pleasures, tastes, and amusements, they enhance each other's value. This kind of marriage is recommended.

They complement one another and make each other shine.

24   Whoever marries someone richer becomes inferior in the home. Neither should one marry anyone inferior. Such unions are condemned by the sages.

Vātsyāyana gives several counsels concerning the life of the couple and married life. He takes exception to free marriage and sexual behavior without barriers, as well as infidelity, and recommends marriage with a young girl according to the rules of the sacred books as contributing to the progress of decent people in virtue and riches.

Yājñavalkya, in his *Smriti*, gives the same advice: "When one speaks of the twice-born marrying shudra women, in my opinion there can be no true bond."

In the *Mitākshara* commentary, it says that marriage can have three aims: pleasure, procreation, or virtue. Of these, the one with progeny in view is of two kinds: one is permanent, while the other is love (kāmya). For a permanent relationship, the essential element is a girl of one's own caste. In a love marriage, by the very permanence of love, the principle of identical caste becomes secondary.

With regard to marriage, Manu says, "The one toward whom he has affection is the one he had best marry."

Under the influence of love, a Brahman may marry the girls of all four castes. A Kshatriya can marry girls from three castes, except a Brahman. A Vaishya those of two castes. Only the Shūdra must marry within his caste. Manu's opinion is, however, refuted by Yājñavalkya, who says, "As you were begotten, so must you in turn beget." The son must be his father's image. Yājñavalkya is firm on this point. Brahmans, Kshatriyas, and Vaishyas may not beget a son with a Shūdra woman.

In order to have progeny, if this is indispensable, a Brahman may marry a Kshatriya or a Vaishya, and a Kshatriya a Vaishya.

Vātsyāyana does not clarify the question of love marriage (kāmya vivāha). Although attaching great importance to the purity of the blood-line, he submits to the instructions of the Scriptures and the ethical regulations concerning marriage.

In such a case, the satisfying of erotic desire is in contradiction with ethical concepts. This is why prudence is required in establishing a marriage. One must assure that the girl belongs to one's own caste, that she is not without guarantors and that, as far back as one can go, among her ancestors there can have been no deceit as to their belonging to the race. Vātsyāyana requires that, over and above belonging to the same social group (jāti), there can be no shadow of doubt that, since her earliest childhood, her virginity cannot be questioned either in word, in thought, or deed. Yājñavalkya, too, declares, "The boy who is still a virgin must marry a woman who has not been deflowered, who is beautiful, younger than he, and has a family relationship allowing them to take part in the same funerary rites."

"A girl who has not had any relation with another man, who is beautiful to see and hear, who is not consanguineous (of the same gotra), is without defect as to her status and physical aspect, is the one whom one should marry."

It is also required, however, that the young suitor himself be still chaste, since otherwise he must look for a woman like himself. This is what Yājñavalkya clearly appears to be saying.

Vātsyāyana, having examined the sacred texts concerning ethics and society, from the points of view of psychology and physiology, is very strict in all matters concerning the marriage bond.

From the point of view of the *Dharma Shāstra*, it is necessary for the girl to be of the same caste, but not consanguineous, and from the social point of view that her parents are alive and that she has good family relations. He examines the girl's qualities and character. From the physical point of view, she must be without blemish or disease.

So that girls can find a suitable husband, Vātsyāyana recommends that they should be made to go out well clothed and ornamented, that they should go to frequented places, in order that, seduced by their beauty, men should seek to marry them. Vātsyāyana explains that, just as buyers in the bazaars will not purchase an object without seeing it, a girl's marriage can only be accomplished if she has been seen and appreciated.

He thus refers to the customs of his own time. It appears that at that time, the practice of svayamvara, whereby the girl would choose from among her suitors, no longer existed. In the Vedic period, there were very few rules concerning marriage. According to the *Rig Veda*, there were numerous girls who, wishing to get married, invited the boys and married them. Beautiful and prosperous girls would themselves choose a husband from the crowd of suitors.

Before marrying a girl, Vātsyāyana recommends examining her nails, teeth, ears, hair, and breasts, which should not be too small nor too large, nor should they be lacking, and verifying that she has no disease.

According to Manu, "one should marry a girl whose ancestors are known for ten generations, whose character and virtue are acknowledged, while one should avoid those who have contagious diseases or belong to families of very high rank."

According to the commentary on the *Yājñavalkya Smriti*, one should avoid a girl some of whose family members are without a profession, without male children, without religion, hairy, suffer from hemorrhoids, phthisis, bad digestion, epilepsy, white leprosy, or leprosy.

Vātsyāyana considers the life of the married couple as the best of lives when cohabitation is continuous. To avoid sexual excesses or unfaithfulness, the girl must be married according to the prescribed rules, it being within the family context that virtue and riches develop.

At that time, it appears that young people gathered together and played all sorts of games. It is then that the ties of love are established and marriage is decided on. However, Vātsyāyana's aim seems to be merely to show off the girl's beauty and attractions, carefully bedecked to attract proposals.

Sometimes the proposal was addressed to the girl's father and, if the family data did not correspond, the father's refusal could drive the girl to despair. Vātsyāyana recommends that as soon as the girl has been seen, her marriage should be arranged without delay. The family had to be consulted and no final answer could be given before examining the suitor's family status. Having obtained information about the boy's family, character, and intelligence, the relations between his parents, his merits, knowledge, and the state of his fortune, the marriage would then be decided on.

According to the *Nīti Shāstra*, the Rules of Behavior, "the girl's hand must be given after having checked seven qualities of the suitor, concerning his family, character, health, knowledge, fortune, antecedents, and age."

According to Ashvalāyana, during the night before the first marriage rite, eight balls (pinda) must be prepared, using earth taken from a stable (goshālā), an anthill (valmīka), a fireplace (dyūtasthāna), the bank of a pond, the fields (kshetra), a crossroads (chatushpatha), and from the cremation ground (shmashāna). The girl is then asked to touch one of these balls. If she touches the one made of stable earth, it is a sign of riches; the anthill ball signifies an abundance of cattle; the fireplace ball, participation in the rites (yajña, agnihotra, etc.); the ball made from earth from the bottom of the pond, wisdom and intelligence; the one from the bank, sickness; the one from the crossroads, unfaithfulness; and the one from the cemetery, widowhood.

Once the marriage has been decided on, the rite must be chosen, in accordance with local custom.

The codes of ethics mention eight forms of marriage:

Priestly (Brāhma): the girl, covered with jewels, is given with nothing received in return.

Royal (prājāpatya): the girl is given by her father, without any counterpart.

Ancestral (ārsha): the girl is exchanged for two bulls.

Astral (daiva): the girl is given to the officiating priest during a yajña (sacrifice).

Of the heavenly musicians (gāndharva): love marriage without ceremony or the agreement of the families.

Of the genies (āsura): the girl is bought from her parents.

Of the incubus (paishācha): the girl is kidnapped without her consent.

Of the demons (rākshasa): the girl is taken as booty, after her family has been destroyed in a war.

The first four are the only ones allowed by the holy books. The other four are forbidden, because they are against the law, are barbarous, impulsive, and antisocial, breaking the barriers of ethics and social order. According to Yājñavalkya, in priestly marriage, the suitor, already chosen, is summoned and the girl, covered with jewels as far as possible, is handed over to him.

According to the *Vivāha Paddhati* (the marriage ritual), the son of the future wife must have twenty paternal and maternal ancestors of noble lineage, and the girl must not have known other men.

In royal marriage (prājāpatya), the father gives his daughter, saying "Both of you must observe morals." For this kind of marriage, there must be proof of six generations on both sides.

In astral marriage, the girl is given to the priest (ritvik) who has performed a yajña, or ritual sacrifice, while in ancestral marriage, she is given in exchange for two bulls.

Friendship and love must be practiced between equals, neither with superiors nor with inferiors.

End of the First Chapter
Forms of Marriage
of the Third Part entitled Acquiring a Wife

Chapter Two

HOW TO RELAX
THE GIRL
[Kanyā Viɟrambhana]

Although the girl has been obtained, she must not be utilized since she is still fearful. An attempt must be made to make her relax. After the marriage ceremony, the way of behaving to bring bliss is as follows.

1   For three days, they must sleep on the ground chastely, side by side, without eating spicy or salty food.

For a whole week, she must go and bathe in the river, accompanied by music, she must attend parties elegantly dressed, see her parents and friends and perform the domestic rites. This is the rule for every caste.

Once they are married and she has come to live in his house, making love is forbidden for three nights. They must not partake of spicy food, but honey, milk, and clarified butter. They must not make love on the morning after the third night, since copulation by day is a grave fault. During the following weeks as during the first three days, she busies herself with household tasks. She takes her meals with him, elegantly dressed, and attends displays of dancing and other kinds of

229

entertainment. She performs the rites of worshiping the gods, the pujah, with offerings of perfume and flowers. Thus the first ten days are spent.

It is said, "Once married, installed in her husband's home, the girl must wait for the tenth day after her menses." She lives with him in his house, but she can also go back to her family.

How does he manage to relax the girl?

2   During the night, when they are alone, they begin to behave in a loving manner.

The girl may be of two kinds, affectionate or shy. In the first case, it is merely a matter of the preliminaries to copulation. In the other case, the girl is embarrassed out of fear and modesty. At night, she is frightened, removed from her dear ones, and would like to go back to her parents. Her modesty must therefore be overcome in a very gentle manner, avoiding all brutality of word or contact.

In what way must one go about it?

3   According to the Bābhravyas, if, during the first three nights, the girl sees the boy lying like a corpse, without talking to her, she may imagine that he is homosexual, belonging to the third nature.

Seeing him silent and motionless, making no attempt, like a village idiot, the girl says to herself, "How stupid I am. He is either homosexual or impotent." She considers his lack of initiative an insult. For this reason, the said prohibitions must be questioned.

4   For Vātsyāyana, amorous games are necessary in order to relax the girl, without, however, deflowering her.

No blame is attached to the attempt. Methods must be used that will relax her, without, however, breaking the vow of chastity since, even if it appears appropriate, breaking a vow is contrary to virtuous conduct.

5   He must show initiative, but without any violence.

Why?

6   A woman is like a flower. She must be treated gently, until she feels secure. If she is violently assaulted, she becomes hostile to any sign of affection. One must therefore strive to pacify her.

All contacts and caresses must be very gentle. The first approaches must all be made with delicacy.

If at any time an approach is too brutal, the woman develops a hostile attitude to the sexual act.

He explains how to take advantage of every opportunity to make progress by contact.

7   Pressing against her, as soon as he feels the possibility, he plucks up courage.

In order to draw near to her when he feels she is well disposed, he begins to talk to her amusingly, like one of her friends. With chatter and games, he manages to conquer her.

Even if she tries to stiffen her limbs, he must seize the chance to touch them.

When she is relaxed, he attempts a first embrace.

8   Gently, he puts his arms around her, but not for too long.

He must not be insistent, since she will allow it for a moment, but will then start to resist.

9   He must only tackle the upper part of the body, so as not to upset her.

He must first busy himself with the parts of the body above the navel, since that is all she can bear. She will resist if the lower part of her body is touched.

10   If he already knows the girl, these approaches can be made in full lamplight, but if he has not known her previously, he must act in the dark.

Light is appropriate for a girl who has come joyously into the house, but for one who has married without having had any relation since her childhood and is frightened and modest, darkness is better.

11 After caressing her breasts, he offers her betel, which he keeps in his mouth. If she refuses, he assuages her with words, vows, and protestations and, falling at her feet, clasps them to him. An embarrassed woman, even if she is angry, will not let him fall at her feet. This is true in all cases.

He takes the betel from his mouth to put it into hers, taking the place of an affectionate kiss. If she refuses, despite his efforts, falling at her feet is the final argument, which always works with all women.

12 Then, after this gift, very gently, after a slight struggle, he takes her lips.

If she will not let herself be touched in a gentle manner, he must do it with passion, touching her without constraint. She will protest confusedly, too shy to speak.

13 After which, they talk openly.

He convinces her to agree to a kiss.
If the girl is satisfied by the kiss, he can start talking with her. *These are the methods:*

14 To make her talk, he asks her questions in a few words, pretending not to know the answer.

15 If he obtains no reply, without getting cross, he gently repeats his questions.

16 If she continues to give no answer, he must not insist.

17 According to Ghotakamukha, a girl who finds herself in a man's possession will in all cases refuse to speak. She will not pronounce a single word or syllable.

It is because he represents the god Eros [Manmatha] that she is paralyzed by her modesty.
So how can one manage to get to talk to the girl?

18 If one insists, the only reply will be a shaking of the

head. If one argues with her, she will not even nod her head.

Without speaking, she will move her head. If she is asked whether she understands, she will move her head up and down to mean yes. In order to say no, she puts her head slantwise so as not to be insolent. If there is an argument, she will lower her head, but if one insists and she is angry, she will not move her head.

In the case of an argument, she must be persuaded with loving words.

19 Do you want me or not? Do you like me or not? He must insist on such questions for some time, until she expresses her agreement by moving her head, or else refuses.

Such questions evoking the past begin to worry her. If he is an old acquaintance, this should be done with a slight insolence. However, if she is embarrassed by the boy's insolence, what happens? Put under pressure in such a way, she hesitates between two courses of action and ends up by surrendering, either signaling yes with her head, or else, considering the boy's intentions vague and needing some explanation, she refuses. Caught by anger, she contradicts him: "No, I don't like you. I don't desire you."

If he persists long enough, she ends up by accepting. Otherwise, she sends him away, in anger.

If they knew each other before, to initiate a conversation presents no problem.

20 All is well if both are relaxed, like friends. But if not, how can they be reconciled?

If she does not lower her head as a sign of acceptance, he starts laughing. With a flood of words, he insults her and argues with her. The silent object of his scorn, she mutters silently to herself. Although she is formulating replies to the boy's words, she remains silent. "You can insist in vain, I will not speak," she says to herself. When he starts laughing, however, she blinks, and a conversation is established.

If there has been no previous friendship between them, he asks himself, "Maybe she doesn't like me." He must therefore examine her behavior, and if he laughingly reports her friends' words, she lowers her head in embarrassment. He says, "This is what your girlfriends say: they do nothing but repeat that you were very much in love and that they had to fight against you." "Is that really what my friends say?" she will wonder. Now that the wedding has taken place, any question of mutual attraction is merely senseless and stupid chit-chat. When the boy starts laughing, she shows that she understands. By blinking and by her expression, she lets him understand that she likes him very much.

He begins talking by quoting a girlfriend who is favorable to him and is trusted by both. After listening to his words, she lowers her head and starts laughing, worried over the gossip of her girlfriend, who is a chatterbox. She contradicts what her friend said, since she had told her fiancé lies as a kind of joke, pretending that she was like this or that.

"Why don't you contradict her?" he asks.

Both husband and girlfriend had agreed to make the girl say, "If you tease me, I won't answer!"; and smilingly she looks sideways at her husband.

This is a good method for establishing a first conversation between husband and wife.

21   Having attempted a rapprochement, he stays silently and imploringly close to her. He offers her betel, ointments, garlands of flowers, until she is obliged to reply.

Having become acquainted through caresses, sucking betel, and talking, the boy courts his wife until she calms down and is forced to answer.

22   Then, delicately, he touches the tip of her breasts.

23   "If you wish to embrace me, I shall not stop you." Having established that, he embraces her and waits no longer to slide his hand further. Gradually, he gets excited and goes further and further, without fearing any opposition.

Once he has been able to touch her, he embraces her. He proceeds to the area around the navel, then, gradually, goes further, but does not seek intercourse immediately. He starts biting and scratching her legs and, if she resists his advances, he threatens her.

If the woman tries to stop him, the boy says, "I am not going to stop." He embraces his wife and slides his hand below her navel. He then raises her and attempts to take her on his knees and, gradually, proceeds with his enterprise. If the woman refuses, he must frighten her a little.

How?

24 "Just now I will mark your lip with my teeth and shall leave the mark of my nails below your breasts. What I do, you will pretend that a girlfriend did to you previously. What else will you say to them?" Arguing like children, they take to the game very quickly.

25 On the second and third night, when she is more relaxed, he touches her sex with his hand.

He starts to let his hand wander over her thighs and pubis and between her legs.

26 And everywhere he leaves a kiss.

Kissing her on her forehead, eyes, and elsewhere, she becomes more malleable and he can undertake everything.
How does he arouse her with his hand?

27 Resting his hand at the top of her legs and caressing her, he reaches the thigh joint. If she protests, he scolds her and calms her down.

First, he passes his hand over the front of her body, going as far as the top of the thigh, then caressing her thigh joint. He calms her, smothering her with kisses and, sliding his hand between her thighs, strokes her secret parts.

28 Without untying her girdle, he loosens the part of the garment that passes between the legs, turning it back and uncovering the base of the thigh. If she does not protest, he takes his pleasure in sliding his instrument [yantra] over it, without, however, breaking her chastity, since it is not the right moment.

He begins by touching her sex, without aiming at fulfillment, since he is bound by his vow for three days. He takes a foretaste of his pleasure on the fourth day. Tormented with desire, he finishes by having an orgasm.

Having untied her garment, he lets his hand wander over her thigh joint. He must do all this to show his love for the girl and to gain her trust, without deflowering her before the time established in a moment of uncontrolled lust.

29   The better to educate her, he shows his passion. He reminds her of pleasant moments in the past, which help to establish favorable feelings. He speaks of the permanence of the true couple. Gradually, after a while, the feelings of the hostile girl begin to awaken. This is the correct way to relax the girl.

Her education must include the sixty-four arts. He shows his passion by his gestures. He recalls to her mind memories of the past and plans for the future. "What I promised you, I will carry out." He seeks to drive away the fears of his wife, who remains cold. In time, the impulses of youth are aroused in the girl who seemed so lacking in feeling. For this, time is necessary: it will not be achieved all at once.

During the first three nights after the wedding, he must teach her the art of loving (kāma kalā). He must promise her, "I have given you my word. You must not be afraid that I will take other wives."

30   In this connection, a quotation:

Having thus pleased the girl with subjects suited to her mind and made himself agreeable, she becomes entirely relaxed.

31   One must not go too far in the direction of the weft or woof. Success with girls is obtained by moderation.

What happens when the girl is relaxed?

32   The girl's state of mind changes as a result of the marks of love. When the girl is relaxed, she gives him signs of affection.

Due to the means employed, the girl allows her womanly nature to appear. During the first encounter, everything must be done with this aim in view. The result is that she becomes amorous.

If one manages to arouse a feeling of love in the young bride, having shown respect and inspired trust in her, one can make oneself loved.

33 If, out of excessive modesty, he does not touch the girl, she, seeing his lack of initiative, will consider him an animal.

Should he remain silent throughout the three nights, she will tend to be hostile to him.

34 If, on the contrary, he suddenly attacks the inexperienced girl, he will only manage to arouse fear and disgust, and she will become hostile to him.

35 A woman who has not received any signs of love is wounded and becomes hostile, an enemy of men. She will either reject them all, or else will go with another.

According to the *Grihya Sūtra*, the marriage must be consummated after twelve, six, or three nights. Some ancient authors say they should wait one year, twelve days, six days, or three days. If consummation does not take place, the girl cannot be considered married, since the sexual act is a part of the rite.

Having embraced his wife, the boy puts a betel nut in his mouth in order to place it in his wife's. If she accepts, it means she accepts his kisses.

Once she has accepted the kiss, he must tell her suggestive stories. Should she not react, he must manage to make her laugh by grimaces, or else search his memory for tales that the girl cannot help protesting about. If she remains deaf and dumb, he must find some intermediary to speak with her.

When they have got to know each other, after embraces, kisses, betel and talking, he must ask for something to drink. Without saying a word, the girl smilingly keeps the cup to herself. When she leans forward to drink, her husband strokes her breasts, letting his hands slide gradually down as far as her navel.

This must all be done during their first encounter on the first night. On the second and third nights, he must caress the girl's whole body, slipping his hand between her thighs. In order not to upset her, he must gently remove his hand from time to time, gradually attaining the sanctuary of Eros. If she allows him to do it, he may untie her garment and, having removed it, take the girl on his knees, without, however, attempting intercourse. They must stay chaste until the third day, and only then may they have their first intercourse. He may only take her when she has fully developed her trust in him, so that her fear will dissolve into pleasure.

In describing the intercourse of Nala and Damayantī, the poet Harsha follows the rules set by Vātsyāyana.

When Nala wants to make love with her, Damayantī refuses. In order to reason with her, he explains to her why she is upset. Not having had any previous experience of this kind, her sweat begins to run. She is afraid, and starts trembling. But when Nala inserts his member into her sanctuary of Eros, Damayantī discovers sensual pleasure unknown before. She realizes that it is a source of wonderful pleasure and they remain for a long time clasped in each other's arms.

After the wedding night, the husband must teach the girl all the techniques of the art of loving and show her unfailing affection. His conduct, treatment of her, and way of talking to her must be such that in the future, the girl's heart knows no fear, doubt, or reproach. She must feel assured that her husband will never leave her for the attractions of another woman. It is a husband's duty to lead his wife along the path of pleasure, without encountering any obstacles, so that their amorous games enjoy increasing success.

It is evident from Vātsyāyana's text that, in order to relax the girl, the boy should know female psychology. Without understanding a woman's feelings, marriage and married life can only be a failure.

End of the Second Chapter
How to Relax the Girl
of the Third Part entitled Acquiring a Wife

Chapter Three

WAYS OF OBTAINING THE GIRL

[*Bālā upakramanā*]

The ways of organizing marriage as well as the ways to relax the girl have been explained above. If the boy cannot obtain the girl he loves, there are four forms of marriage, beginning with mutual agreement, called gāndharva.

If marriage in its accepted forms cannot be carried out, there are four other kinds of marriage. If the girl cannot be obtained by one of the forms of marriage contemplated previously, she must be secured by one of the following four kinds of marriage: either by the form of mutual agreement (gāndharva), or one of the other three. This means that if the girl's parents, despite her agreement, refuse to give her away, marriage will take the form of flight and mutual agreement (gāndharva), by kidnapping (paishācha), or by capture (rākshasa).

1 Honest but poor, of an average but ignorant family, or because he is merely a rich neighbor, he cannot obtain her due to the opposition of her father, mother, and brothers, on whom she depends, but since he has desired her from childhood, he must find a way of marrying her despite everything.

239

Notwithstanding his merits, the boy cannot obtain the girl due to lack of money, because his family is poor, or else, even if he is moderately prosperous in appearance and character and is of good family, because he lacks education. He may also be a neighbor of good standing, who cannot obtain her due to disputes about property boundaries, or for reasons of pride or money, or else because he is dependent on his parents and brothers and is without any means of his own, or because he has frequented the house since childhood and is considered a youngster and not to be taken seriously.

Also, if he is thought to be impotent or homosexual (janakhāpana), it is not deemed desirable to give him a girl of a good and virtuous family.

If he cannot marry her, what must he do?

2   Having been in love with her since his childhood, it is up to him to contrive something.

If she has also loved him since childhood, they will decide to marry according to the gāndharva formula, meaning marriage by mutual agreement, as being the only way of obtaining the girl he desires.

In countries where such arrangements are accepted, one of the procedures is as follows:

3   A boy who has been separated from his paternal or maternal family since childhood and obliged to live with a maternal uncle, according to southern custom, finds himself in a humiliating position. In the hope of acquiring riches, he strives to seduce his uncle's daughter, even if she has already been promised to another.

Being without resources, he contrives to go and live with his rich maternal uncle, in the hope of marrying his daughter, as is the custom in the south, but, being an orphan, he risks a refusal. Whether or not she is promised to another, he manages to seduce her.

4   Or else he seeks to seduce another girl outside the family.

If he cannot have his uncle's daughter, he will look for another outside the family group. He strives to win the girl's love and organize an elopement with her to his own country or another.

So long as she is not of his uncle's or his own gotra (genetic group), he can marry any girl of his caste according to the gāndharva rite, which consists of an elopement and a declaration of mutual love.

5 According to Ghotakamukha, "If they have had a relationship of true affection since their earliest years, to take possession of her is legitimate."

If they have known each other since childhood, whether virtuously or not, an agreement to go away with her, with a view to amorous relations, is allowable. This is one of the situations contemplated by ethical texts. Marriage by mutual agreement (gāndharva) is morally acceptable. It belongs to the four forms of legitimate marriage previously mentioned.

Elopement may be of two kinds, according to whether it is caused by the boy or the girl, as a conclusion to a previously established affection.

6 Since their childhood, they had talked together about flowers, ways of making garlands, housework, ways of making money, the reasons for being faithful. They described to one another the people they knew.

Since childhood, they had gathered flowers together to make garlands, and built toy houses of wood or mud, imitating dishes of rice with sand, and speaking of the people that one or the other knew. As children or adolescents, they played together according to their fantasies. They used to build paper houses, make rag dolls, make imitation food with mud and dust and other games proper to their age, whether invented or learned.

7 They would play together at the game of pulling strings, their hands overlapping, at hiding dice in their fist, clinging to the middle finger, or at the six pebble game, as well as others that they played at home with their chums or servants.

8 They would play at finding an object blindfolded, at the saltseller, at turning their hands around forward, at finding a coin in a stock of corn, at the game of the blindman and the thief, and other village games.

Vātsyāyana gives this advice to a boy in love: if the boy's family status is lower than the girl's, if he is not as rich, or belongs to another social group (vijāti), or if he is a neighbor or has ties of friendship with her family, he must avoid running away with the girl. That being said, if he is in love with a girl and they have been friends since childhood, and, notwithstanding everything, he wants to make her his wife, it is advisable for them to elope.

Under such conditions, the master describes local customs concerning the relationships of love and friendship. He suggests that, if the boy has neither father nor mother and lives with his maternal uncle, he must strive to establish amorous relations with the latter's daughter in order to marry her, since in the countries of the south, and Mahārāshtra in particular, marriage with one's uncle's daughter is permissible. From Vātsyāyana's sayings, it is clear that love marriages are a very ancient custom in India. The books of ethics, or Smriti, mention marriage by flight (gāndharva), by gift (daiva), by capture (paishācha) and as booty of war (rākshasa). This opinion is confirmed herein.

In this chapter, the quotation from Ghotakamukha, who is one of the authorities on the subject, does not consider the mutual attraction of boy and girl since childhood to be immoral, and furthermore, the gāndharva, paishācha, rākshasa, and āsura forms of marriage are accepted as well as approved by the texts on ethics. This, however, poses a question.

If children playing together find the awakening of feelings of love, how can they understand that for a certain time they could be friends but that later on, marriage would be denied them? This seems contradictory. We know that the notion of intercourse exists among children, and that it is there since birth, without their even being aware of it. Boys and girls play sexual games. The question is at what moment does the idea evolve that they will marry.

Children's games leading to a mutual attraction between boys and girls, as described, form part of a long tradition. Gathering flowers, making garlands, building toy houses: such games are encountered in every country. Pulling a string, placing hands one over the other, hiding something in one's hand, catching hold of a finger, and the six pebble game are, however, not innocent pastimes. It is strange that this tradition has continued since Vātsyāyana's time, since such games can be seen in villages even today.

Thus, the girl who plays hand games with boys will end up by being kidnapped. The game in which an object is hidden in the fist is still played in every village. Tamarind fruit pips or such tokens are hidden thus, and the one asks the other, "Even or odd?" The loser has to pay. In the game of the middle finger, the winner's skill is put to the test.

9 Those who gain each other's trust end up by becoming attached to one another, out of habit.

Having continual trust, they also become fond of one another. Furthermore, she lets herself be masturbated [matkārya] by the daughter of the boy's nurse, creating a closeness. How could she fall in love with someone else?

The boy behaves like an intimate female friend of the girl with whom he is in love. Their love and closeness can only grow stronger.

10 The daughter of the boy's nurse can also serve to win the girl's affection and friendship. Once she has taken her for a friend, if she sees that the girl has doubts about the boy's qualities, she will remove them and make her well disposed and fearless.

If the nurse's daughter knows how to make herself agreeable, she can soothe the worries of the beloved. She examines the girl's state of mind and lets her know that the boy is in love with her. She eliminates any worries due to shyness and modesty. She strives to put the girl into a favorable frame of mind, so that the boy's initiatives will find her with no fear. In stroking the girl's clitoris without the boy's knowledge, she prepares her for sexual games.

The nurse's daughter must show she is fond of the girl's doll. Once the girl is in her power and she has understood her state of mind, the nurse's daughter will persuade her to join her lover.

11 Even if the girl does not realize her attraction for him, or his qualities, the nurse's daughter will make known to her the violence of his feelings and will strive to make her fall in love.

If the girl does not realize that the boy desires her, the nurse's daughter [dhātreyikā] will show the boy's qualities to his best advantage and try to make her fall in love with him.

12   Wherever she discerns curiosity, she manages to seize the opportunity.

Whenever she sees a chance, the nurse's daughter worms her way in, makes herself understood and is successful.

When the nurse's daughter sees that the girl has doubts, she incites her curiosity about the boy.

13   The boy sends her the playthings mentioned previously, or others that are new and rare, and unknown to the girl.

If his beloved is very young, he buys playthings and gives them to her. Such toys must be expensive and difficult to obtain, so that she has never seen anything like them.

14   He gives her balls decorated with changing colors, and dolls made of cloth, wood, horn, or ivory, wax, or porcelain.

In order to amuse his beloved, the lover must show her balls covered with colored stripes which, after a moment, change color, or else he brings her miniature characters made of various materials.

15   He teaches her to cook rice and other things according to recipe, since this is the principal science of women.

16   When he finds the opportunity, either openly or secretly, he gives his girlfriend a pair of wooden sheep, a wooden nanny goat and billy goat and, symbolically, a pair of earthenware or bamboo cattle, as well as images of the gods and little shrines, or cages with china parrots, since they represent the bird of Eros. Also amusingly shaped water vessels, made with pieces of conch, oyster shells, clay, wood, or stone, or a small doll representing a musician playing a miniature vīnā, shells containing offerings, powdered carbon (rājāvarta) for drawing, and betel made with leaves with instructions for use. According to his means, he must offer whatever may be pleasing to her, giving her whatever shines. If he deems that it may serve his purpose, he offers her everything that can please her.

For what purpose?

17   Seeing that she is well disposed toward him, he speaks of a meeting.

Seeing she is happy, he hesitates no longer. In order to prevent her looking elsewhere, he speaks of their marriage.
When the girl has accepted secret and hidden meetings, he can speak to her of other things.

18   If the gifts he has made secretly are discovered, afraid of her parents, she pretends that they are intended for someone else.

If her parents angrily demand where the gifts come from, she says she accepted them because someone else wanted them.

19   He ponders on tales that might inspire passion. He quotes famous accounts to her, which interest and seduce her.

He charms her mind with romantic stories, such as the tale of Princess Shakuntalā and others.

20   If she likes to be astonished, he surprises her with conjuring tricks. If she is interested in the arts, he shows his skill, and if she loves music, he sings songs that enchant her ear.
On the eighth day of the moon of the month of Ashvin (May), and other festivals of the moon, on days of pilgrimage, eclipses, on returning from a journey, when she is in grief, or the day on which her ears are pierced, he offers her clothes and jewels, being careful not to put her in the wrong.

He must do it without anyone knowing.

21   Once she has assured him, through the offices of the nurse's daughter, that she does not wish to know any other man, and that she is in love with him, he can teach her the sixty-four kinds of amorous games.

22   Having received this message and in order to put it
into practice, he demonstrates to her his skills as a lover.

23   He shows himself to her without his belly garment
and seeks to reveal his feelings, gauging her expression at
the sight of the shape of his penis.

Why does he show himself unclothed [anupahata]?

24   Since her childhood, the girl has constantly seen the
men of her family, but without ever having erotic relations
with them. She now becomes enamored of the first man
who desires her.

*She desires the boys she sees often, but her modesty prevents her
from showing it.*
It is clear that the girl desires the boys of her neighborhood or of
her own family, but even if she desires them, she may not have relations
with them.
How does she show her feelings at seeing him undressed?

25   One must know how to interpret the signs and apparent manifestations of her feelings.

*Her reactions are indicated by her facial expression and appear-
ance. These should therefore be taken further into account.*

26   When he faces her, she does not look at him. When he
looks at her, she shows embarrassment. She lets him catch
a glimpse of some parts of her pretty limbs and watches to
see whether the boy is amorously attentive and is not looking elsewhere.

*She lowers her head out of modesty. She shows her breasts and
armpits, while undoing her clothes.*
When in front of her beloved, out of modesty, a young girl does
not look at him but, turning her head, looks at him out of the corner
of her eye. In one way or another, she will let the beauty of her body
be seen and will note whether the boy seems attracted by her or whether
he is inattentive and looks elsewhere.

27   When questioned, she replies with a half-smile, in a

low voice, with indistinct words, while lowering her head.
If she is near him, she takes pleasure in staying there for
a long moment. If he is far off, with the idea of "he must
look at me," she speaks with those close to her without
looking at them and does not leave the place.

*If the boy makes a proposal, she shows her agreement with a smile
and by her expression and speaks in a shy manner.*

28   If he looks at her for an instant, she laughs and starts
chatting so that he will not go away. Sitting on the young
man's knees, she puts her arms around him and embraces
him. She gets a maidservant to adjust the marks on her
brow. She becomes vivacious with those next to her.

*Whenever he looks in her direction, she laughs and winks at him.
If her girlfriends annoy her, she repulses them. Curled up on the knees
of the boy [bālaka], who caresses her and kisses her deeply, making a
maidservant redo the red marks on her forehead, she looks at her hero
[nāyaka]. Surrounded by her relations, she arranges her hair, moving
her limbs to show them off.*

29   She questions his friends and sets great store by their
assertions. She confides in the servants with whom she
plays and chats. She evaluates her suitor according to what
they say. She listens attentively to the gossip of her servants and others.

*She lets her suitor's friends see her feelings and talks a lot. She
seeks to establish his character through what his servants have to say.*
The beloved confides in her lover's friends. She respects their
opinions. She behaves affectionately with his servants and plays cards
and other games with them and gives orders authoritatively to the boy's
servants. And if they speak about him, she listens carefully.

30   Going to the boy's house, she plays dice with him, and
speaks of their desire to form a couple. She avoids showing
herself without being well adorned. If he asks her to wear
ear or hand ornaments or other jewels, she borrows them
from a girlfriend. She always wears the ones he has given
her. Any mention of another suitor displeases her, and she

refuses the company of those who want to claim her hand.

Chaperoned by her nurse, she goes to his house. She needs such cover to go outdoors. She likes playing with the boy and stays with him a long time, flattered by his compliments. Out of modesty, she makes him transmit his presents through a girlfriend. She clasps him in long embraces and refuses to frequent people sent by another party.

Informed by a maidservant, the boy goes to the dwelling of his beloved. Seconded by the maidservant, they play games and talk together. She is always elegantly dressed. If he asks her to wear earrings, a jewel, or a necklace, she immediately gets a girlfriend to lend them to her. She always wears the jewels he has offered her. Any mention of other boys displeases her, and she refuses to see those who speak of them.

Here are two quotations to terminate this second subject dealt with:

31   "Having interpreted the state of her feelings from spontaneous signs, he must contemplate the ways of marrying the girl."

Stimulated by all these signs and with his sex [linga] changing its state, the boy, a prey of his passion, commences amorous games [samprayoga], having decided to marry her in the gāndharva fashion, by simple mutual agreement, in order to end in complete copulation.

There are three kinds of girl: the young girl [bālā], the adolescent [tarunī], and the young woman [praudā], who are respectively the three kinds of mistress.

32   The young girl plays children's games; the adolescent is interested in the arts; the young woman seeks affection. Their trust must be won in order to seduce them.

The astute boy seduces the young girl with playthings, the adolescent by his skill in the arts. To obtain the young woman, he needs the assistance of persons she trusts.

This chapter describes the attempts made by the very young lover to attract the girl he loves and to make her enamored of him. The ways and means employed can be divided into two parts. One is through her circle, by gifts of clothes and wonderfully attractive jewels, as a means of managing to get to know his heroine and of gradually nurturing her love. The other way lies in offering her things that let her know his feelings, so that the young girl realizes the boy's intentions.

Much prudence and intelligence is required to begin with in choosing the means. The trust and affection of the girl's circle must be won over. And if they become go-betweens, they must be convinced to act in such a way that the girl's love for the boy will grow. For his go-between, he must choose someone who has access to the girl's intimate circle and whom she considers as a close friend. Their intimacy and promiscuity must be such as to encourage the young girl's sexual desires and, if the opportunity arises, to arrange a pleasant encounter. Vātsyāyana recommends choosing as a go-between the nurse's daughter or a close girlfriend. These assistants should be able to understand fully the girl's state of mind and be capable of helping bring her desires to fruition and make things easy for her. Moreover, with their understanding of the boy's feelings, they should inform the girl of them without arousing in her any fear for her reputation. By means of these confidential go-betweens, the boy can make himself known to the girl, send her messages and, when her heart is inflamed, he can take advantage of it. The boy must contrive that her companions sympathize and confide in him, and must make himself appreciated by them so that they praise him to such an extent that the girl becomes madly desirous of seeing him and loves him before even having set her eyes on him.

It is her companions' task to make her passion grow.

The hero must take care that all the gifts he sends his heroine are marvelous and out of the ordinary, such as she has never seen before and are not possessed by any of her girlfriends. The girl is proud to receive such objects and gets a good impression of her hero. In making use of these things and in showing them to her friends, she considers herself favored. The reservations of her mind relax and, little by little, she gives herself to him mentally.

If the jewels are to her taste, they put into her mind ideas about married life, erotic feelings, a desire for amorous games. On seeing them, the girl starts making wonderful plans for her future. With excitation, she imagines amorous relations with the boy. She appreciates his taste and his choices. At the same time, useful and pleasant things she may desire must be taken into account. One must collect gifts which are to her taste.

Thus, when the girl has been informed of his amorous feelings by the go-between in her circle, the boy must strive to express the same, while taking care to remain prudent. Always dressed with seductive elegance, he does his best to meet the girl and present himself before her. During such meetings, the boy can get an idea of the girl's state of mind and evaluate her feelings according to her behavior.

Nothing must be overlooked in evaluating the signs that reveal the girl's feelings toward the boy. For this reason, in this chapter, Vātsyāyana studies the female character with great subtleness. He says that with most women, while showing strength, one should behave gently. The girl will quickly realize it, but her desire is never clear or evident. Even if she wishes to, she cannot, out of modesty and decency, greet the one she loves. This is why young men must know how to evaluate a woman's feelings from signs, her facial expressions, or the movements of her hands and feet.

A woman's way of seeing things is bizarre and secretive. When they say "no," it means "yes." Their efforts to be contrary hide their agreement. When a girl does not look at the boy in front of her, and turns her head away, her wink must be caught. If the boy chances to look at her, she immediately lowers her head. She reveals her feelings in adjusting her sari, by moving her limbs, passing her hand over her jewels, fidgeting with her fingers, scratching the ground with her fingers, and so on. If the boy does not look at her, she is furious and remains impassible, her gaze fixed in the distance. She does not lower her eyes. If the girl chances to meet the boy and he addresses her, she has difficulty in replying, uses imprecise words, while smiling with indifference and lowering her head. If by chance she meets him while she is surrounded by her friends or members of her family, she turns toward her girlfriends and argues with them, while making sure that the boy looks at her. In all cases, she wants the boy to stay where he is.

When she sees the boy, the girl's behavior is usually modest and shy, and sometimes very odd. If she is carrying a baby in her arms, she will caress it and kiss it ceaselessly. She gets her girlfriends or maidservants to adjust her jewels and, with their assistance, practices all kinds of pretenses and games. The astute boy must study shrewdly all ways in which he can amuse the girl.

End of the Third Chapter
Ways of Obtaining the Girl
of the Third Part entitled Acquiring a Wife

Chapter Four

HOW TO
MANAGE ALONE
[Ekapuruṣha abhiyoga]

1 Having marked all the favorable signs, he turns his attention to the means of uniting with her.

Since no one assists him, he must manage alone, although he may well be able to find some support.

When it is clear that the girl is enamored, the young man seeks to establish relations with her.

Such relations may be of two kinds, external or internal. The former is described first.

2 Playing at dice or other games, when they argue, he takes her hand lovingly.

Saying to her, "You claim I am cheating," he takes her hand tenderly, "but it is I who have caught you."

When they argue, while playing chess or other games, the hero seizes the heroine's hand, in such a way as to cause a strong sensation in her.

3   He puts his arm lightly [sprishtaka] around her, as previously described.

Seizing favorable opportunities and moments, he practices the four kinds of embrace: light, penetrating [viddhaka], stirring [uddhrishtaka], and tight [pīditaka].

4   To make her understand his intentions, he shows her cut-outs representing copulation.

He shows her geese and other animals making love.

5   Sometimes, he also shows her other things.

Such as erotic paintings and other objects. Gradually, her curiosity is aroused and she is no longer bothered by their obscenity.

6   When bathing, he dives some way off and then draws near to her and touches her before emerging.

While underwater, he touches her and then comes up beside her.

7   He describes the nature of his feelings by writing on fresh palm leaves, or other substances.

In accordance with the popular game, in order to let her know his feelings and to show her his intentions, he writes them down on palm leaves.

8   He talks to her endlessly about his heartache: "You cannot imagine how much I suffer." He reaches his goal by sheer force of saying these things.

9   He also tells her his dreams, revealing his feelings.

On the pretext of making a comparison with reality, he tells her that it came to him in a dream.
It is useful to recount dreams, if it aids your plans.

10   At the theater, or during family reunions, he comes and sits next to her and finds some pretext for touching her.

At receptions or family reunions, he places himself close to the girl. He is always beside her at the theater and takes advantage of the fact in order to touch her.

11   She finds herself with no defense, squeezed against him. He presses his leg against hers.

12   Then, gradually, he touches one of her fingers.

Very gently, after a while.

13   He scratches the tip of her big toenail.

14   Having done this, he draws his leg higher up hers.

Having scratched her with his nail, he gently goes higher up her leg, as far as the groin.

15   He does it gradually, so that she should not resist.

To get her used to it, he must press against her limbs the whole time.

16   Leaning thus on her thigh, he takes hold of her toes and squeezes them.

17   Things given or received must always be an odd number.

Whether objects or bunches of flowers, but even when he takes hold of her with his nails.

18   After drinking, he lets a few drops of water fall on her.

19   If they are seated in an isolated place or in the dark, she forgives him easily, likewise when they are lying down next to each other.

While strolling, sitting down at times when the girl is not frightened, she will allow him to touch her nails; likewise if they are seated or lying on the same bed.

In an isolated place in the dark, sitting close to one another, he gently caresses the girl, who resists no longer. When seated or lying on the same bed, he scratches her gently.

20   At such moments, he can learn her feelings, if she puts up no resistance.

And does not protest.

21   When they are alone, he says, "I have something to tell you." From her reply, "What is it about?," he can deduce her state of mind. This will be explained in the part entitled "Other Men's Wives."

From her manner of closing the conversation, he can tell her state of mind. Her kind of reply is a test of her mood. In deducing her state of mind from these spontaneous signs, he can tell up to what point she is in love.
After which, the boy says what is on his mind and can thus verify its effect on the girl.

22   Finding her in a favorable mood, when she claims to have a headache, he seizes the opportunity to take her back to his home for a short talk.

23   Once they are in the house, in order to get rid of her headache, he takes her hand, and affectionately strokes her eyes and brow.

24   He explains that this action is the most efficacious remedy.

She says, "Your hand is the best of remedies. At the touch of your hand, my headache vanished."

25   "I am the one who must give you this treatment. It would not be seemly for a young girl to have it done by another." Continuing in this way, the bond of affection grows between them.

When they leave each other, she intimates that he should return.

26   This treatment is recommended for three nights, three evenings.

The result is as follows:

27   Seeing her go to his home, rumors increase.

Since she is interested in the arts and in legends, she always stays a long time.

28   She tries to justify herself with those who question her, but without revealing anything.

29   According to Ghotakamukha, even if one has the idea of going far away afterward, girls must not be dishonored.

Ghotakamukha, who is an expert on the subject, explains that, however much trust you may have in her, and she in you, she must not be placed in any difficulty.

30   When one's approaches have met with success, one must finish by acting and by mounting her [upakrama].

31   In the evening or in the darkness of the night, a woman is defenseless if amorous advances are made to her. She is ready for the act of love, and the man is not unaware of it. For this reason, at such a moment, one must change over to action, which is what normally happens.

At night, when no one can see them, women desire to make love, and to have themselves taken. They do not defend themselves, and are perfect partners in copulation. They must therefore be satisfied by means of the act desired.

32   A single man, living apart from the woman he loves, needs the assistance of her nurse or a girlfriend to go and visit her and bring her back to his own home. After which, he acts as described above.

33   To begin with, he sends one of his own maidservants, pretending to be a girlfriend, to her house.

34   He observes her reactions during religious ceremonies [yajña], weddings, journeys, festivals, or when a funeral cortège is passing by, and it is by taking into account her state of mind at these different times that he manages to possess her.

Meaning, to accomplish a gāndharva marriage by mutual agreement.
Under such circumstances, people are easily put off the scent (vyagra). These are good opportunities for the lover to carry out a

gāndharva marriage (free union) with his beloved, inasmuch as he is already assured of her feelings, having observed the same for a long time.

35 According to Vātsyāyana, at times and places when women show they are ready to surrender, one should never retract.

After having tested the woman's feelings many times, when, during a religious or other kind of festival, she gives you the sign, you must not reverse your policy (nata).

If due to lack of money or for some other reason, you are unable to manage, alone, to unite with a girl who is enamored of you, she, in turn, will change her mind. It is known as a change of direction: in changing her attitude, she will turn her back on you.

What are the reasons for breaking off?

36 An honest girl, but with a doubtful reputation, without wealth, coming from a good family but not having found a husband, or else an orphan of unknown origin, must herself attend to catching a boy to marry her.

What means are employed in such an initiative?

37 She can marry a good boy, sturdy and handsome, with whom she has been pledged since childhood.

It all depends on the boy's attitude.

38 She must not reject a simpleton who appears to be wholly under his parents' influence, or one who lacks sexual drive. By showing kindness and seeing him often, she will end up by attracting him.

By pretending she loves him, she establishes a relationship. By means of behavior that pleases him, she makes him happy and turns him in her favor.

A girl who thinks that a sexually deficient young man, who remains at home with his parents, could be captured by her, takes an interest in his moods and, in various ways, manages to attract him.

39   The girl's mother, nurse, and friends must collaborate
in making the boy malleable.

*To overcome the boy's shyness, they say nice things to him both in
public and in private.*

40   When he is alone, or at unwonted times, they visit
him, bringing flowers, scents, and betel in their hands. They
show him skillful applications of the arts, stay with him
while he is being massaged or has a headache, telling him
pleasing things, all the while seeking to arouse his interest
in the girl.

*The girl must flatter the boy she has in mind, when he is alone
or at unexpected moments. She brings him flowers, perfumes, betel, or
garlands. She shows him her skill at some of the sixty-four arts. She
tells him things that please him. She uses the means described above.*

41   However, she herself must not invite a man to her
house. The Master says that a young girl who offers herself
destroys her own chances.

However anxious she may be to find a husband, a girl must never
take the initiative. A woman who is excited, enterprising in love, destroys any chance she has with men.

42   If he takes the initiative in uniting with her, she must
then seize the opportunity and let him do what he wants.

She should not resist.

43   When he takes her in his arms, she should not show
her passion. She gently offers no resistance, with a stupid
air, so that he takes her lips by force.

*The boy should not be aware of her excitation. She must not allow
her feelings to be guessed from her behavior. She must not give him
like for like, but be submissive and gentle, all the while being ready for
him to embrace her by force.*
When the boy clasps, embraces, and caresses her, she must not

show her own desire. She must play the fool, as though she did not understand the boy's movements, which she accepts, while contriving to get him to embrace her by force.

44   Even if she is intensely excited, she must make difficulties if he wishes to touch her sex.

Even if she is excited when the boy tries to touch her secret parts, she restrains his hand from attempting to reach them.

45   Even if she wishes to, she must not uncover herself until the marriage date is certain.

Although they have a reciprocal desire to see each other's sexual parts, the girl must not, whatever the boy's efforts, let him touch them or examine her sex, since it is never certain that he will finally marry her.

46   If she is convinced that his feelings for her will not change, she may give herself to him, foregoing her virginity.

According to the gāndharva practice of free marriage, she allows him to break her hymen.

47   Once free of the state of virginity, she confides to highly trusted girlfriends that she has made a gāndharva marriage.

Here ends the subject of reversing roles [prayojyasya upāvartana].

She confides to her friends, "I have made a gāndharva marriage, by mutual agreement." This way of attaining one's goal is practiced by many. Cohabitation with a girl is allowed, cohabitation being an acknowledged status.
Here ends the subject of the girl who, through her own skill, manages to take possession of a boy who wanted nothing to do with her. In this connection, here are a few quotations:

48   One must marry a girl who is desirous of being united, who dreams of the happiness of being protected, who is obliging and submissive.

This is the best woman for a free union.

An independent girl may, with her own means, find herself a husband whom she can dominate.

49 Without worrying about his qualities, appearance, or abilities, she takes him as husband out of love of money, even if he has other wives.

Simply because he is rich.

50 A girl must never fail to take for a husband a young man who is full of qualities, skillful in business, whom she has been able to meet due to her intrigues and can keep in her power.

If he is rich, but already has other wives, there are nevertheless certain risks.

51 It is better to take control over a husband who is a devoted young man, even poor and uninteresting, but who has just enough to live on, rather than another full of qualities but inconstant.

It is better to be content with a boy who can only just manage to earn a living for his family, rather than catch a libertine, even if the latter is rich and charming.

52 The wives of the rich are often numerous and ill-controlled. They then look elsewhere for the satisfactions they cannot find at home.

The rich take many wives and are unable to control them.

53 It is not advisable to marry a man of lowly status, even if he is cultured, or an old man, or someone who travels abroad.

54 One should not marry anyone who only wants his own way, is violent, a trickster and gamester, or who has other wives and children.

55. If she has to choose among several suitors of equal merit, she should choose the one she likes the best.

"Marry the one you love," as the saying goes.

After explaining in the previous chapter the employment of go-betweens in order to obtain the beloved, Vātsyāyana describes the case of those who, without being in any condition to obtain assistance, wish to establish a permanent relationship.

How can a man, without assistance, seduce a girl from a good family, in order to make her his mistress and marry her by simple reciprocal commitment according to the gāndharva rite? How, without assistance, can a girl attract a boy of superior status and of serious mind, in order to make him her husband? The main subject of this chapter is the description of the ways of doing so. In this connection, the means to be employed are those that a man acting alone may utilize. This is why it is known as initiative of a man managing alone (ekapurusha abhiyoga).

Vātsyāyana suggests various ways, which are of two kinds, external and internal. In describing external means, the author suggests that when the lover and his beloved are playing chess, during the game, the lover should start off some difference of opinion, giving rise to a violent argument. In this case, the way in which he seizes the girl's hand is the same as when the betrothed takes his wife's hand during the marriage rite. When he takes her hand in this way, the girl realizes that he wishes to marry her acording to the gāndharva rite.

When the young man has been successful in all his external enterprises, he must make use of external and internal means. Wherever he meets the girl, he must begin to tease her, offer her things she has indicated she would like to have. When they have the opportunity of being alone together, or of sitting one next to the other in the darkness, he must pinch her buttocks and breasts as much as she can bear.

Alone, or in darkness, women lose their modesty. For this reason, such circumstances are very useful for amorous games and copulation. It is one of the principles of the *Kāma Shāstra* that, during the night or in a solitary place, erotic desire is easily awakened in women. No great effort is called for. When the boy and girl find themselves side by side in some place, he must give her physical signs of his intentions. Words serve no purpose, because the girl can always object to the words by shaking her head. If words appear to be necessary, they should always be very allusive. One should always express oneself very briefly, so as to arouse the woman's curiosity and, if she asks for an explanation, this is the right moment to put the thing clearly before her.

Thus, having studied the woman's feelings by both external and internal means, the boy can invite her to his house under some pretext. If she claims to have a headache, he explains that the touch of his hands is better than any remedy, thus winning her affection and trust. She gradually becomes fond of him, but he should leave her in doubt for a long time.

He goes with her to the theater or to receptions, at which they greatly amuse themselves. At no time, however, should he pronounce the word marriage, since Ghotakamukha, who knows the subject well, considers that, whatever their love for their lover, women are apt to break away in the event of sudden difficulties, repeated failure, or if they get bored, and then no effort can get them back.

Great means and great effort are needed to make a girl wholly favorable. It is only after repeated attempts that the boy can be certain that the one he loves is ready for whatever he may desire. Only when she is totally in his power should he venture to make sexual approaches.

In indicating favorable moments and places for amorous relations between the lover and his beloved, Vātsyāyana explains that, if one tries to possess a girl in the evening, at night, or in the darkness, she cannot refuse, since she prefers a time and place when no one can see her. Moreover, at such times and on such occasions, passion (rāga) rises in the woman's heart. Although her sexual desire increases, she will not take the initiative, but if the man does so, she will not stop him.

Vātsyāyana opines that, when a young man (yuvaka), poor and with no family, wishes to marry a girl of his own or better class, but cannot obtain her, he should strive to catch her by the means indicated in the previous chapter. Likewise, when a girl has no family, or is the daughter of poor parents, and marriage with a desirable party is impossible, she herself must manage to catch the suitor she desires. For a girl, too, external and internal efforts are involved. When she meets the person whom she wishes to marry by mutual agreement (gāndharva) in an isolated place, or in the dark, she should greet him in such a way as to demonstrate her skill in one of the sixty-four arts of the *Kāma Shāstra*. She should discourse pleasantly with the boy she wishes to seduce. All her remarks should delight him. She should show that she agrees with him about everything, but in no case should she, by her bodily conduct or signs, commit the error of letting him know that she wants intercourse. However desirous she may be to make love, she must make no attempt to do so, nor show any eagerness.

Vātsyāyana considers that a woman who makes advances destroys any chance she has. The man would thus take her for an abandoned woman who sleeps with everybody. He would despise her and turn away from her. A woman should never show her willingness until her lover is ready for action. She should not resist too much, however. During the preliminaries, when her lover takes her in his arms, she should examine the boy's feelings, while not showing excitement or agitation. She must take his state of mind into account and not anticipate his desires. She must submit to the boy's enterprises, showing ignorance and foolishness. She must not resist, but when her lover seeks to take her lips, she must show a slight reticence, so that he must embrace her by force.

A very young girl (taruṇī) must always take care not to uncover herself in front of her lover, until she is fully convinced that he will not leave her at any price.

In no case should she, for love of money, marry a man who is rich but no longer young and has other wives, nor a stranger, or one who is ugly, violent, cunning, a gamester, or unstable. A girl should find a husband whose character matches her own.

End of the Fourth Chapter
How to Manage Alone
of the Third Part entitled Acquiring a Wife

Chapter Five

UNION BY MARRIAGE

[Vivāha Yoga]

Those who wish to choose a spouse [svayamvara] to their liking marry according to the gāndharva rite, by mutual agreement.

There exist other forms of marriage, however, such as the āsura [by bride purchase]. The ways of contributing to their success are explained. The gāndharva form is the one most frequently encountered.

1 Because the young girl lives isolated from the world and sees no one, her nurse undertakes to assist her out of affection.

Without saying anything, the nurse undertakes to seek a boy in the neighborhood.

By rendering small services to someone, the nurse skillfully engages his sympathy.

2 She concerns herself with a boy of her choice and assesses his merits. To make the girl interested in him, she describes his qualities, with some exaggeration.

She then embarks on capturing the boy she has chosen.
Although she hardly knows the boy, the nurse seeks to make the girl interested in his qualities. To do so, she chatters ceaselessly on the subject, exaggerating his merits, so that the girl's interest is aroused.

3   She points out the defects of any other suitors who might run counter to her goal.

4   She tells her that her father and mother take no account of the suitors' merits and that it is only for love of money that they heedlessly wish to marry her off.

Her parents, knowing nothing of her suitors' merits, reject the one who is meritorious, giving preference to one who is insignificant but rich.

5   In order to persuade her, the nurse gives her as an example other girls of her caste, or famous heroines such as Shakuntalā, who themselves chose their own husband.

She describes to her those who have chosen a husband for themselves against their parents' will, and takes as an example the tale of Shakuntalā.
In seeing the nymph Menakā, sent by Indra, the King of Heaven, to hinder his austere practices, the sage Kaushika succumbs to desire. But he subsequently abandons the daughter born of his seed in the forest, when Menakā returns to heaven. This daughter is fed by a variety of birds, called shakuntā, which is why she is called Shakuntalā in the tale. Taken, out of kindness, into the hermitage of the sage Kanva, she grows up there. Seen by King Dushyanta, who has come to hunt wild animals, she marries him of her own will. The nurse also names the king's daughters as an example.

6   In the greatest families, one sees women secluded and ill-treated as a result of the hostility and intrigues of the other wives.

She explains to her that, even in the best families, the father, out of greed, sometimes gives his daughter to a polygamous man whose other wives will detest her. There, abandoned by her own family, she suffers cruelly.

7   The nurse describes to her what she risks.

What might happen to her in the future.

8   She tells her of the happiness awaiting her with a man who has only one wife and praises the boy she recommends.

Thus she will not be made to suffer by other wives.

9   Once she feels the girl is interested, she strives to soothe her fears, shyness, and modesty.

Once her interest is aroused, the girl becomes uneasy: "Am I making a mistake? Is my virtue in danger?" Then, gradually, she frees herself from her qualms concerning her virtue, her fear of her seniors, and her modesty with regard to her family.

10   It remains for the nurse to lead her enterprise as go-between to a successful conclusion.

The messenger is known as a go-between only in a manner of speaking.
The nurse must then put into practice all the means indicated in the chapter on go-betweens.

11   Even if the hero takes you by force, without your consent, you will become his wife and the marriage is valid.

If he takes you by force, you are not to blame. Even in such a manner, the marriage is regular.
The nurse tells her, "If the hero abducts you as if you were not responsible, people will have nothing to reproach you for and your desire will be fulfillled."

12   It is decided to act and, at the right moment, the hero, bearing the sacred fire taken from a priest's house, scattering the sacred herb and pronouncing the prescribed words, will take you thrice around the hearth.

Being convinced, she waits, as agreed, in an isolated place.

Having been informed, the heroine waits for him outside her father's house. She no longer has fears or doubts. He goes to look for consecrated fire in a priest's house and, according to the rites, hero and heroine circle the hearth three times.

13 After which she informs her father and mother.

14 According to the religious authorities, the marriage, to which the sacred fire is witness, is irreversible.

15 She must then explain everything to her family, who accuse her.

Not only to put things in order, but in her own interest.
However, she reveals to her family what has really happened only after she has lost her virginity.
The Master explains why she must inform her parents:

16 The family is dishonored by such a marriage. They fear sanctions after an abduction and thus prefer to give their consent.

When the hero has taken her to his house, if her parents do not agree to give her to him, the crime of abduction dishonors the whole family, and they fear punishment. If the king hears what has happened, the boy also risks punishment.
The girl's parents, scared by the stain on the family's honor, hasten to adopt the boy into their clan. This is the best solution.

17 Thus, the young woman has obtained her hero by skillful intrigues. By affectionate behavior, beautiful gifts ,and civilities, she has him accepted by her family.

18 A gāndharva marriage, by simple mutual agreement, would have been preferable.

Instead of this twisted way of going about it. Another kind of marriage will be described.

19 When the boy is unable to reach his goal on his own, he uses as go-between a woman of good family who has access to the girl's home, having been intimately acquainted with and appreciated by her parents for a long time and

friendly toward himself. She brings them money and, using some pretext, takes the girl to his house.

Not being able to obtain the girl's hand by his own means, he employs a woman of good family, who is able to enter the girl's house, has been acquainted with her parents for many years, and is kindly disposed toward him. She makes them accept some money and, using some pretext, brings him the girl he wishes to marry.

Knowing that the girl's parents' intend to marry her for a price, it is by taking advantage of their lust for gain that the girl is brought to him by devious ways.

20 Then, as above, bringing sacred fire from a priest's house, he marries her.

21 When the marriage rite has taken place, he receives her officially from the hands of her mother, who gives her consent from fear of scandal.

If the girl's parents have already concluded her betrothal to another and the date of the marriage is close, the go-between must then, by describing to the girl's mother the defects of the chosen suitor, sow doubt in her mind and make her realize that her daughter will never accept this marriage. She describes the qualities of her suitor, comparing them with the defects of the man to whom they wanted to sell her. It is thus, by perfidious means, that she obtains the mother's agreement for the daughter to marry her hero.

22 With his agreement, during the night, she leads the boy to a neighbor's house and brings fire from a priest's house to accomplish the rite.

This occurs at a neighbor's house so that the money can be handed over discreetly.

When the go-between is assured that the girl's mother has renounced the chosen fiancé and has told her that the other boy is ready to marry the girl, then, at her intimation, she makes the boy come discreetly to a neighbor's house and sends to a priest's dwelling for the sacred fire. The girl is then married discreetly.

23 If the young man is attracted by a courtesan or a

married woman, it is better to win the friendship of one of her brothers of his own age and, by services rendered and kindnesses, make him finally come to understand his aim.

Since such women are difficult to obtain, he must gain the friendship of her brother by means of small gifts or other advantages, to assure his aid in obtaining the woman desired.

24   Young men of the same age and character are often ready to give even their life for their friend, and help each other's enterprises, if the opportunity arises. This is why he will help him reach his goal.

Thus, with the brother of his heroine as go-between, he lures the sister into an isolated spot and, taking the fire to witness, marries her.

Lying with a sleeping or drunken girl is called the marriage of the paishācha, or succubus. Describing the same, he says:

25   In circumstances such as the eighth day festival dedicated to the moon, the nurse contrives to let the girl drink and, having made her drunk, under the pretext of having something to do, leads her to an isolated place where the boy is to be found. The latter, raping her while she is unconscious, thus accomplishes the marriage.

For the eighth day festival of the moon, at the end of the day, people stay awake all night to perform rites in honor of the moon, as they also do on other occasions. The nurse, being devoted to the boy, intoxicates the girl by making her drink wine or some drug. Then, on the pretext that she has something to do, such as, "I have lost a ring," leads her unconscious to an isolated place where she lets her be raped by the boy. Afterwards, she reveals the fact to her family and her whole circle. This is one of the ways of performing a marriage.

26   When she is half-asleep, the nurse leads her to an isolated place where the marriage is consummated while she is unconscious. Then, having compromised her, the union is made official.

She is dishonored while sleeping. Here there is no question of the sacred fire, since it is an act contrary to ethics.

The rākshasa marriage, "of the demons," carried out by brutal abduction, is now considered.

27 Having seen her in the village or in the garden, the boy abducts her with the aid of his companions, killing her guardians or making them run away, as do the demons. This is also one of the forms of marriage.

A stranger in the village, with the aid of his numerous companions, abducts the girl after killing or putting her guardians to flight, as Krishna did for Rukminī. Being unethical, there is no question of the sacred fire as in gāndharva marriage.

Of these kinds of marriage, which are the ones to be avoided and which are normal?

28 In order of importance, the best marriage is the one in accordance with ethics. Where the sacred fire is lacking, there is no hierarchy among the others.

First are those sanctioned by moral law, which are four in number. From this point of view, the Brāhma marriage, by gift with dowry, is preferable to the gāndharva, by mutual agreement. For the others, nevertheless, there is an order. The gāndharva marriage is better than the āsura, by purchase.

Although, according to certain opinions, both conform to law, one is nevertheless preferable to the other. The gāndharva rite is not on the same level as the āsura. However, the āsura rite, by purchase, is better than the paishācha rite, by rape, and the latter, although unethical, is better than the rākshasa, by brutal abduction. The rākshasa rite is an act of violence, and cannot be compared with the others. It is quite another matter.

29 Love is the goal of the marriage union, and although the gāndharva marriage is not the most recommended, it remains the best.

Although but little appreciated, it is the one in which love tri-

umphs. This is why, being a harmonious union, it is considered as the form of marriage of the heavenly musicians (gāndharva).
Without love, marriage has no purpose. Although considered with indifference, the gāndharva marriage is the most just, the one in which love and sexuality are harmoniously combined.

Its importance is explained:

30 Marriage can bring many joys and sorrows. Because it is based on love, the gāndharva marriage is the best.

Marriage may bring many sorrows, often due to lack of savoir faire, wrong choice, or a mistaken way of life.
Because it is desired, the gāndharva marriage causes least problems. It is a love marriage, without conflicts or disputes. This is why it is the best.

The four kinds of marriage have been described above. Of these, Brāhma, by free gift, and ārsha, the archaic form, by cattle barter, are considered well omened, although in both these forms, the decisions of bride and groom have nothing to do with it.

If the boy or girl is not in favor of these sacred forms, however, Vātsyāyana recommends that they should seek a love marriage and find the means to accomplish it. Under such circumstances, the Master advises the young man and girl to perform a gāndharva marriage.

A marriage based on love is a source of happiness, requiring little effort, and causes little suffering and few quarrels over behavior and ways of doing things.

A boy who is unable to inspire love in the girl of his choice therefore proposes to her parents to grant him an āsura marriage: by purchase. If he cannot obtain the girl for money, the boy must therefore abduct her in order to marry her. Such forms of marriage are attributed to succubus or nightmares (paishācha) and to the demons (rākshasa).

Since in the Brāhma (free gift) and daiva (gift to the officiating priest) forms of marriage, the girl's consent is not considered, the author of the *Kāma Sūtra* considers it preferable to contract a gāndharva marriage, according to the girl's will, while totally abhoring marriage by purchase, rape, or abduction. For the gāndharva marriage, the girl's agreement is required before anything else, since without it, the gāndharva marriage is not possible.

In this chapter concerning the forms of marital union, the Master describes the ways of obtaining the girl's consent, with the aid of a go-between. The first essential for such go-betweens is that they should be disinterested messengers. The characteristics of the disinterested messenger are described in the fourth chapter of the part dealing with servants. For the success of the messenger's enterprise in uniting lover and beloved, it suffices that the boy should tell him simply, "I must win the favors of such a girl," after which the messenger acts on his own initiative to bring the enterprise to a successful conclusion. The boy need not intrigue or worry. In the play *Mālatī Mādhava* by Bhavabhūti, the author, praising Kāmandakī, a religious acting as messenger, and declaring the confidence one can have in her success, writes that, "the success of the scheme depends on the skill of the messenger."

For this job, the girl's nurse's daughter or other assistant of her household can be utilized. The boy cannot know what the messenger tells the girl about him. She must so arrange matters and the situation that, while keeping the boy's desires in mind and singing his praises, the girl may not suspect that the go-between has any connection with the boy. Furthermore, if the messenger learns that the heroine is interested in some other young man, she will disparage him with such dexterity that the girl, although he had pleased her, will begin to despise him.

If her parents are strongly opposed to the boy whose praises the messenger is singing and of whom the girl is enamored, by intriguing, the adroit messenger places the parents in such embarrassment that they end by consenting to a gāndharva marriage. In *Mālatī Mādhava*, the nun Kāmandakī, in similar circumstances, forcefully condemns Mālatī's father:

"How can you favor till now someone who has no merit and look with disfavor on the side of love? It is merely because he is the king's companion in pleasure that you wish to give your daughter to Nandana, his friend."

If the girl's parents wish to marry her to another at any price, the messenger, quoting Shakuntalā or some other tale as an example, explains to them the importance of choosing a husband to their daughter's taste. By telling them such tales, she manages to make the parents change their mind and accept the love marriage.

Thus, following the messengers' instructions, the heroine, hiding herself, reaches the house of the one she loves. Vātsyāyana recognizes the validity of such a marriage. Due to his acknowledgement, the sacred rules can be disregarded, requiring that the marriage, according to the rites prescribed in the texts, be celebrated in the suitor's house. Once the marriage has taken place, taking the fire as witness, the public authorities and society are disarmed. Neither parents nor the law can declare the marriage invalid.

Gāndharva marriage has been widely practiced since most ancient times, and this kind of marriage is recognized everywhere as being popular and valid. The "svayamvara" of a princess, when she puts the nuptial necklace around the neck of one of her assembled suitors, is a form of gāndharva marriage. The husband was elected, after which, according to the rules for domestic rituals, or *Grihya Sūtra*, the sacrament of marriage took place before the fire, taken as witness. The weddings of Nala and Damayantī, Aja and Indumatī, Rāma and Sītā, and Udayana and Vāsavadattā, all took place in this fashion.

Vātsyāyana's opinion is that, after celebrating a marriage of this kind, the parents must be informed, not only to give them pleasure, but for practical reasons. The purpose of the gāndharva marriage is not to separate the girl from her family and friends. This is why Vātsyāyana considers it the best. After describing the gāndharva marriage of the first category, the Master also considers the second category in which, while the girl becomes attracted to the boy as a result of the messenger's efforts, her parents are still opposed. The emissary must obtain the mother's consent by giving her money and, under some pretext, leading the girl out of the house, marry her to the boy in front of the fire.

In its third form, the lowest kind of gāndharva marriage, it is the girl's brother whose cooperation is acquired by satisfying his whims. After this, the hero says to him, "I am in love with your sister and want to marry her."

Then, with his complicity and under some pretext or other, his sister enters and the marriage is arranged.

In connection with the paishācha marriage, the *Manu Smriti* says, "He who, out of licentiousness, dishonors any girl, deserves immediate death. But the man who, out of licentiousness, dishonors a girl of his own caste is not put to death."

Raping the girl after her abduction is the rākshasa marriage. This too is condemned by religion, since the rites and offerings in the fire do not occur.

Vātsyāyana prefers the rākshasa marriage, by abduction, to the paishācha rite, by rape, since in such a marriage, courage and audacity predominate. From his point of view, although the gāndharva marriage belongs to the medium category, it is more widespread because the final goal of the marriage is the love of the couple, and because love, from the very beginning, is the basis of the gāndharva marriage.

Vātsyāyana has a sympathetic attitude toward the gāndharva marriage. However, from a religious point of view, the four forms—Brāhma, prājāpatya, daiva, and ārsha—conform more to religious law and are thus considered superior.

Here ends the Fifth Chapter
Union by Marriage
and the Third Part entitled Acquiring a Wife
of the Kāma Sūtra *by Vātsyāyana*

———— Part Four ————
Duties and Privileges of the Wife
[Bhāryā adhikārika]

Chapter One

CONDUCT OF THE
ONLY WIFE

*Once married to the man, how should the wife behave toward him?
This is what is known as the duties and privileges of the wife. According to the situation, the man who possesses the girl either has no other
wives, or else has a certain number of other wives dependent on him.*

*A wife may therefore be of two kinds: the only wife, or wife among
others.*

We shall first describe the conduct of the only wife.

1   The only wife is totally trusting, considering her husband as a god and completely devoted to him.

*If there are other wives, there is a risk of unpleasant situations.
It is said that, "The one that feeds them is the women's god," but this
does not concern their physical condition.*

A devoted wife (pativratā) puts all her trust in her husband, considering him in her heart as a god. She conforms at all points to his
wishes.

2   She takes responsibility for the household, and so on.

With her husband's consent, she takes care of the house. Eschewing the outside world, she involves herself entirely in the household and takes on the domestic tasks.

3   She attends to cleaning the clothes, tidying the rooms, flower arrangements, cleaning the floor, being attractive to look at, performing the three daily rites of offering to the gods and of worshiping them at their domestic shrine.

She makes the various tasks of cleaning and ordering the house a strict rule. She does the flower arrangements, polishes the floors, while being always pleasant to the eye. She also performs the three daily offerings [in the sacred fire] and worships the gods at the domestic shrine.

4   According to Gonardīya, there is no state happier than the state of marriage.

It all depends on the way of envisaging things.

5   The wife must behave suitably to her husband's elderly parents, servants, his sisters, and their husbands.

She must accept her parents-in-law, her sisters-in-law, and their husbands as her own, and speak to them in a seemly manner.

6   On carefully prepared ground, she must sow aromatic plants [harita] and vegetables [shāka], plant sugarcane [ikshu] in clumps, mustard [sarshapa], cumin [jīraka], ajamodā [hingu, asafetida], cinnamon [tamāla], fennel [shatapushpa], and small cardamoms [gulma].

Aromatic plants [harita], such as coriander [dhanyāka], ginger [ārdraka], and vegetables [shāka], spinach [palankiya] and others, must be planted in well ordered rows.
Sugarcane [ikshu] is planted in clumps.

7   She must plant on a single plot rows of: āmalaka [myrobalan, *Emblica officinalis*, gulābāsa], mallika [jasmine,

Jaʃminum ʃambac], jātī [*Jaʃminum gran∂iflorum*], kurantaka [yellow amaranth, *Barleria prionitiʃ nevari*], navamālikā [red jasmine, chameli, *Plumeria rubra*], tagara [valerian], nandyavarta [kadamba, *Anthocephaluʃ ca∂amba*], japāgulma [China rose] and other ornamental plants. In the grove of trees, she should also plant: bālakoshīraka [khasha, *Saccharum ʃpontaneum*] and pātalika [*Stereoʃpermum ʃuavolenʃ*] with abundant blossoms.

8 In the middle of the garden, a well, a reservoir, and a tank must be dug.

9 She must keep beggars out of the way, also wandering Buddhist or Jaina monks, women of bad reputation, mountebanks, and magicians.

She must have no contact, under pretext of charity, with beggars, Buddhist or Jaina nuns, old men, red-robed religious, bad-living women, mountebanks, fortunetellers, magicians, and so on.

10 With regard to food, she must reflect, "This he likes, that he doesn't, he drinks this and not that."

11 Hearing his voice outside, when he returns home, she comes to the threshold, well dressed, saying, "What must I do?"

Elegantly dressed, at the entrance to the house courtyard, she says "What are your orders? What must I do?"

12 Sending the servants away, she bows at her husband's feet.

13 Even when alone with her master, she never shows herself without her jewels.

14 In the case of his making excessive or useless expenditure, she scolds him when they are alone.

She remains shy in front of other people.

15 She must ask her husband's permission to attend marriage ceremonies with her girlfriends, or to go to receptions or to the temples. Otherwise she will be suspected of improper behavior.

16   It is only with his approval that she takes part in games.

To take part in the games on the Night of Yaksha, she must have her husband's consent.

17   She must go to sleep after him and awaken before him.

18   The kitchen must be apart, far from inquisitive eyes.

The kitchen must be clean, well kept and ordered, and located where no stranger's glance can penetrate.

19   If her husband behaves badly, she must show her displeasure, without exaggerating her reproaches.

Reprove him without insistence, saying, "Do not do that again. Let it not happen any more."

20   When she has any reproach to make him, she does it without dramatizing, when he is alone or perhaps in front of his friends, if the opportunity arises. She must never have recourse to magic practices.

She must not attempt to control him by magic practices.

21   Gonardīya says that this is the main cause of loss of trust between a married couple.

Magic practices are forbidden, because they destroy trust and the feeling of security.

22   She must avoid disagreeable words, turning her glance aside, speaking with a pout, sitting on the threshold of the house, watching the door when given instructions, or staying alone for a long time in one room of the house.

Going into the garden of the house, listening to someone's advice, or staying alone a long time, are bad habits.

23   She must be careful of bad smells from sweat, or residue between her teeth, since they quench amorous desire.

24   For amorous encounters, she must dress luxuriously
with many jewels, many flowers, and ointments.

*Wearing brightly colored garments according to the occasion, choos-
ing the colors he prefers. To give her husband pleasure, when he is
disposed to make love, she puts on her numerous jewels to appear more
beautiful, when the time comes, in the "chamber of colors," the chamber of love [raktāvāsa].*

25   On going out to amusements, she must wear elegant
but unpretentious garments, only a few jewels, discreet scent
and makeup, white flowers in her hair.

Pretty but simple clothes, simple earrings, no colors that are too flashy.

26   If her husband practices periodic abstinence or fasting, she does the same. She tells him, "We are bound to one
another. I am not independent."

*She does as he does, in order to demonstrate her devotion. She is
bound to her master for fasting. If he forbids her to, she replies, "I am
not independent." Thus, she shows him her affection.*

27   She takes advantage of opportunities for buying earthenware, bamboo, wooden, leather, iron, and copper utensils
cheaply.

28   She also purchases salt, oil, and spices, which she keeps
in containers for normal use, but she hides the pots containing rare products.

*Seasalt, clarified butter [ghee], oil and other liquids, spices such as
valerian [tagara] and the fifty-two medical roots, placed in wooden
bowls and kept in a hidden place where they do not spoil.*
*As well as achcharīlā, dāruhaladī [Berberis asiatica], and other
aromatic substances in current use; gourd and pumpkin seeds. Ingredients that cost twice, three, or ten times ordinary prices, and those that
are difficult to find, are placed in bottles in a hidden spot.*

29   In order to sow them in season, she gathers the seeds
of: radish [mūlaka], sweet potatoes [ālu], beetroot [pālanki],

absinthe [damanaka], rātaka [myrobalan, *Emblica officinalis mongiferas*], cucumber [enva], aubergines [kapusavarta], marrows [kushmānda], gourds [alābu or tumbī], sūrana or kunda [*Amorphophallus campanulatus*], bignonia [shukanāsa, sarvato bhadra], svayamgupta or kapikachu [*Mucunia pruriens*], yellow grapes [tiliparnika or kashmari, *Gyrandropsis pentaphylla*], and sundry plants such as agnimanthala [*Premna spinata*], garlic [lashuna], onions [palāndu], and other plants in current use, as well as medicinal herbs, in order to sow them in due season.

30   She must never speak to anyone about what she possesses, or of what she knows about her husband.

Never speak of money put aside. "Money piled up must remain secret." Likewise any secrets that her husband may have confided in her.

31   In comparison with women of the same age, she should excel them by her accomplishments in the kitchen and her behavior.

As compared to other women of her age and condition, the wife should excel them all by her dexterity, her devotion to her husband, her skill in cooking various dishes, her pride, and other behavior.

32   She must regulate her spending by calculating her annual income.

33   A good wife should always take care to make butter with leftover milk; prepare molasses with sugarcane and oil with colza, etc., spin cotton and make cloth with the thread; stow away pieces of string, cord, thread, or bark; check stores of wheat and rice; supervise the servants; set aside the rice water, wheat bran, and burnt charcoal for reuse; take care of the domestic animals, the sheep, chickens, quails, parrots, mynahs, nightingales, peacocks; and each day make accounts of entries and expenses. These are the things with which a good wife should busy herself.

34   Dirty or worn garments must be collected for washing or redyeing. Those that are no longer of any use may be

given to deserving servants; the others can be used for rags.

They are given to good servants in appreciation of their work. With the rest, wicks can be made for lamps, or other uses can be found.

35 She lays in stocks of wine in jars and jars of liquors, ready in case of need, and keeps track of the rise and fall of prices.

She lays up stores to have on hand in case of need. She makes sure that prices are low, since in trade prices rise and fall.

Wine and liquors in jars must be kept in reserve for use, or eventually for selling in order to buy others. In such transactions, care must be taken about profits and losses.

36 According to custom, the husband's friends must be welcomed with flower garlands, sandalwood, and betel.

As is the custom in decent houses.

37 In her relations with her father-in-law and mother-in-law, she must be submissive and not contradict them, speak gently in front of them and not laugh too loudly, show that she agrees with what pleases them and, as far as what displeases them, act so as not to contradict them.

38 She must not get excited at amusements and games.

At games, whatever her excitement, she must behave with moderation and not lose her temper.

At amusements, she must not seek to assert herself.

39 She must be adroit with family members.

Show skill in dealing with kinsmen and avoid quarrels.

40 Never give anything without her husband's knowledge.

Even if to her child, or to get rid of something.

41 Make sure that the servants do their work properly, but also see to their comfort.

The work required of the servants must be done regularly. Their food and drink must be adequate.

See that the servants are conscientious in their work. Respect their days off and their holidays.

Such is the conduct of a woman married to a monogamous man. What must she do, however, if her husband lives abroad, leaving her alone while he amuses himself on the trip?

42   When her husband departs on a journey abroad, she removes the married woman's marks and her jewels, dedicates herself to devotion, and looks after the house according to the rules established by her husband.

She attends to worshiping the gods, praying, fasting, and must behave as her husband has taught her.

43   She must sleep beside her parents-in-law and obey their instructions. She must carefully look after whatever belongs to her husband.

44   She must appropriately perform all her daily tasks and carry through whatever he has undertaken.

Her daily occupations include the children's parties, and checking the expenses foreseen by her husband.

45   She does not go to visit her own family, except in case of sickness or for religious festivals, and always accompanied by someone of her husband's family as witness to the purity of her trip. She must not absent herself for long. She must never go out without being accompanied.

She must not visit her parents without a reason, except for a bereavement or religious ceremony. For the sake of her reputation, she must be accompanied by someone from her husband's family, and must not stay long for fear of the anger of her parents-in-law. If she is invited to a party, she says, "I cannot accept unless I am accompanied."

In merrymaking or at weddings, she behaves like a woman abandoned by her husband: she does not take part in the amusements.

46 She practices fasting according to her parents-in-law's instructions. She must supervise the servants so that they are clean and obedient. She must content herself with the minimum in buying and selling, and must seek to reduce expenditure.

Since trade is a sin, agricultural products must not be accumulated but, to avoid excessive expenditure, the essentials of agriculture must be obtained.

For purchasing, she should use responsible and trustworthy servants who know how to bargain, so as to limit expenditure as far as possible.

47 When her husband returns, he must first see what state she is in. Together, they make an offering to the gods, after which she greets him.

When the hero returns from his journey, she stays as she is, in her garments of absence, so that he can see how she has been behaving. She must not make herself beautiful in order to welcome him. Together they worship the gods, after which she welcomes him.

To conclude the second subject dealt with, he quotes:

48 Two verses in this connection:

"She who wishes the hero's well-being leads an irreproachable life as suits a single wife, whether she comes from a good family or is an ex-courtesan. Women protected by good conduct obtain respectability, riches and love, a social status as well as a protector [bhartāra] without other wives."

An honest woman must avoid all deceit to make herself well considered. Such a woman realizes the three aims of life. By "woman coming from a good family" is meant "untouched by other men."

According to Vātsyāyana, the main aim of this chapter is to define the behavior and attitude toward her husband of a young woman who has married according to her wish. Vātsyāyana distinguishes two kinds of wife: the only wife, and the one who has to put up with other wives. This chapter describes the attitudes and behavior of the only wife. Her first duty is to inspire total trust in her husband. She must adjust her conduct and ways of behaving to her husband's ideas and, as far as possible, make it so that their two bodies have a single soul. To attain such a goal, their attitudes must be disinterested and identical. This is why the texts suggest that the woman should consider her husband a god and worship him. The husband, too, should consider his wife as the goddess of fortune in his house and respect her. The codes of ethics, the *Dharma Shāstra*, tell us that prosperity and bliss dwell in the house where the wife is respected. In order to enjoy her husband's constant esteem, the wife should conform to his ethical convictions and follow him in everything. It is by renouncing herself, by giving herself entirely to her husband, that such a high aim can be reached. Whether a child, a girl, or an adult, the wife should always be submissive to her husband.

The wife, who is called the goddess of the house, must set up an inner garden, planted in pretty rows with spices and vegetables, such as coriander (dhaniyā), chili (adarakhamīrcha), henna (medhi), as well as trees and, for their beauty, scented flowering shrubs.

According to the *Koka Shāstra*, highly scented plants must be set in the garden, as well as trees with delicious fruit and flowering bushes.

Paths must be traced between the flowerbeds, passages, and square spaces and, in the middle, a well, reservoirs, and a pond must be dug.

The *Koka Shāstra* says that "the wife must avoid contact, even in the case of a distant kinswoman, with women who lead a bad life, with ascetics, beggars, dancers, and fortunetellers, and women with disheveled hair."

To give her husband confidence, if he has any doubts, and to satisfy him fully, a well-born woman must always be attentive to what he says. She must observe the signs that allow her to guess what he wants. She must support him in all his worries and difficulties.

"When she hears him approach, she comes to greet him on the threshold and makes him enter the house" (*Koka Shāstra*).

"He likes this kind of thing. He does not appreciate this drink. Every day he must be given the desire to eat" (*Koka Shāstra*).

When her husband returns and the meal is ready, she does not send the servants, but seeks him herself to wash his feet. On all occasions, the wife must take care not to appear before her husband with dirty or crumpled clothing, with her hair in disorder or badly combed. Whenever she appears before her husband, she must wear fresh clothes and approach him smiling. Thus, her husband's affection can only grow. If she is annoyed with him, she does not let it appear, and if her husband is annoyed, she does not allow bad feelings to take root in her heart. If her husband overspends, or buys useless things, she tries to reason lovingly with him, when they are alone. In front of other people, she never speaks of money matters, remaining discreet and avoiding arguments. She skillfully attempts to make her husband shed any extravagant habits. In the house, she keeps every little thing in order and makes sure that everything is clean and well ordered.

"Always with good humor, she must perform her household tasks, be refined in seasoning, have a firm hand in spending, if she sees that he is a spendthrift" (*Koka Shāstra*).

When the marriage is celebrated according to religious rules, it includes a rite called Saptapadi, in which husband and wife make a reciprocal vow. According to the *Kāma Sūtra*, this vow implies that the wife, wherever she may go, to weddings, ceremonies, or festivals, must do so with her husband's permission, even if it is only a matter of going to visit her mother. If the wife is guilty of going without permission, her husband will consider that she acts according to whim and will begin to have doubts. When doubts appear, married life loses its flavor and ends by breaking up. This is why the wife should strive to adjust her ways to her husband's wishes. The scholar Koka goes so far as suggesting that even with her husband's permission, the wife should be accompanied by a trustworthy person and should never go out alone.

"Even with permission, she should go out chaperoned" (*Koka Shāstra*).

When they go to bed, with loving words she massages her husband's legs to make him go to sleep, affectionately, like a mother putting her baby to sleep. She must go to sleep after him and awaken before him. The kitchen is the place that reveals a wife's qualities and character. This is why a wife should always be very careful about the cleanliness of the kitchen. The kitchen must be built so that those who are eating cannot see inside. The kitchen must glitter with cleanliness.

Vātsyāyana says that, wherever the goddess of the house goes, whatever work she performs, she must not show herself in a sweat. If she speaks, it is with a soft voice, her looks are full of affection, innocent looks. She does not gossip in the doorway, she does not ask advice of anyone in secret. She answers questions politely and modestly.

She does not seek to hide herself to talk to a man.

Even without being seen, she must not stay on the threshold, or gossip or argue. "She does not go to other people's houses, nor does she call them to her door. Never must she see a man to ask his advice"

(*Koka Shāstra*). If someone's attitude annoys her, she takes refuge in her husband's affection and respect.

For a decent woman, cleanliness of body and mind are the most important things. At every moment, she must strive to keep her body clean and beautiful. She does not allow her sweat to spread a bad smell, nor her mouth to taste unpleasant. If she does not pay attention to these body odors, her mind too will be soiled and her attraction for her husband will decrease, her health will be affected, and her beauty decline. To take care of her health and beauty is a wife's first duty. It is a very important form of discipline (sādhanā) and of yoga. A woman who is always careful of her beauty chooses her clothes and ornaments with care, according to place, occasion, and season. By wearing them according to circumstances, she becomes attractive and beautiful to see. In which season should one wear a sari of such and such a color? What flowers should she put in her hair? What scent should she use? These are the questions to which an intelligent woman pays attention. Thus, in conquering her husband, she truly becomes the goddess of the house.

Vātsyāyana does not pretend that her domestic tasks and control of expenditure should be neglected to attend to her beauty care. But, according to the principles of the *Artha Shāstra*, he gives practical advice.

End of the First Chapter
Conduct of the Only Wife
of the Fourth Part entitled Duties and Privileges of the Wife

Chapter Two

CONDUCT OF THE
CHIEF WIFE
AND OTHER WIVES

If the young married woman finds herself among other wives, how must she behave toward them and, in particular, toward the chief wife?

1   Because his wife is stupid, not serious-minded, or unable to have children due to barrenness, or simply because he wants a change, the hero wishes to remarry. The fact that she only produces daughters may also incite him to take another wife.

2   Despite the first wife's devotion and conduct, he wishes to leave her and seeks a pretext, or else she herself, unable to have children, advises him to take another wife.

Under pretext that she is stupid, frivolous, or barren, he wishes to leave her. A man who likes change seizes one of these pretexts. Otherwise, it is the duty of the wife who cannot have children to suggest a new wife, another marriage. But also, if she only has daughters, he takes another wife in order to have sons.

3   The new wife, if she is capable of doing so, strives to impose her prerogatives.

She seeks every means to dominate the first wife. This is because she is at war with her. A rivalry is established between them. What must the first wife do?

4   She shows comprehension toward the hero and treats the new wife like a younger sister. She helps her prepare for the night and does not take offense at the vanity which the happiness of being fertile causes in the other.

Understanding the hero's reasons for interesting himself with the other, even if she has no desire to do so, she dresses the new wife so as to make her more attractive. She must take no account of the latter's behavior or her presumptuousness, due to the vanity of having been chosen, for fear of causing hostility.

Vātsyāyana explains how to avoid rivalry between wives.

The first wife must behave with the new one as if she were her younger sister and not a rival. She must prepare her and make her beautiful for the night's love games. This will develop complicity between them. If the new wife says disagreeable things to her, the elder must not take offense.

5   If the younger one neglects her duties toward her husband, she takes responsibility for it and covers up for her. The younger will then respect her and treat her favorably.

If she sees the other make some mistake with her husband, she strives to cover her so as to win her trust.

If the new wife makes some blunder with her husband, the older wife will hide it from him. If, however, it is a matter of something that may in the future affect her health, she explains to her that she must not do it again.

6 She teaches her the various erotic techniques on the quiet, in a place where the husband can hear them.

Where no one else is apt to hear them and out of the hero's sight, while arranging that the husband can hear them.

7 She is very affectionate with the other's children, amiable with the members of her family, pleasant with her friends. She is full of attention for the other's kin, without showing any preference for her own.

When the new wife has children, the elder treats them with affection. She behaves amiably toward the other's sisters, even if their husbands are disagreeable. She shows affability toward the other's friends, in order to win her affection. She shows no preference for her own acquaintance, nor speaks badly of the other's.

She shows a lively affection for the new wife's children, and is benevolent toward her servants. She treats the other's brothers- and sisters-in-law with greater respect than she does her own.

8 The first wife must welcome the new wife warmly.

And be tolerant with her.

9 If the husband shows greater affection toward one of the wives, it causes fights with the others.

10 The chief wife must show comprehension.

She sympathizes with the others, but tries to stir up quarrels. She seeks to inspire trust, the better to propagate conflict.

11 If the favorite wife seeks to dominate the elder one, the latter makes no opposition, but gives her a bad reputation.

Among the wives, one sometimes tries to dominate the other, without respecting the rules of cohabitation, and takes advantage of being closer to the husband to denigrate her in front of him when the other is absent, or for quite another reason.

If the husband tries to give importance or superior status to one of the wives, the chief wife, without herself joining in the fray, calls the other wives together to fight her.

12 The ones who importune the husband to take sides only stir up conflict.

The quarrelers who come and expose their wrongs to the husband so that he should take sides, exaggerating problems, only magnify the conflict.

After which, it is he who must arrange a peace treaty.

13 But the hostilities only grow more.

When the husband intervenes.

14 And if the conflict dies down, the chief wife does her best to revive it.

Having decided to set at variance, she seizes every opportunity to revive the conflicts instead of quelling them.

15 If the husband decides that he wants peace immediately, he himself must organize the reconciliation.

Taking the chief wife aside and speaking to her without the others, he flatters her by assuring her that he appreciates no one as much as her.

When she realizes that her husband still loves her, the first wife herself tries to make peace.

Now the subject is the attitude of the younger wife.

16 The younger wife must consider the elder as a mother.

17 Without the other's knowledge, she does not utilize the gifts she receives from her family or acquaintance.

Even clothing.

18 In everything she has to do, she stays under her control.

She considers her own initiative forbidden, being dependent on the other.

19 She informs her when she is the one to sleep with the husband.

She informs the chief wife, who has lived virtuously with him, when she herself sleeps with their husband.

20 She does not repeat to anyone what she has told her.

She does not repeat the elder's words to anyone, whether true or false, to avoid quarrels.

21 She looks after the other wives' children better than she does her own.

This involves all the children of the older wives.

22 But secretly, she takes the greatest care of the husband.

When they are alone in bed, she seeks to satisfy him better than the others.

23 If the other wives make trouble for her, she does not complain to her husband.

24 When they are alone, she tries to obtain signs of affection from the husband.

When the other wives are absent, she seeks signs of love from her husband.

25 She says to him, "You are my whole life."

Wishing to obtain special favors from him, she tells him, "Your affection is my reason for living."

26 But she does not boast of the favors or signs of affection she obtains.

From fear of arousing the fury of the other wives.

27 She who reveals secrets ends by being snubbed by her husband and causes him to humiliate her.

28   According to Gonardīya, out of fear of the chief wife, the younger wife must see that her husband's signs of affection take place in secret.

29   She must have compassion for the first wife, who has remained barren. The husband must also pity her.

She must be understanding in word and deed to demonstrate her good feelings.

30   By thus flattering the elder a little, she behaves like a loyal wife.

Such are the younger wife's relations with the eldest of the wives who, being barren, has no children.

Relations among all the wives are now envisaged, whether older or younger.

After the description of the virgin bride comes that of the remarried women. Remarried women are of two kinds, those who are no longer virgin, and those who still are. The latter are entitled to the sacrament of marriage and are therefore counted as young girls. It is said, "One must make sure in a seemly way that she is a virgin." If she is secondhand, there is no sacrament, and she is simply accepted. In the world, she is known as "soiled" (aparuddhiketi). Such a woman is not recognized as a legitimate wife by the sacred books.

According to Vasishtha, "If she has been given only in intent or in word and she is still a vigin, even if the water rite has been performed, she is marriable. She who has passed in front of the fire, or has children, is considered a widow."

The cases of those who are no longer virgin and those who have children are considered.

31   Of a woman who is a widow, or has suffered due to her husband's impotence, but is desirable and full of qualities, who remarries, it is said that she has a new existence.

Because her husband is dead, or because he was impotent, she has suffered, in not being able to have sexual relations, but she is still desirable and, according to Gonardīya's opinion, she can remarry with a man of a good family and lead a new existence.

When a widow who is unable to control her sexuality meets a sensualist (bhogī) and takes as a husband an individual endowed with strong sexuality, she is born to a new life (punar-bhava) and is called punarbhū, reborn or remarried.

32 According to the Bābhravyas, a woman must leave an unsatisfactory husband and choose another to her taste.

Quitting her husband's dwelling, she leaves, not being satisfied with him.

33 For her own satisfaction, she becomes intimate with another man. Many women procure themselves another man for amorous relations.

34 It is by experiencing their erotic qualities that a woman makes her choice, Gonardīya explains.

Comparing the amorous qualities of their erotic experiences, a woman makes her choice according to whether the man is a good or bad lover, but if she changes several times, she becomes similar to a prostitute.

According to Gonardīya, after leaving the second for the third who is more expert in love, a widow finds her current lover without interest, goes on to a fourth and then, finding a better one, gives herself to him. Thus, incessantly leaving lovers of little talent for better ones, a widow enters into the prostitutes' category.

35 She follows her own fancy, says Vātsyāyana.

If the one whose qualities the sensual woman found to her taste no longer satisfies her, she passes on to another. She can thus be seen passing from one to the other, seeking pleasure.

36 She strives to obtain the means of meeting her expenses from her family, from what she receives from her lover for her domestic tasks, and from the gifts of friends who value her.

A widow of good social standing seeks to obtain from her family, or from the jobs she does for her lover, and from what she is offered by people who value her, whatever she needs to receive those who come to her parties [madya goshthi—drink meetings], as well as the fruits and flowers she needs for her garden. She also receives clothes offered by her friends or family.

It is with such means that she arranges to live and provide for her needs.

And also for her beauty care, gifts, tips, and drinks for the parties at which she meets her friends.

37 Otherwise, she makes do with her savings, or the jewels she has been offered.

Widows of the middle or lower classes must defray their expenses with what they have been able to save. They wear old clothes or else, in case of need, what their lover has been kind enough to give them.

38 There are no rules about what her lover gives her.

39 When she leaves her keeper's house, she leaves behind whatever her lover had given her out of affection, in order to live on what her new lover gives her. If she is thrown out, she receives nothing.

She leaves of her own will, tired of her lover, abandoning the gifts she has received. She must therefore live on what her new partner gives her.

40 She goes to him whose household she can dominate.

Desiring to dominate, and to be important, she installs herself as mistress in her lover's house, for an indefinite period of time.

41 She behaves affectionately with her lover's other wives, who are virtuous and respectable.

42 She is amiable with the staff and merry with her lover's friends. If she is skilled in the arts, she teaches them to the other wives.

She is always amiable with the people of her lover's family. She laughs and amuses herself with them. Skillful in the arts, she instructs the other wives.

43 She herself reports to the husband any misconduct of those living in the house.

She reports to him any irregular conduct on the part of his other wives, such as being absent for two nights, going out elegantly dressed for a love meeting, or having relations with lesbians.

44 The widow's role consists of secretly demonstrating the sixty-four arts of pleasure, of assisting the other wives in them herself, of making gifts to their children, of behaving maternally with them, decking them out and dressing them with care. She shows great patience with servants and friends and willingly takes part in parties, drinking bouts, walks, and amusements.

She continues to sleep with the hero and practices the postures, embraces, and other practices that stimulate men.

She assists the other wives, the women of the family, with their dress, jewels, and makeup. She treats them with respect since they are of good family. She treats the servants like friends, with patience and gifts.

She merrily takes part in parties, drinks willingly, and also likes going for walks.

In a hidden place, she demonstrates the sixty-four arts, according to the hero's desire. She is well-disposed toward the other wives, without being prompted to do so. She places herself humbly at their service, with great respect and affection.

45 If one of the other wives suffers from barrenness, the widow shows more attention to her than to those that have children, and protects her. If she so desires, she teaches her the arts.

Certain women are unhappy because they are barren. Conduct with them must be the same as with those that have children. According to the husband's instructions, the widow behaves with them as she does with the other wives. Taking them under her protection, she teaches them to be skillful in arts such as paper cutouts. In showing their skill, they lose the feeling of being unfortunate.

Among married women, some are persecuted by the other wives because they are barren. The widow must aid these unfortunates, without taking the side of the other wives, in such a way that the husband will grant them his favors. She teaches them the arts that are worth showing, because in showing their ability, their melancholy vanishes.

46   The husband employs his childless wives as dry nurses.

They take care of and feed the children of the others.

47   They show their attachment by the welcome they give to the master's friends.

48   A barren woman must attend to religious rites and also sleep with the husband.

For religious duties such as the ceremonies in memory of the dead, she must take the initiative and see that the hero's fast days are observed.

49   She must be amiable with the family, without attempting to give herself importance.

With the other wives, as also with the members of the family. Because she is barren, her position is that of an excluded person. In other respects,

50   In sleeping with him, by her skill she stirs up again the attraction he feels for her.

Knowing his temperament, in her relations with him, even if he is not inspired, she proves to him the attraction he feels for her.

51   She makes no reproaches to him, nor does she reveal her wiles.

She does not reproach him for not loving her, nor does she pride herself on her skill in manipulating the man's penis.

52   When there is strife, he turns away from her.

If she is in conflict with the other wives, he is annoyed with her, and if she approaches him for love, under some pretext he turns her away.

On the other hand, the hero seeks to draw to himself the wife who quarrels with the widow.

53 The widow seeks to let him meet, in hiding, the girls he secretly desires.

Performing the job of messenger, she arranges meetings and keeps matters secret.

54 She must contrive that the hero considers her devoted and without treachery.

She must accommodate herself to the situation. Frigidity is often the cause of barrenness.

The more numerous the wives, the more the hero considers them as a weekly fatigue. Often, he refuses to couple with the one whose turn it is, and sends her away.

The hero is of two kinds: royal or boorish.

In describing the first, it is a matter of the harem. The atmosphere of a gynoecium is such as described, and can be compared to a prison.

With regard to royal customs and the affairs of the harem.

55 The environment and organization of the harem are described.

The description deals with the inner chambers of the harem, the women who live there, and matters concerning them. The case of the sole wife and of the first wife with the others must be considered separately.

The conduct of the eldest and youngest wife have been described. The behavior of queens in the harem is the same.

56 The queens must have servants or eunuchs to bring the king flower garlands, ointments, and clothes as gifts.

The messenger shall say, "This is from this or that queen."

57   On accepting them, the king gives his own necklace in exchange.

To express his affection.

58   Elegantly dressed, in the afternoon he comes to see each of the inhabitants of the harem, who are covered with jewels.

Elegantly dressed, the king, carrying the objects received, pays them a visit, with an amiable word for each.

59   He makes them sit for a moment, according to their rank, and chats jestingly with them.

He makes them sit down, taking into account their family rank, since this is a requirement of etiquette. He converses laughingly with all the women who are his wives.

60   After which, he goes to see the widow.

After having paid his wives a visit, he goes to see the widow alone, because she can have no rank.

61   He then goes to see the courtesans and dancers who live in the harem.

62   Widows have a place apart in the harem.

Among the queens, but in the outer harem, where the dancers also live. First comes the residence of the queens, his legitimate wives. Then, in the outer part of the harem, the kept women, after which, outside, the courtesans, and further outside, the residence for actresses and dancers.

63   The assistants of the king's pleasures choose those who are ready for love, sending away with the servants those of whom it is not the turn and those who are menstruating. In the afternoon, after the king has arisen, they prepare the love chamber and send him those of the queens whose turn it is, who have sent him ointments marked with their name.

Discarding those who are not in condition for sexual relations, the assistant chooses from among the wives in turn for the love chamber the one who is just at the right moment of her cycle, whose gift of perfumes he has accepted, and who wears his ring on her finger.

The assistant who organizes the king's pleasures in the harem smears the one who has received his ring with saffron and, after the king has breakfasted and had his siesta, arranges the encounter in the love chamber.

64   The king invites the one he has chosen to the love-chamber.

To whom he has given his ring.

The queen whose gifts the king had accepted and who has received his ring is advised through a maidservant of the harem that the king awaits her in the bedchamber.

65   For festivals, concerts, and theater spectacles they are all invited, according to rank.

The noble ones like the others take part in drinking bouts.

At harem festivals, the king honors all the queens and offers them wine to drink. Furthermore, they are all invited to receptions and concerts.

66   Harem residents must not go out. People from outside may not enter, except the women who come to work there, on condition that they are not loose-living or sick.

Those who are well behaved; the others are not employed, nor are the sick. Only those who are apt for work, with goodwill and pleasant relations.

67   In this connection, a quotation:
"The man who has several wives must treat them equally. He may not neglect some and put up with the short-comings of others."

He must not show that he is enamored of one of them in particular, nor overlook the ill-conduct of those who behave badly by putting up with their defects. He must keep the peace between them.

68   If he is particularly excited by sexual games with one of them and is especially attached to her, he must not say so to the others.

So that the others are not offended by it.

69   He must not let strife due to cohabitation develop among his wives, and must know how to reprimand those who deserve it.

He must not allow rivalries to establish themselves, due to the women's coexistence, and must reprimand the ones that deserve it, and not the others.

When there is strife among the wives, he must not stir them up, and must scold and accuse the one who starts the quarrels.

70   In secret he shows trust in one, while publicly praising another. He shows great respect for yet another. Thus he pleases all his women.

He secretly gives confidence to those who are shy. He publicly showers praise on those who are anxious to mark their rank among the wives and flatters those who are vain.

In such a way must he strive to please all his wives.

71   He gives pleasure to one by strolling in the garden, to another by making love, to a third by gifts, by praising those who are cultured, by giving secret appointments. Thus he keeps them all satisfied.

As a conclusion to this chapter,

72   A young woman who has conquered her husband's initial shyness and behaves according to the established rule takes him into her power and dominates the other wives.

Whether she is sole wife or under the thumb of an older one, with whom she has to bear the arduous aspects of cohabitation,

The wife who, knowing how to check her anger, behaves according to the rules of the *Kāma Shāstra*, holds her husband in her power and dominates the other wives.

This chapter is the continuation of the previous one, describing the behavior of the sole wife. This one deals with her conduct in the presence of other wives.

First she wishes to know the reason for the other wives. Vātsāyana explains that the causes are her stupidity, her lack of seriousness, her barrenness, or the fact that she only gives birth to daughters, provoking her husband's desire to have other wives.

Vātsyāyana gives these reasons for polygamy among ordinary men, since the powerful, the rich townspeople, kings, and so on, do it to show off. From a social point of view, Vātsyāyana generally conceives of two wives for the ordinary citizen and explains the duties of the chief and younger wife. When a man is unwise enough to take more than two wives into his house, what is their relative position, and the conduct of a wife toward her seniors and juniors?

In the case of two wives, what must be the conduct of the elder? According to Vātsyāyana, she must behave as if the younger were her little sister. She must always be attentive to her happiness, to the point of organizing her love meetings for her, teaching her erotic skills, showing great affection for her children, and being more amiable with the members of her family than with her own brothers and other kin. If there are several co-wives, the senior one must behave in this way with the younger ones. If they are too numerous, however, she cannot avoid strife. Due to questions of rivalry, enmities develop among them. If the husband prefers one of them, those who were the former favorites make war on her. When strife breaks out, the chief wife must strive to calm the others, since otherwise, by means of such conflicts, the house becomes a battlefield. However, in the midst of a crowd of wives, an intelligent and honest woman can cleverly organize her life. Such a wife respects the chief wife and considers the latter's children as her own. She does not throw remarks here and there about the great wife. When she has the chance of sleeping tranquilly with the husband, she contrives that he continues to be attracted by her, by giving him pleasurable treatment. When her co-wives make trouble for her, she does not tell it to her husband, who, in her soul, is a god, although she may sometimes mention it to others.

Vātsyāyana explains that an astute co-wife must remember that if she manages to gain influence over her husband by her skill, she must not be proud of it or treat the others with contempt. She does not reveal the secret bonds that exist between her and the husband, since she would lose his trust and would be despised by him.

Vātsyāyana explains that, if the chief wife has the misfortune to be barren, the others must have compassion for her and the husband must be prompted to treat her with kindness.

In this chapter, Vātsyāyana also contemplates the case of a remarried widow, whom he mentions among the wives. One may marry a young girl who becomes a widow after her first marriage. The remarried widow is of two kinds: the one a virgin, the other not. The *Vasishtha Smriti* says that the girl who has remained virgin, if she had only been betrothed and given, but without consummation of the marriage, may, with her own agreement, be remarried according to the rites. Since, according to circumstances, she has been married twice, she is called reborn (punarbhū).

According to the Scriptures, remarried widows are of six kinds: virgins; those who are not; those who have had children; etc. A woman who, being unable to control her feelings, has had sexual relations with a man, is also called punarbhū (remarried). The second marriage of a virgin widow is permitted by Scripture, but for one who is no longer virgin, the rites are forbidden. She is taken for what she is and considered as a kept woman (rakhela).

In this chapter, Vātsyāyana also mentions divorce. He explains that when a woman leaves her husband and, to satisfy her desires, sets herself up in another's dwelling, then again leaves him, she can do this without any problem. If she claims that he lacks temperament, that he is impotent, and so on, Vātsyāyana says that a woman who, driven by her sensuality, leaves a man whom she has married, not only leaves one man, but may do so with a thousand.

This is why she is not respected. When she has managed to catch and has left two, three, or four, she is no longer counted as a wife, but as a whore. On the other hand, Vātsyāyana explains that the best sort of remarried widow is one who, once established in the dwelling of someone she esteems, places herself at the family's service, as if it were her own. She busies herself by welcoming guests, with charities and religious offerings, expenses for the garden and for receptions. If she abandons one lover, on a whim, to go with another, she must give back all the things that he had given her.

The duties of the numerous wives dwelling in the king's harem are special, since among them some are considered to be of high rank, or else of middle or low extraction. For kings, the wise author of the *Kāma Sūtra* explains that, whatever the number of wives, he must treat them all with the same consideration. He explains that a woman's success among the other wives depends on whether she knows how to check her anger and set an example by her behavior. She also gains ascendency over her co-wives and over her husband.

Here ends the Second Chapter
Concerning the Conduct of Wives
and the Fourth Part entitled
Duties and Privileges of the Wife
of the Kāmā Sūtra *by Vātsyayana*

Part Five

Other Men's Wives

[Paradārīka]

Chapter One

BEHAVIOR
[Shīla]
OF WOMAN AND MAN

The ways in which a man has sexual relations with a girl or a widow have been explained in detail. The matter now is those who behave like prostitutes. Love with other men's wives is a matter of pleasure and money. In explaining the means of reaching sexual relations, the question of prostitution is taken before that of adultery. Vātsyāyana explains why sexual relations with women married to other men are forbidden.

1 The reasons for not sleeping with other men's wives have already been explained.

Since sexual relations with women married to another will not bring the joy of having children, this question has been correctly explained in the general remarks on women.

2 In this connection, the possibilities of success must first be examined. What risks are involved? Does she want to make love? And so on.

309

One should reflect deeply before having relations with married women. If it works, what do I risk? Is success possible without taking too many risks? When I have possessed her, what are the risks for the reputation of either of us? What will be the effect of our union? My own reaction? And what will remain?

Before allowing oneself the desire for relations with another man's wife, one should reflect: Shall I obtain the one I desire or not? If I am successful, shall I have problems? Is it worthwhile? Once I have conquered her, will our relationship last? And what shall I gain thereby?

3   When he realizes that his passion is passing from one stage to another, in order to avoid destroying himself as a result of this passion, he proceeds to take possession of another man's wife.

At the sight of the woman, passion is aroused in the form of violent desire to possess her and, passing from one stage of passion to another, he is deeply affected by it. Seeing the state of his feelings, he must contrive to possess her, since he cannot renounce it.

If he reaches the conclusion that "without this woman I cannot live," he must arrange for them to sleep together.

What are the stages [sthāna] of passion?

4   The stages of development of passion number ten.

Considering the madness of love that, not reaching its goal, grows continuously and ends by leading a man to renounce life, the Master forewarns against the extremes of behavior that result from it. The stages of amorous passion are ten in number:

5   A vision gives rise to a desire, which takes hold of the mind and becomes an obsession. He can no longer sleep, his body weakens, he loses interest in everything, loses all sense of propriety, loses his reason, loses consciousness, and ends by dying. These are the ten characteristic stages of amorous passion.

Having glimpsed the woman, he feels a burning desire to unite with her. His passion then grows and he tries ceaselessly to see her again. Not being able to implement his desire, it becomes a fixation. From this fixation arises the will to find the means of obtaining her, which becomes an obsession. He loses his sleep. Not sleeping, he gets thinner. He loses interest in everything. Being wholly preoccupied, he ends up by burning with fever. Losing all sense of propriety and all fear, he goes mad. He has fainting fits and, having ruined his health, he ends by dying. Such are the stages of a passion that commence with a simple glance.

6 According to the authorities [ācharya] on the subject, in such a case, one must first examine the physique and character of the young woman, her virtue, faithfulness, purity, and availability, and measure the violence of one's own passion.

Before letting amorous desire take hold, he must first examine the woman's character, her physical aspect, the signs of love games on her body, which are indicative of her behavior, her faithfulness, purity, life, her blameless conduct, so as to decide whether the enterprise is worth the while.

According to the masters of the *Kāma Shāstra*, before attempting to sleep with another man's wife, an intelligent person will strive to tell from her appearance, beauty, and peculiarities which woman is virtuous, honest, and faithful, and which could be attracted by adultery.

7 According to Vātsyāyana, a woman's nature can be known from the indices of seduction, by which she reveals her behavior and her tendency to unfaithfulness and sexual union.

Examining the possibilities of sexual relations from her appearance, beauty, character, faithfulness, and purity, before going ahead, he must consider whether or not she is attainable by violence or gentleness. After this, he decides to pursue his enterprise according to the indices of seduction. The reasons for excluding the same are three, as concerns a man and woman who are greatly attached to each other, and are faithfulness, virtue, and purity.

Vātsyāyana's opinion is that, by examining a woman's body and the marks on it, one can know whether she is faithful or dissolute.

8 It happens that a woman desires a man whose excitation she sees and that the man also desires her. As a result of some impediment, however, as Gonardīya explains, they cannot fulfill their desire.

It happens that a married woman is attracted by another man. She desires him, excited by his fortune or his appearance. Thus, passion is born. On his side, seeing the woman excited, the man desires her. An obstacle, for some reason, arises, preventing them from uniting. Full of erotic ardor for each other, they are thus both in a state of frustration. Gonikāputra speaks of this to teach them to be more skillful.

9 Although the feeling is similar for both, it is stronger in the woman.

Although they are both in the same state, the feeling is stronger in the woman.
Women who tend to fall in love with someone else are more often encountered than fickle men.

10 A woman in love takes no account of what is good or bad. If there is an obstacle on the path to her goal, however, she will not persevere.

If she has an inclination, she does not care to know whether it is good or bad. She desires things too intensely. If, however, as a result of some obstacle, she does not reach her objective, she immediately sees the error and, realizing her mistake, makes up her mind what to do, since it is women's nature not to see a mistake till after the attempt.

11 By nature, she refuses a man what he desires.

Although she wishes to make love with him, she refuses to give herself, but seeks a reason to unite with him. To seek a pretext is her nature.

12 Approached many a time and oft, she eventually gives way.

Because she wishes to.

After the man has made repeated attempts, she ends by sleeping with him.

13 For reasons of ethics or responsibility, some men prefer to give up, although they are in love and are awaited.

Due to the prohibition of the sacred books and the Aryan rules of conduct, although he desires it, he renounces the idea, the reasons for his behavior being either concrete or intangible.

14 Even if she is set on uniting with him, she will not manage to do so.

Because of the obstacle of virtue, or because of her good reputation, the woman who desires to unite with him does not manage to. This is due to her moral sense, since there is a step to be taken between desiring an act and committing it.

Although the woman seeks to lure him into the trap of her love, she does not succeed in catching him.

15 In an occasional relationship, after the act of love, the woman wants a repetition. He, having obtained it, becomes indifferent.

Not attaching great importance to it, after making love, he is not interested in repeating the act. This is characteristic of a man who seeks only erotic pleasure. His business having succeeded, he becomes indifferent, and does not seek to repeat the act, because it is a matter of pure eroticism.

Women make love to establish a pleasant relationship. But a man, once he has ejaculated, becomes melancholy.

16 He does not esteem a woman who is easy to have, but is interested in one who is difficult to obtain. This is a general rule.

Out of a spirit of contrariness, he disdains a woman who is easy, and falls in love with one who makes difficulties.

17 The causes of refusal.

The reasons for which a woman does not desire another man are as follows:

18 Because she loves her husband.

Her husband's love is the cause of her refusal, even if she likes the other.

19 Because of her children.

Out of regard for her children, whether she is nursing them or from mere affection.

20 Because she has passed this stage.

Because she has matured, she is ashamed to give her body to another man.

21 Because she has troubles.

Full of sorrow as a result of the death of a loved one, even if she wishes to, she refuses.

22 She cannot manage to free herself.

Since her husband is always close to her, she does not see how she can get away from him.

23 If she is invited to, without the proper forms, she gets angry.

Put suddenly to the question, without any sign of respect, fear is the reason for her anger.

24 He gives up the enterprise if it appears without a solution.

Desperate at not succeeding, he gives up.
Realizing that she will never give herself to a man, he renounces the idea of sleeping with her.

**25   She is seeing someone else or is in love with another:
he withdraws.**

*She is going with another, so there is no possibility for the time
being. There is no hope of enticing her for a long time if she is in love
with someone and is not, for the moment, available.*

26   Because he lacks discretion, she flies from him.

*"He does not hide his feelings in public. He will make me everyone's
laughing stock." And she runs away from him.*

**27   He speaks of his intentions with his friends and fol-
lows their advice.**

*He reveals his intentions to his friends and suits his behavior to
their suggestions. He follows their advice instead of seeking to understand the woman's feelings.*
This is why she does not want him.

28   She suspects that he is without financial means.

Thinking that he is penniless, she avoids going with him.

29   She fears his violence.

*He does not know how to control his temper and causes distress.
She stays out of his way.*

30   The hind fears sexual ardor.

*The hind has a weak character. The hind is afraid of being subject
to one who is capable of sexual brutality.*
Women of the hind category do not want to sleep with a man
endowed with a large instrument, or whose temper they fear.

**31   She distrusts a townsman who is too skillful in erotic
technique.**

*Townspeople are too cunning, too expert in love: the innocent
peasant girl is frightened of it.*

If the man is from the town and is highly skilled in erotic technique, she refuses to sleep with him out of modesty.

32 She prefers they should remain friends.

He behaves to me like a friend. I fear what his attitude may be afterward.

33 She is shocked by his ignorance of the customs of the country and period.

He is not informed about local habits.

34 She despises him because he is of low extraction.

Due to his inferior status, she fears that her girlfriends and other people will leave her.

35 He is stupid because he does not understand when he is given a sign.

When he is presented with an opportunity, he does not seize it: he understands nothing.

36 For an elephant woman, a hare is insufficient.

For an impassioned cow-elephant, the hare appears to lack the means. The elephant woman, when she realizes that the man belongs to the hare category, that his instrument is small and that he lacks temperament, has no desire to sleep with him.

37 Out of compassion, she fears to hurt him.

"Because of me, in wishing to mount me, he risks hurting himself." She takes pity on him and does not desire to sleep with him.

38 Stating her own defects, she refuses.

Considering her own defects, sicknesses, unpleasant smells, she avoids sleeping with him.

39 She refuses likewise, fearing for her future, since if it were known, her parents would throw her out.

Fearful that on learning of the affair, her family would reject her.

40 Because he is old, she has no consideration for him.

Finding him old, she does not respect him.

41 She asks herself whether he is not a connection of her husband's.

She reflects, "Has he been sent by my husband?" With this idea, she refuses to meet him.

42 For ethical reasons.

There are a few women who pay attention to what is good or bad. Because she has religious principles, she refuses to commit an evil act.
For the one who seeks to seduce her, the following is suggested:

43 Among the reasons for refusal, he must first determine which can be attributed to his person.

Among the causes of refusal, he must first of all consider the ones of which he is the cause and, having determined these, eliminate them so as to avoid a refusal.
What must a man do, who wishes to seduce other men's wives? The procedure is clear: he must astutely hide his own weaknesses and defects from them.
If his defects have already been perceived by the women, what must he do?

44 Moral objections do not resist the mounting of passion.

Moral objections, her husband's love, the fact of expecting a baby, of having passed the age, because she is in mourning, religious convictions, and all those barriers connected with Aryan ethics, are broken down by the growing of passion. This is why it is necessary for love to grow.

45 The means of counteracting failures are indicated below.

"In order not to be rejected by her, I must be conscious of my own defects."

46 Familiarity overcomes excessive pride.

A citizen who is skilled in the arts, when at loss for arguments, should behave as a friend. Familiarity will overcome the pride of a married woman.

A woman draws away from too enterprising a man, but her fear decreases when she knows him better.

47 He must skillfully avoid shocking people.

If he makes blunders from ignorance of local customs, he must acknowledge his errors. He must know how to bear humiliations due to social rank, gray hair, and other things that diminish him. He must skillfully obtain forgiveness for any humiliations borne by the heroine, which may have affected her vanity in front of others, drawing his inspiration from the techniques taught by the treatise.

He must adroitly remedy reticences borne of a feeling of humiliation.

48 He contends with the effects of his mistakes by his humility.

Scolded for his ignorance and for not having hidden his feelings from his friends, he develops an inferiority complex. He makes his excuses when he is alone with her.

By his humility, he removes any doubts that the woman had about him.

49 It is the same with doubts arising from fear. It is necessary to inspire trust.

If highly excited, he is capable of violence; if he is a hare, he lacks temperament; if he is of another sphere, what will become of him in the future? He must remedy all these fears by inspiring trust.

If he knows how to control his behavior, success is in sight. Otherwise, union is impossible. The question is now to know which men are appreciated by women.

50 Generally, the characteristics of a successful man are as follows: he knows the *Kāma Sūtra*; he knows how to tell tales; he has been known by her since childhood. Being of the same circle, they have grown up together and their mutual trust derives from their games and other contacts. He does what he is asked. He speaks well. He knows how to make himself agreeable. She has obtained information about him beforehand through competent messengers. Having heard the praises of his friends, she knows he is charming. He has already had amorous experiences. He is a neighbor, and they have been children together. He has an erotic temperament. He is popular with the servants, with her nurse, and with the newly wed couple. He likes strolling in the garden. Proud as a bull, he is patient, courageous. From the point of view of culture, aspect, and qualities, he is better than her husband, greatly superior also in his ways of doing things.

Men who have success are usually those who know the Kāma Sūtra, *who know how to tell a story. If they are also expert in love, they have success with women.*

Those who have frequented each other's houses since childhood develop a reciprocal affection and are successful. A young man who is already adult, knowing how to treat women, is successful.

He who has become a confidant in games, cutting paper, etc., meets with success; he who does what she asks of him is successful; he who expresses himself in a seemly manner, with moderation, succeeds; he procures what she wants and gives it to her; sent as messenger for another whose praises he should sing, it is he who manages to seduce her.

He ends by succeeding from having courted her much; because he has already had amorous relations with girls, he succeeds; if he has a reputation for getting women pregnant, he succeeds.

They have grown up together, in the same house: he succeeds; neighbors reveal that he is of a libidinous temperament: he succeeds.

Making friends with the nurse, what he learns through her about the husband makes him succeed. In houses with newly married couples, he succeeds with the women. He loves shows, dancing, theater, strolling, and journeys. He behaves amorously with women: he succeeds. He has a reputation for being a bull, which women like.

Audaciously, he reacts immediately when women call him. Courageous, knowing no fear, he is ready to seduce other men's wives. With those who are tired of sleeping with their husband, even though he is their support, he succeeds in making love for the sake of pleasure.

Coming from a good family, he is greatly superior to the husband, in culture, appearance, and manners. In any case, a man of amorous temperament pleases women.

51   He must contemplate the means of obtaining the woman he likes.

While thinking over the means of implementing his enterprise, he must reflect, "What kind of woman is she? Is it possible to conquer her or not?"

52   The women that can be obtained without any effort are as follows: one it suffices to set one's hand to in order to have her; one who is always on the doorstep, looking along the street leading to her house; one who goes to indoor receptions dressed very scantily; one who always looks at men; one who, when she is looked at, looks around her; one on whom a co-wife is imposed for no particular reason; one who is visibly hostile to her husband, or without family, or without a husband.

The ones that can be obtained without effort or difficulty are those that stand at the door looking at men; those who usually stay beside the door can be obtained with a few jokes. Those who find themselves with another wife, through no fault of their own, and out of revenge desire another man. Those who detest their husband and want nothing to do with him, even if he has qualities. When there is such hostility toward the husband, the couple is generally unstable.

A woman without a family is generally shameless. One who has no husband needs to depend on someone else.

53 One who boasts incessantly of her high birth, whose children are dead, who likes parties, who is friendly with everyone, who frequents loose-living persons, who is a virgin, whose husband is dead, who has suffered greatly from poverty, whose husband has a first wife, whose husband has many brothers, who is vain but scorned by her husband, who is proud of her talents, which her stupid husband denigrates, who is neglected by her husband: such women look elsewhere.

Born of a well-known family and being always reminded of it, her attachments are elsewhere.

Her children dying, leaving her husband without offspring, she thinks that with another man she will be fruitful.

Fond of parties at home, or at the homes of her girlfriends, she looks for distraction.

She falls head over heels in love with people and adopts them, frequents loose-living women, actresses, dancers, and often prostitutes.

A widow, though still a child, whether or not a virgin, her innocence is already lost.

Having suffered poverty, she is attracted by those who can spend.

She has learned everything from her numerous brothers, or from an older wife, or from her brothers-in-law.

Saddened at being ignored and neglected by her husband, out of a wish to be appreciated, but not being desired, she no longer takes pleasure in his company.

54 Women who become dissolute are those who, while adolescents, have been married by force and have not been allowed to marry the man they wanted. One who is a man's equal in mind, intelligence, character, and aptitude. One with a quarrelsome nature, who takes sides, blamed without having any fault, humiliated in front of her equals, whose husband is on a journey, whose husband is irascible, dirty, impotent, lazy, fearful, hunchbacked, dwarfish, deformed, dissolute, loutish, evil-smelling, sick, or old.

Married by force when still a child, by freak of chance, she has never made love with him. She is in love with another, whom she desires, out of long-standing love.

One who is his equal in intelligence and ability, by her knowledge of the arts and her capacity for learning, becomes a rival.

If they are of the same circle, the same country, have the same sort of behavior and same nature, she becomes a rival. Scolded by her husband without having done anything wrong, she will not bear it. She desires someone else. He treats her as inferior to her equals, humiliating her as compared to other wives of similar status: out of spite, she desires another man.

If her husband is unfaithful to her while traveling, who would not look for another? If a man gets annoyed for no reason, his wife will soon take a gigolo [vita] as a lover.

He has a bad smell, he does not wash: his disgusted wife turns away from him.

He belongs to the gypsy caste, so his wife usually works as a prostitute.

He is impotent [klība].

Being lazy, he neglects his work, and she does not trust him. If he is fearful, his wife will seek another who is courageous.

If he is hunchbacked, dwarfish, or deformed, or uses crutches, since she has a horror of his deformities, his wife takes no pleasure with him.

If he has two or more wives, she knows that with two wives happiness is at an end. A peasant woman cannot bear a husband who is a townsman.

If his body smells bad, there is nothing stimulating about it.

Likewise if he is sick for a long time, if he is old or at death's door. In order to terminate the three subjects of this chapter,

55   Here is a quotation:

"A desire that arises spontaneously increases with experience. From mutual understanding comes ardor, which, gradually, becomes a permanent feeling."

Excited on seeing her, he desires her. Once he has made contact, with a view to amorous relations, his desire increases. The longer he knows her, the more his ardor becomes explicit. Seeing that relations are possible, he becomes excited. When he sees the possibility of fulfillment, he is seized with ardor and his passion becomes a reality, becomes permanent.

It is normal for a woman to desire any handsome man and for a man to desire any beautiful woman. In attempting to establish relations, these desires become explicit and occupy their whole mind. The intention thus becomes an obsession.

56 Knowing that he has reached his goal, he unites his rod with the woman. A man who knows how to remove obstacles succeeds in possessing women.

Feeling that he has succeeded, he thinks, "This is the moment to possess her." His rod indicates his readiness. The shape of the sex is always an indication. It can be seen, if it rises from increased desire, while they are still apart. It reaches its goal when it penetrates the woman.

Realizing that he has brought his enterprise to a successful conclusion, deducing the woman's state of mind from her glances, and finding the means to set aside any difficulties, the man then manages to sleep with other men's wives.

The *Dharma Shāstra*, or codes of ethics, saying that "other men's wives are like your mother," imply that one should respect other men's wives, whereas the *Kāma Shāstra* explains the ways to seduce them. It should not be deduced from this that the *Kāma Sūtra* is contrary to ethics: it has nothing to do with ethics. Indeed, virtue, prosperity, and love are interdependent. They are mixed up with the life of mankind like the warp and woof of cloth. Eroticism is just as important in this world as in the next, but the author of this treatise does not let his eyes wander from the substance of his subject. He looks at good and evil in the same way.

The *Kāma Sūtra* is not a treatise on ethics, but it does not transgress the bounds of ethics and social convention. The *Kāma Sūtra* represents a philosophy, a point of view about the world. It constitutes a code of behavior.

Man's inclinations and tendencies are described in detail, with the aim of ensuring happiness. The treatise gives advice about good things as well as about bad, and one should behave so as to make oneself as happy as possible. From the point of view of the author of the *Kāma Sūtra*, sleeping with other men's wives is a sin. But how could he hide such a reality? How could he ignore this aspect of human nature, since it has been practiced from age to age, throughout the history of mankind? It is in following this principle that Vātsyāyana has included a chapter on "eloping with another man's wife." For the same reason, in the *Upanishads*, copulation with other men's wives is indicated in connection with the practices of the left hand (vāmadevya).

In the *Āyur Veda*, the treatise on medicine, copulation with other men's wives is indicated as a remedy for erotic fever (kāma-jvara). Vātsyāyana is not only the author of a treatise, but also a theoretician and reformer of the state and of society. He states clearly that his description of good or evil acts is made from the point of view of studying his subject, from the point of view of science. It is the task of thoughful persons to use their discernment and take the good aspects, separating water from milk. Just as medical science explains that for certain diseases one should eat dog meat, similarly, in special circumstances, an individual may find himself in need of sleeping with other men's wives, and he should put it into practice only after a serious study of the *Kāma Sūtra*.

There is nothing shocking in this. If, however, everyone considered it part of normal ethical conduct, social barriers would no longer exist, the mixture of castes would affect the children, the ethics of the state would collapse, and the result would be the decline of the human race. The dominion of ethics would disappear. The state and society, no longer having any rules, would become like animal societies.

With this intent, Vātsyāyana describes the ten situations that arise at the moment of sexual union. There is no shame involved in describing these ten erotic situations, such as, for example, relations with other men's wives. Such desires comprise ten erotic situations that are universal. The essence of what Vātsyāyana says is that, in order to fulfill one's heart's desires, whether it is a question of a young girl or a young boy, of one's own wife or the wife of another, or of any other person, the solution can be found in these ten general situations, which are the aim of this chapter and which concern not only other men's wives.

The ten erotic situations of which Vātsyāyana speaks do not only concern men, but are also applicable to women. Just as men seek to go with other men's wives, women also go with other women's husbands. Just as a man who wishes to sleep with another man's wife strives to reach his goal, a woman who wishes to sleep with another woman's husband also exerts herself. Another factor is that a man knows neither shyness nor hesitation and has great daring, while a woman lacks audacity and impudence. Her desire, however, is not less than the man's. This reality should not be ignored. Proof is given by the dialogue between Yama (the god of the infernal world) and his sister Yamī, in the *Rig Veda*. Yama's sister, agitated by desire, says to him:

"This place is totally uninhabited: here one can never meet or see anyone. I am now nubile: sleep with me and beget a son in my belly. This is my desire."

Hearing these words of his sister's, immodest and against the law, Yama replies:

"You are my sister. I cannot commit with you an act that is against the law. What you say and what you want to do are not right for a sister, even though, as a game, the equinoxes do it. But those brothers and sisters who practice such perverse behavior are no longer brothers and sisters, but sinners who attract the thunderbolt and, through their own fault, go to their destruction."

In praising unions of the left hand, the *Chandogya Upanishad* says that the woman's call is the prelude, lying beside her the hymn, penetrating her sex the offertory, and ejaculation the final hymn. Thus copulation is based on the hymns of the *Sāma Veda*. "For the man who puts these hymns into practice, such coupling is fruitful. The man becomes more active, he lives his whole life, he prospers in children, cattle, and fame. He has numerous wives, he abandons no one, if such is his vow. This means he never abandons a woman who has shared his couch," explains Shankara Āchārya, in commenting on the text.

In his commentary, Rānānuja Āchārya writes, "He who suffers intensely from his adulterous desires should consider that they form part of the rites of the *Sāma Veda*, of the left hand, which does not forbid sleeping with other men's wives."

Apart from this, in the *Purānas*, in connection with the stories of Ahalyā and Indra, of Kuntīs and the sun, and in literature, those of Dushyanta and Shakuntalā, of Mālatī and Mādhava, and innumerable other love stories, no barriers are encountered to prevent one from sleeping with another man's wife.

The author of this treatise is not limited by the conventions of a period or a country. He composes a work that is valid for the whole world. He must keep in sight the happiness of mankind at all times and in all countries. It may be that in certain countries, sleeping with another man's wife is a sin, while in others it is an admissible social custom. Thus, to marry the daughter of a maternal uncle is condemned in northern India, and recommended in the south. Nowadays, for a woman to have several husbands is considered bad behavior and contrary to proper morals, yet even today in Nepal, in the Jvaunasāra tribe, it is considered a sign of nobility for a girl to have five husbands. In Kerala, among the Nambudiri Brahmans, with the exception of the eldest son, all the other sons are married to Naiyyar (Shūdra) girls, and their children belong to the mother's caste and inherit from their uncles and elder brothers, which is a fall in status elsewhere in India. In Western countries, sleeping with married women is habitual, and it cannot be said to be otherwise in virtuous India.

It may be that, prior to Vātsyāyana or his time, in some part of the earth, or among particular groups, the practice of sleeping with other men's wives was part of civilization, as proved by the *Purānas*, the lyrical works, and the *Upanishads*. This is why, if they had not been mentioned in the *Kāma Sūtra*, it would have meant ignoring an important aspect of human nature and of society, which a man of Vātsyāyana's culture could not overlook.

End of the First Chapter
Concerning the Character of Men and Women
of the Fifth Part entitled Other Men's Wives

Chapter Two

ENCOUNTERS TO GET ACQUAINTED

[Parichaya Kāranam Abhiyoga Prakarana]

Union is reached after a long association.
The ways of attaining a union with married women are described.

1 According to the ancient authors of the *Kāma Shāstra,*
if one manages to seduce a woman by one's own means,
there is no need of an intermediary. Usually, however, one
gets to possess a woman thanks to the subtle intrigues of a
messenger.

*According to the opinion of the masters, a boy can himself establish
relations with an independent woman. On the other hand, in the case
of a woman married to a monogamous man, who secretly desires to
unite with another man, whether or not she shows her desire, a go-
between is necessary for success.*

2 According to Vātsyāyana, if one can, it is better to do
things by oneself in all cases. However, if there are difficulties, a go-between should be used.

327

As far as other men's wives are concerned, one must strive to reach one's goal by one's own means. If one cannot manage, a go-between must be made use of.

From a general point of view:

3 One must speak boldly to her without reserve, when she accepts an encounter. If she makes difficulties, it is the go-between's job to convince her.

If he shows sufficient boldness, the hero may overcome her virtue without an intermediary. If the hero can talk freely to her, without taboos, what need would he have of an intermediary from the moment she shows she is disposed to discuss the situation? If she makes difficulties, one should remember the saying, "Often those who refuse have already lost their innocence. They make difficulties only with words."

Sometimes women who have already lost their virtue and have had several experiences are nevertheless difficult to approach. If the hero has no opportunity to speak to them, he does it through an emissary, since otherwise they cannot be easily conquered.

It is not recommended to take action during the first encounter, for fear of lack of hygiene or of the body's being affected by some sickness. To examine her oneself at the moment of union would be uncouth. It is by acting with full knowledge that relations are established. It is said:

4 "If one wishes to copulate, before all else, one must know with whom one is involved."

It is better to have her examined by a messenger.

If the hero wishes to make sure himself, he must first get to know her in brief meetings.

5 Meetings may be spontaneous or planned.

6 Occasional meetings take place near her own house. When arranged, they take place in the dwelling of a friend, an acquaintance, a teacher, a doctor, at weddings, religious ceremonies, archery, or walks in the gardens.

Meetings near the home may be accidental, but are often intentional. In a friend's house, while visiting a neighbor, at weddings, etc., they are the result of planning.

There are two kinds of meeting, according to whether they take place indoors or outside. The first kind is described thus:

7 To understand a woman's mentality, her behavior must be studied constantly: the way she undoes her hair, cuts her nails, adorns herself with jewels, bites her lower lip. It is by studying all these attitudes that one learns to know her. One should also listen to what her kin say about her; the gifts she receives; whether she sits on a friend's knees; whether she sometimes interrupts a conversation by yawning with a frown; whether she quietly gives advice to those listening to her; whether, out of a spirit of contradiction, she says the opposite when a young man says something, just to please herself; whether she lets the boys kiss her and embrace her; whether she takes betel from their mouth; whether she lets strangers scratch her chin [pubis]. This means that a woman behaving thus can be obtained if the opportunity arises.

One's behavior to her must be based on a study of her nature, through her appearance, expressions, glances revealing her state of mind, the way in which she does and undoes her hair, cuts her nails, looks after her body and adorns it with jewels, bites her lower lip, puts her finger in her sex to scratch it, listens willingly to the flattering words of her friends. He also examines her kin, the gifts she accepts from strangers so that the donor can take advantage of her, the way in which she sits on a friend's knees or interrupts a conversation with a yawn and a frown, saying in a low and hesitant voice, "Who was it who was talking to me?" Whether she allows herself to be touched by young people or lets herself be masturbated, rather than do it herself. Bivalent, she is attached to a boy and is the mistress of another. Behaving thus, she is clearly only interested in whatever pleases her. Receiving advice or scoldings from others, she does not bother about what might be the outcome of her bad conduct. Such a woman, who has experienced boys' kisses and caresses, sucking their tongue, who is young and scratches her pubic area, is always ready for an amorous adventure with one or another. If a boy seeks to have relations with her, he may touch her body, breast, thighs, and back as much as he pleases, caressing her or making her suffer.

She gives a double meaning to what people say to her; what she thinks of one, she attributes to another. She sucks the lips of the boy she has chosen and embraces him. She sucks the boy's tongue. With her little finger, she scratches below the pubic area. Considering both time and place, a capable boy will reach his goal.

8   Relations are easy with a boy who has been close to her since childhood, playing amorous games and children's games; whose gifts she has received; and who told her tales when she was with him: "He who is skillful with words wins people's friendship and establishes a bond with them." Hiding himself, but in such a way that she can hear him, he recites the *Kāma Sūtra*.

He has been close to the girl. While playing together, he treated her with gentleness and affection, lending her children's playthings, balls, etc. Giving and returning things creates a bond. On reaching intimate terms, he would speak to her of love and, when she has fallen in love with him, he establishes amorous relations with her. In order to create a bond, pretending that he had something to do, he would come and go to her house. Being interested in what he was doing and by going to-and-fro, she would never think of anyone else. Hiding in some place within earshot of her, he would recite the Kāma Sūtra in such a way as to let her understand the meaning. He would do it while pretending not to have seen her. Otherwise, if she had seen him, she would have treated him as a deceiver.

In this connection:

9   When their mutual acquaintance develops, he lends her objects and takes them back. Each day, at every moment, she keeps something, such as, for example, scented betel nuts.

When their familiarity increases, he leaves with her things that he has collected for her to look after and then give back to him. Leaving something and taking something back every day, she keeps a part of what she finds useful, such as scented things. In this way, in the daily giving and taking back of things she keeps for a little while, he manages to see her frequently.

10   Then, at family gatherings with the other women of his family, they find themselves together, sitting on separate seats.

With the agreement of the other women of his house, he invites her for a meal with them in order to chat with her.

11 By seeing her frequently, he manages to win her confidence.

And strengthens their amorous relationship.

12 He has whatever ornamental objects she may desire made by the goldsmith, the jeweler, the makers of flower garlands, and others. He procures them to give to her either with the aid of his people, or else procures them by himself.

He has the objects she desires made by the jeweler, goldsmith, florist, dressmaker, and others.

13 Thus, by means of constant attention over a long time, to the knowledge of all, he ends by being accepted.

He has been noted by everyone for a long time. On seeing him, they immediately understand.

14 After which, he undertakes other activities to please her.

Having finished one job, he takes on another, so as to see her constantly.

15 Anything she needs in the form of work, objects, skills, he shows his devotion by fulfilling or by finding the means to procure them for her.

He fulfills her every need, or teaches her to do so, by bringing competent people.

16 He converses with her and her servants to show her ancient customs and practices, and judge the quality of products.

17 When she consults him about some transaction, he explains how she should go about it.

Thus, in connection with the purchase of things, he gets the girl used to consulting him.

18   When discussing with her, he declares she is wonder-ful and clever, which facilitates relations.

In this connection, the author quotes:

19   "Once mutual acquaintance has been established, not-ing her signs and expressions, he approaches the girl with a view to uniting with her. Such sexual relations are per-formed secretly if the girl is a virgin. Thus she is opened by him when he unites with her."

Once they know one another, according to her signs and expres-sions, seeing she is ready, he unites with her.

He takes her as indicated in the chapter "Union with the Girl," in which the necessary approaches are indicated for seducing the girl. Girls are dissimulating, so discretion is necessary in order to possess them, while those who amuse themselves openly can be pursued with-out hesitation.

20   With a woman whose nature one knows and with whom feelings are reciprocal, whatever one possesses is shared: everything is held in common.

There is no longer any difference in their feelings and she shows what she feels. Thus they share whatever they possess: he utilizes the woman's objects and she takes his.

21   This involves precious perfumes, scarves, flowers, and also rings. Then, accepting betel from his hand, when she is getting ready to go to a reception, he asks her for the flower she has put in her hair.

When she has changed her attitude, he offers her rare perfumes with a strong scent, flowers from the north that he has found, rings of great value. After this, she accepts some betel from the boy's hand and, when she consents to accompany him to a reception or for a walk, he begs her to give him the flower fixed in her hair. In such a way, he reaches his goal.

22 He marks the expensive perfumes or precious objects
he gives her with his nails or teeth, as a souvenir.

*When the boy gives her perfumes and precious objects, if he has
them delivered by someone else, he marks them with his nails or teeth
as a souvenir, to remind her that it comes from him. By this special
means, he shows his feelings.*

23 By means of repeated encounters, an indestructible
relationship is created.

*Often, a faithful liaison is created between a married woman and
a man.*
Quoting another author:

24 "Gradually, he touches different parts of her body,
caresses her, embraces her. Then he offers her some betel.
When she gives him back the borrowed objects, he caresses
her secret parts, after which, he possesses her."

*When they find themselves in a solitary place, he caresses the
various parts of her body. She allows him to do so; he embraces her, and
so on. . . . He caresses the area of her sex, the lower part of the body,
the springing of the thighs: then he mounts her.*

25 Having made love once, he need not attempt to recommence.

Having taken her, he does not start on a second copulation.

26 She was taken in such a way as to make the copulation pleasant for her. Such an experience must not be
repeated.

*By the pleasure she found in it, the fact of having been taken is
dear to her. She does not desire another experience.*

27 According to an ancient saying, "In the house where
the husband sees or hears speak of the misconduct of other
women, it is difficult to find one who is easily accessible."
28 An intelligent man, careful of his own interests, does

not try to seduce a woman of doubtful origin, who is over-protected, fearful, or endowed with a stepmother.

Doubtful means of badly defined origins, protected by weapons, fearful of her husband. It is better not to seduce her. He does not let himself be attracted, since it would not be a sure blow.

An individual who is careful of his own interests should not seek to have, even by accident, relations with a woman who is undecided, protected, fearful, or endowed with a stepmother.

There are two aspects to the desire to sleep with another man's wife: if she is a girl whose virginity has never been taken, the man needs no go-between. He should boldly see to it himself with his own means. Since the girl has no experience, she can easily be caught in the net. An astute expenditure in this connection does not go without results.

To attract women who have experience of these games, however, it is better to use the services of a messenger, serving as an intermediary, who will know how to interpret the signs and clues, to know whether the girl is innocent or experienced.

In both cases, if one can do without an intermediary, it is better to trust to one's own efforts. It is only if obstacles are encountered during the enterprise that the aid of an intermediary is useful.

In any attempt to attract someone, acquaintance must first be made and love allowed to develop during the encounters. One must strive to see her and to be seen by her. While walking, as if by chance, their glances meet, but also on special occasions, festivals, etc., meetings can be arranged. One must know how to hug children and take them in one's arms, which are outward ways of getting acquainted. Gradually, they start speaking to each other and a bond is established. Once this first contact has been made, occasions for meeting will be found, and by coming and going to her house, a certain familiarity is established. She must be brought betel, nutmegs, sugarcane, which she can keep at home, thus getting into the habit of giving and taking. In this way, permanent relations are established and there are occasions for speaking together. One must gradually take over the burden of certain tasks, attend to what she desires at the jeweler's, the goldsmith's, and so on, and order jewels for her. One must always cut a fine figure in front of her and loudly praise her knowledge.

He starts talking to her concerning nothing in particular and strives to include her servants in the discussion. Women are very quickly caught up in the vortex of a discussion. One must praise their ability and presence of mind.

In order to trap other men's wives, the author of the *Kāma Sūtra* indicates above all the importance of a language code. Thus, the man, instead of being called by his name, is known as "the fruit," the woman "the flower," and the family "the root."

The use of these conventional signs must not be revealed to anyone. The messenger teaches them to the heroine, to be used by her when people are present. They can also be employed when writing letters.

Besides the spoken language, there is also a language of parts of the body (anga sanketa), of flowers (pushpabhāshā sanketa), of betel, of clothing, and of small packages (potali), which form five secret codes.

In the language of flowers: red flowers are used to indicate love; orange to indicate separation; if love is not reciprocal, a black ribbon; if the lover wears a necklace of this sort when leaving her, the girl knows that she is no longer loved. The beloved gets to know her lover's state of mind by means of flowers. Instead of bringing them themselves, lover and beloved send flower garlands to each other by messenger.

The ways of communicating by signs are not possible without learning them. They serve for citizens who have studied the art of love. For peasants or simple people they have no meaning. In love, they behave like animals. In practice, sign language, whether or not learned, becomes established between lovers.

Meetings are occasions on which lover and beloved can be together, but this does not imply an opportunity for misconduct. By means of various signs, attracting the beloved and inspiring trust in her, he strives to meet her. One should not hurry with this kind of activity. Patience and precautions are needed, as well as exchanges and gifts. Through his gifts, the lover shows his feeling, his good taste, and his qualities. Then he must conquer the woman's doubts, hesitation, and fears.

Once her hesitation and fears have been removed, one may commence with kisses and caresses. A place must be found, however, where they can set up their nest. Women who keep a house of call are rapacious, and have to be paid. In large towns, there are many specialized houses where women go to meet their lover, on the pretext of visiting a temple. Besides such places, the authors of the treatise speak of others that are convenient for adulterers, which are: barns, fields thick with rye, the inner courtyard of a house, ruined and deconsecrated temples, ruins, the gardener's house, the house of the dove breeder, cemeteries, riverbanks.

According to the *Sāhitya Darpana*, "There are eight places where one can hide for love meetings. These are fields, gardens, ruined temples, the courtyard of the go-between, a caravansery, cemeteries, the bank of a river."

Best of all is the dwelling of a known and trusted go-between. If such a house cannot be found, it is better to find an isolated spot in the forest. "The young girl was entranced to see the unmoving lotus leaves, of a pure emerald color, spread out for her to rest her brow" (*Kāvya Prakāsha*).

End of the Second Chapter
Encounters to Get Acquainted
of the Fifth Part entitled Other Men's Wives

Chapter Three

EXAMINATION OF SENTIMENTS

[Bhāva Parīkshā]

Once contact has been established, feelings must be examined to see whether she shows initiative and whether her resolution is certain, and to assure that she has no other amorous liaison.

1 Once contact has been made, the woman's state of mind must be studied, her feelings examined, ascertaining whether she is sure of herself and her resolution is firm, whether she has amorous relations with anyone else or lives with him as his concubine.

He examines the character of the one he desires and, having studied her feelings, embarks on action.

2 He succeeds in doing so, thanks to the advice of the go-between.

He utilizes a messenger to ascertain her feelings prior to deciding. He must make use of an astute intermediary, who does not show her preferences.

> 3 If he cannot obtain a meeting, he realizes that although
> she desires him, she is of two minds. He must therefore
> operate gradually in order to make up her mind.

*Not obtaining a rendezvous despite repeated attempts, after some
days, the hero understands that although she would like to meet him,
her mind is divided. He thus considers what he must do to succeed.*

Since she refuses to meet the hero, he concludes that, living as she
does with someone else, she finds herself in a dilemma. He must gradually find the means of getting her out of her dilemma.

In this connection, he explains:

> 4 Although not granting him the encounter, she neverthe-
> less shows herself to him, carefully dressed and adorned
> with jewels. From this he deduces that, although she is
> uncertain about coming to see him, she could be taken by
> force.

*Covered with necklaces, she shows herself to the hero. From this
he concludes that, although divided in mind, the heroine is accessible
and that he must take her by force.*

> 5 If, notwithstanding a great deal of effort and time, he
> fails to reach his aim, he must realize that the enterprise is
> fruitless and that the liaison must be broken off.

*After patiently making every effort over a long period of time, he
realizes that the enterprise is fruitless and will never lead to sexual
relations. What she is looking for is a relationship without conse-
quences. She puts his patience to the test and then breaks off the liaison.*

He must understand that the meetings have no point and that, if
he is to manage to sleep with her, it will cost him endless complica-
tions.

He may however succeed, because:

> 6 The human mind is inconstant.

*The spirit of the human race is like that. The human mind is incon-
stant, its ideas unstable. Often, after a break, the liaison recommences.*

7 After having been attached to him, she leaves him. She does not give herself, but does not reject him. She thinks that in so doing she is testing his pride, and is unable to bring the liaison to success. At such a point, an adroit go-between may manage to assist him in possessing her.

She breaks off the liaison, but keeps contact. Out of pride, she refuses to yield. There is no question of her desiring another. Indeed, she is proud of her hero and he can, in the long run, succeed with her. Through reciprocal acquaintance, her shyness, vanity, and pride fall to pieces. A go-between who thoroughly understands matters manages to help him finally possess her.

Some women are made in such a way that, after meeting their lover several times, they refuse to see him. They will not accept copulation, but do not insult him. In this they see an expression of their dignity. It is through constant attention that the lover manages to persuade them to sleep with him. Success can often be obtained with the aid of a skillful go-between.

In this connection, it is said:

8 "It is better to drop a woman who insults you when you make advances to her."

If she rejects you with abuse, it is better not to have anything to do with her.

It is better not to run after a girl who shows her lack of interest in the hero and, if he speaks to her, replies with abuse.

Nevertheless, on this subject:

9 There are women who, after having insulted you, will unite lovingly with you. These are the ones whom one must try to have.

There are those who insult you but have a loving nature. If one conquers them, one can unite with them when they have repented.

10 If, for some reason, he touches her and she allows him to do so without paying attention to it, it must be understood that she is divided between refusing and consenting.

For some reason, he touches her and she puts up with it, makes no absolute opposition. She pays no attention to it, as if she were unaware of his intentions. As a result, realizing that she is uncertain, he reaches his goal. If she allows him to touch her without stopping, her consent has been acquired.

Realizing that she is seized by doubt, the hero will manage to sleep with her if he takes her boldly.

11   Stretched out beside her while she dozes, he places his hand on her. She pretends to be asleep. If, on awaking, she removes his hand, it means that she wishes to unite with him.

Lying beside the sleeping girl, he seeks to find out whether she is disposed to have intimate relations. She pretends to sleep. Why? Because she wants to have sexual intercourse. Otherwise, why would she pretend to sleep? There can be no doubt as to the fact that she is only pretending to sleep with the aim of copulation.

12   At this point, he should rest his leg on the girl's leg.

As he did with his hand.

13   Having begun thus, he caresses the sleeping girl.

Having first slid his hand then his leg against hers, and seeing that she is disposed to have intercourse, he begins to make love to the sleeping girl, caressing her, embracing her, etc.

14   Then, on the following day, he sees whether she is still interested in intimate relations. He also gets news about it secretly from the go-between.

After having arisen, if she does not appear to be annoyed, it means she is disposed toward copulation. She is inclined to continue their relationship. She does not behave as though she were outraged, so that he knows she is ready to unite with him without standing on ceremony. He instructs the go-between to make sure of it.

If the girl is proud, however, and if she shuns a meeting the next day, he must arrange matters through the go-between.

15 If she does not show herself for some time, she is nevertheless still sentimentally attached to him. As soon as she gives him a sign, he sees from her behavior that he may try again.

If, after having been together and then remaining for a long time without seeing each other, she comes to him once more, without resentment, in the same spirit, finds him and gives him the sign, he seizes the opportunity and, understanding her state of mind, mounts her and unites with her, since she will not stand on her dignity.

16 When she is close to him, she is nervous. When they are alone, she exposes her body, her voice trembles when she speaks, her face, feet, and hands perspire. She caresses his head and massages it, then, throwing herself on the ground, she shows her passion for the hero.

This is how she expresses her feelings: she speaks in a trembling voice; her fingers and toes are wet with sweat, as well as her face, which shows her emotion when they are alone together.

When they are apart, she is agitated; when they are alone, she bares her limbs; when she speaks, her voice trembles, her words are unclear; sweat appears on her hands, feet, and face. She attempts to knead the hero's head and feet. From this, it can be deduced that the heroine is enamored of the hero.

17 Overcome with passion, she caresses him with one hand; with the other arm, she arouses him by touching him and massaging him, as though by chance.

Made bold by her excitation, when they are alone, after the go-between has brought them together, she shows her intentions by her caresses. With one hand she excites him, letting the hero see—to his seeming surprise—that she has decided to provoke an erection, considering that, if she does not touch him he will not understand. With her other hand, she caresses him.

Excited by desire, she sets about massaging his feet. With one hand she kneads his foot and with the other, she underlines her intentions, even if the boy seems surprised.

18   While sleeping, she places both her arms on him and
rests her forehead on several places on his thighs. Caressing the top of his thighs, she stops there without proceeding downward again. She leaves one of her hands there
without moving it; seizing his member, she squeezes it, and
after some time, lets it go.

*She leans on the area of the boy's sex, close to the thigh joint,
for some time and then lets it go. This should not be done against
his will.*

19   If the boy accepts her performance, the next day she
comes back to caress him again.

*Taking advantage of his state of mind, she attempts to caress him
again, having encountered no obstacles.*

20   She does not touch him excessively, but neither does
she stop doing it.

*Sometimes, out of excessive boldness, she allows her deepest feelings
to be seen.*

21   When they are alone she shows her feelings, but does
not let other people know them. She dissimulates in public,
guarding her secret from others.

22   Close to him, seeking to serve him, she is ready for
love, but if he is not aware of it, she may get the assistance
of an understanding go-between.

Seeing that he stays there, despite her signs, suggestions, and winks,
she uses a messenger to reach her goal.

23   During their conversations, she must determine the
boy's state of mind, to find out if he is interested in another.

*Despite clear signs, sleeping together remains a far-off prospect.
She must then reflect well about what he wants, whether he is interested in another girl, whether he is in love.*

24 A quotation on the subject:

"They must first get acquainted and then speak. It is by talking together that they can appreciate their feelings and understand their mutual attitudes."

25 If, by her attitude, she shows she agrees, the man can without any fear prepare to unite with the woman.

26 If, by her behavior or her feelings, a woman shows in advance that she is favorably disposed, it means that one can sleep with her without delay, even at the first meeting.

27 When a woman gives proof of friendly behavior and gives clear answers, he should understand that she is desirous of amorous relations and can be obtained instantly.

28 If an enterprising and subtle woman astutely seeks information about a boy, it is certain that she can be obtained, even if she breaks off relations.

A man who wishes to sleep with other men's wives must, in order to attract them, arrange frequent encounters. A woman with a strong character will not allow her feelings to be read immediately and will not furnish any opportunity to sleep with her.

When he meets a woman of this kind, a man should carefully examine her behavior. If she gives no favorable sign, the hero must persuade her through the medium of a go-between.

On seeing the heroine's attitude, he should understand whether his feelings are shared, and, if she will not grant him any possibility of sleeping with her, whether he should then act violently with her. A woman who is caught in the trap of having to choose cleverly puts an end to their meetings only to take them up again. She herself is undecided, "Do I really want to sleep with him or not?" With a woman in this state of mind, the boy should not give up his desire. He should not renounce sleeping with her, but just as the girl studies the boy's nature, he too should examine hers. He should ceaselessly watch her state of mind, and gradually, the girl will end by being ready for sexual congress.

Some young girls who do not usually mix with boys fall in love after a first meeting with a boy and show him that they are full of admiration. Understanding the state of mind of such girls, the boy should quietly stay close to them and, when they are alone together, even if she says no, he should take her by force.

Some women are very enterprising, but lack temperament. For the boy, it is useless to amuse himself with such women, caressing them and embracing them: a woman who lacks sensuality is of no interest. This can be realized by sleeping with her. If her interest is not aroused, one can nevertheless attempt to persevere and, when one gets to know her better, she sometimes ends by giving herself entirely.

Vātsyāyana warns the boy that the feelings of human beings are changeable. Reversals of behavior are continually encountered. A woman's nature is even more changeable than a man's, which is why they are inconsistant in their deeds and words. It is due to this instability that after breaking off a liaison, they can become attached once again.

Philosophic writings mention the instability of man's feelings. Indeed, the Yoga system was created to control the instability of the human mind.

Philosophy (darshana shāstra) is considered to be the basis for controlling thought and the instrument of liberation. The *Bhagavad Gītā* says in clear terms that man's mind is both unstable and obstinate: to control it is as difficult as controlling the wind.

Not all women, or even most women, but only some women desire to attach themselves to other men, or are even capable of being aroused by this desire. Even when they desire to do so, they find satisfaction in making those who lust after them appear stupid. For this reason, an understanding of a woman's state of mind is of the utmost importance. There can be no question of treating it as if it were twenty-two quintals of wheat: one must apply one's intelligence.

If a woman is not loose-living, and a man finds no response to his appeals, signals, and attempts, receiving, on the contrary, hard and contemptuous words, he should understand that it is useless to run after her, since this woman has no desire to go with another man. There are those who, although disposed by nature to desire to do so, are not inclined to sleep with someone, due to modesty or hesitation. This is why an astute man manages to get his hands on another man's wife after developing mutual acquaintance, attaining a certain familiarity, and studying her mentality.

End of the Third Chapter
Examination of Sentiments
of the Fifth Part entitled Other Men's Wives

Chapter Four

THE TASK OF THE GO‑BETWEEN

[Dūtī Karma]

In order to arrange a meeting, the messenger must decide on the possibilities of a rendezvous after studying the girl's behavior. Her usefulness lies in this. How does she manage it?

1 A woman whose attitudes and favorable behavior have been observed, but whom one cannot meet alone, can only be approached through the mediation of a messenger.

By certain indications and behavior, she lets it be understood that she is favorable, but remains aloof. It would not have been possible to meet her previously, or make her acquaintance. It is therefore necessary to put oneself into the hands of a messenger who will approach her and bring her gifts.

The three main virtues of the messenger are to be adroit, moderate, and enterprising.

2 She must present herself as a virtuous person and please the girl with astute chatter, telling her tales taken from

literature concerning the amorous relations of famous
women and men's adventures with other men's wives. Furthermore, she flatters the girl, praising her beauty, knowledge, her generosity, and virtues.

*To begin with, she introduces herself as a virtuous person. To
inspire trust, she must appear to be decent. Little by little, she perfidi-
ously tells her tales taken from selected texts, the* Purānas, *and literary
works recounting the adventures of women otherwise happily married,
such as Indumatī and other legendary characters. She also tells her
tales of adultery, as for example of Gautama or Brihaspati with married
women, tales of abduction, such as that of Indrachandra and others.
Once she has been accepted, what does she do? She sings the praises of
the heroine's beauty, her speech, knowledge, generosity, her skill in the
arts, her virtue, and her character.*

3   "With so many qualities, how did you manage to fall for
such a husband?" In such a manner, she inspires regrets.

*"Given your qualities, how did you get such an ugly husband?,"
and so on. The woman is then caught by regret and becomes hostile to
her husband. It would be better not to be married than to be saddled
with him.*

4   She tells her, "You wonderful woman! Your husband
doesn't even deserve to be your slave!"

5   She declares that he is without temperament, irascible,
unfaithful, a liar, mean, unstable, and suggests he has other
bad habits hidden, in order to alienate his wife.

*The go-between tells her that her husband is lacking in ardor,
while she is passionate. As she has seen, he is too quick, ejaculates too
rapidly, and is unable to bring her to orgasm. He is mean and leaves
her without money. He is coarse with people, despicable, treacherous.
Thus convincing her, staying close beside the heroine when no one can
hear her, she seeks to convince her and lead her astray and, by means
of her exaggerated talk, she finally manages to do so.*

Whatever good intentions he has, the messenger changes them
into bad intentions.

6 Noting which faults upset her, she insists particularly on those very ones.

Of the defects she exposes, she insists on those that can incite the woman to lose her virtue. She insists that the faults she describes are all real defects of the husband.

7 If the woman is a hind, she accuses the husband of being a hare.

If he has not the defect of being a hare, she accuses him of being a stallion.

8 The same applies for a mare or elephant woman.

In their case, it is not a fault to be a bull or stallion, but it is a defect to be a hare. If the woman is narrow, it is not a defect if the man has a small organ. It would be a mistake to accuse the husband of having a large sexual organ. On the other hand, for a mare or cow-elephant, the husband must not be described as a bull or stallion, but as a hare.

According to Gonikāputra, the messenger should insist on the importance of matching organs in sexual relations.

9 According to Gonikāputra's work, once the messenger has won the heroine's trust, she must speak to her about sexual relations [upasarpa], first in a subtle manner, and then boldly.

Having gained her confidence, the messenger prepares her to sleep with the boy. How does she manage it? Prudently at first, if it is the first time that she has lost her virtue. She employs indirect arguments and, with perfidious words, ends by obtaining her consent.

In order to lead the enterprise with which she has been entrusted to a successful conclusion, the messenger entices her to her own home but, if it is the first time that the heroine has been bold enough to meet a man, the messenger should not reveal her hidden purpose.

10 Describing the boy's character in a complimentary manner, she mentions his prowess in love.

She mentions how he behaves at the beginning of the act, during the act, and at the end.

She commends his simplicity and describes to the girl his wonderful performance, explaining the various sensations felt during coition, and how it proceeds at the beginning and also at the end.

11 If the woman is impeded by her concept of conjugal fidelity, the woman only speaks to her about the physical act.

If the girl is reticent as a result of virtuous feelings of conjugal fidelity, since having intercourse with another is a sin and she has never had any amorous experience, the messenger describes the physical act to her and speaks to her as follows:

12 Lucky woman! Let me tell you something strange. Someone, a young man of good social position, was overwhelmed on seeing you. The boy has lost his head and gone mad. Being of a delicate nature and never having formerly known any suffering, he is a true saint. It is to be feared that, being as he is, he will end up by dying.

He was seized with passion on seeing you and has lost his head over it. He absolutely wants to get to know you, and has asked me to arrange a secret interview with you in order to meet.

He is a young man of good social position, not a nobody. He wants to meet you whatever the cost, but he told me that he fears you may have set your eyes elsewhere, on another man, using words full of sorrow about women, inflamed by his passion. He is capable of dying of it, of destroying himself.

He is a real saint. If he cannot have you, he will die of despair.

13 Having convinced her, the following day, seeing she is caught in the snare of her words, the messenger leaves the house and then returns.

Then, satisfied at having convinced the girl, since she has not protested either in words, nor by her expression or look, she speaks openly to her.

Seeing she is interested, the messenger summons her the following day and if she sees that her face is smiling, her eyes bright with satisfaction, she takes up the conversation again without reticence.

14 She speaks to her of Ahalyā, Avimāraka, Shakuntalā, and other legendary figures and their adventures.

She makes her listen to tales like the one about Ahalyā, Gautama's wife, and her abduction by the amorous king of heaven, while the sage was walking around the sacred fire with his spouse. Ahalyā is the object of desire of the fire god, who issues from the sacred hearth in human form. Having become pregnant, she is repudiated by her father-in-law for fear of family dishonor. The child to which she gives birth is considered to be the son of the chief of the savage tribe of the Shabaras.
Roaming with the tribe of thieves [Ajāvika], he performs many noble deeds. Nourished with milk, he becomes very strong. His son, who is Ajāvika by marriage, becomes their general. Similar, too, is the story of Avimāraka: having grown up, one day while camping in the forest of the kingdom, he kills an elephant in order to save a woman whom the animal was threatening. He falls in love and marries her.

15 She describes in exaggerated terms the boy's ability in the sixty-four arts and his success with women. She intrigues her and tells her of his affairs with women with or without previous experience.

With some exaggeration, she describes his knowledge of the sixty-four arts, such as music, etc., and of the five techniques. She mentions his successes in love, the fact that he is also desired by men, admired by women, his secret successes with virgins and nonvirgins.
She mentions celebrated beauties and women of great virtue, whom he has already conquered.

16 The messenger then marks her expression.

She ascertains the effect of her words from the girl's expression.
How does the woman behave toward the messenger?

17 On seeing her, she greets her smilingly.

And asks her questions.

18   She invites her to be seated.

Calling her, she says, "Sit down on that chair."

19   She asks her, "Are you comfortable? How did you sleep? Was the food good? What are you looking for? What do you want?"

"I don't understand why you are making such efforts. What is your purpose?" she asks. In so doing, she incites her to talk about the boy.

20   When they are alone together, she unmasks her.

She gradually leads her to reveal her secret.

21   Finally, the messenger admits she is acting under orders.

The go-between does what the boy has asked of her, and reveals everything.

22   The woman then remains pensive, sighs, and yawns.

With troubled mind, she sighs and yawns, desiring the god of Love.

23   She gives the messenger gifts as a mark of affection.

She gives her a gold bracelet and a scarf.

24   She also invites her on all pleasant occasions.

For every festival, or every interesting occasion, she tells her, "Why don't you come today?"

25   Then, having established friendly relations, she dismisses her.

Hoping to see her again.

26 "You talk nicely. Why do you do nasty things and tell stories?" After which, why does she send her away in such an unfriendly manner?

She tells her, "I like seeing you and talking to you," but, challenging her stories, she adds, "Why do you do this nasty job? I welcomed you well enough. Why do you tell me such tall stories?"

27 She accuses the boy of being treacherous and faithless.

This boy is a traitor, who does not behave honestly. He is faithless and makes love to more than one girl.

28 On examining his previous conduct and the tales of his amorous escapades, which he himself has recounted, she begins to have doubts about the flattering remarks of the messenger.

Faced with the reality of him whose description she has heard, and given the list of his repeated adventures, which he himself recounts and which are too modestly described in the messenger's praises, she is seized with doubts that paralyze the positive feelings she had toward him.

29 She ridicules and throws doubt on the hero's state of mind as told to her, but she does not contradict.

Laughing, she challenges the desires of the hero who will one day fall at her feet in admiration, and also the other gossip of the messenger, which she considers as perfidious and treacherous. Unbelieving, she entertains doubts about the fulfillment of her desire.

30 Seeing her expression, the messenger reminds her of her former relations with the hero.

Speaking again about the hero and his previous contacts with her, while exaggerating them, she excites her anew.

31   By praising him and describing his qualities, without forgetting the stories of love, she revives the girl's interest.

In singing his praise, since verification is unlikely, she does not forget to recall the boy's amorous adventures, besides praising his merits. Here the authors' opinions differ.

32   According to Auddālaki, the go-between's task is impossible if they have neither spoken nor seen each other.

If they do not know one another and have never seen each other, nothing will come of it, nor any result be reached by the go-between's efforts. In this connection, it is said, "Without having made acquaintance, or having observed the other's gestures and expressions," between people who do not know each other and who have not exchanged meaningful gestures and expressions, the intermediary's task has no point. It is said that it is only after having made acquaintance and exchanged gestures and glances that the task of bringing them together can be undertaken.

According to the opinion of Shvetaketu Auddālaki, if the girl has never met the boy, the go-between's job is impossible.

33   For the Bābhravyas, however, even if they do not know one another, indirect signals may arouse interest.

If they exchange signs, even without knowing each other, the messenger can serve as a contact. As already stated, if the woman had previously given signs and indicated her state of mind, they can even have intercourse from the very first meeting.

If any agitation of the feelings appears, the messenger can do her job.

34   For Gonikāputra, even without knowing each other, without even knowing what they look like, it is possible.

Not knowing the other's appearance, without having ever met, one can still manage to imagine the other's aspect. This is why it is spoken of as "picturing at a distance."

35   For Vātsyāyana, the go-between's business may be carried out without their knowing each other and without
having seen what they look like.

*In praising the go-between's efforts, although she is merely a third
party in the business, he says, "By means of rapidly describing the one
and the other, she unites them in advance."*

36   Staying in his own home the while, he shows his good
intentions by beautiful gifts, betel, ointments, clothes, jewels, scents.

*Without any direct contact, a boy and girl who wish to meet
exchange rare things, such as betel, saffron, flower garlands, jewels,
and beautiful clothes, as a sign of friendship.*

37   Here and there on these presents, the boy leaves the
mark of his nails or teeth.

*Because of their purpose, the marks on these presents should indi-
cate their origin, indicating the hero's feelings to the heroine.*

38   The clothes are marked with stains and saffron imprints.

*Which reflect his personality, so as to remind her that it is a sign
of admiration.*

39   Having inscribed some leaves with the feelings that
perturb him, he uses them to wrap the earrings that he
sends his beloved.

*Various feelings, such as desire, sadness, anger, astonishment, mixed
with compliments, are written in the form of riddles on these leaves
with which, without damaging them, he wraps his gifts.*

40   When she receives his gifts, she thus knows the boy's
feelings.

*Having written down his states of mind, she is aware of them and,
in exchange, sends him a friendly message.*

41   Having established this bond between them, the go-
between accomplishes her role.

*Once they have accepted each other, the go-between has fulfilled
the mission with which she had been entrusted.*

42   According to the Bābhravyas, the meetings are arranged
by going to a temple or on a pilgrimage, for a walk, or in
the gardens, going to look for water, during weddings, ritual
ceremonies, walks, bathing, funerals, carriage drives in the
country, and other opportunities for meeting.

*Even if women are reticent for reasons of seemliness, boys take
advantage of any opportunity, whether in a crowd or alone: during
visits to temples, pilgrimages, going to bathe among the crowd, and not
while looking for water when it is lacking, in the case of fire in the
house that one must thus leave, when there are thieves and one pursues
them, by accepting to enter a carriage for a country drive.*
The famous authors of the Bābhravya group say that such meetings are also possible at weddings, important ritual ceremonies, festivals, funerals, civil uprisings, and fairs.

43   According to Gonikāputra, the dwellings of girlfriends,
nuns, female beggars, hermits, or ascetics are the right places
for love meetings.

Whoever seeks a place for pleasure finds it easily.

44   According to Vātsyāyana, a permanent facility is the
dwelling of the woman herself, if he knows the exits and
considers the ways of getting out. When he has managed to
enter, without any time limit for leaving, it gives them the
possibility of finding long-lasting bliss.

*Knowing the entrances and exits of the heroine's house and which
way he can enter and leave, if the times of entering and leaving are
not restricted, he can stay with her without limitations. This is not the
case in a house belonging to a girlfriend, which supplies an opportunity
for his pleasure, but is risky from the point of view of a way out.*

As a general rule, according to the task, there are several kinds of go-between.

45 Independent [nisrishtārthā], specialized [parimitārthā], letter carrier [patrahāri], acting on her own authority [svayamdūtī], messenger to an idiot [mūdhadūtī], sent by the wife [bhāryādūtī], mute [mūkadūtī], or as ungraspable as the wind [vātadūtī]: such are the eight kinds of messenger women of the adulterer.

46 The independent [nisrishtārthā] is so-called because she carries out the task she has been charged with by the hero or heroine in her own way.

As she pleases, she describes the two to each other, employing three ways of drawing them together, according to what is pleasing to the one and the other, so that they manage to make love together. For this, she uses three methods. In order to accomplish her mission, the messenger employs means that are appropriate to her mandate.

In connection with her, it is said:

47 She usually commences with flattering remarks.

In conversations with one or the other, she sings their praises and, by talking to them both, she changes their opinion. She sees them often. If the girl seems to be enamored of another man, she clears up the matter through her insistence.

The messenger, who is well known to both hero and heroine and lives familiarly with them, acts in their interest.

48 One employed by the heroine acts without paying compliments.

Hired by the heroine, she does not make use of flattering discourses, but simply arranges their meetings, without much talk. In this connection, it is said, "First make acquaintance, talk about it afterward." Sometimes, the hero, who has been spoken to, only sees flattery in it. This is not the case of the girl.

49 If they are of the same type and same character, they

will appreciate each other immediately, without needing anyone to praise them.

Having a similar character, they understand each other at once. The mandate is fulfilled at their meeting. Since their understanding is immediate, they do not need to hear flattering descriptions in order to understand each other. Sometimes, this is the best way to succeed.

50   Specialized [parimitārthā] is the name given to one who acts in a limited sphere, arranges a preliminary meeting, and does not attend to the rest.

She accomplishes her work, which is to arrange a meeting, in a limited manner and leaves the rest to fate. Thus she has a limited role. In this connection:

51   When they have seen each other's outer appearance, she leaves the rest to their spirit of enterprise.

When she has seen from their appearance that they seem to be well matched, the rest is for them to discuss. Their union depends on their boldness.
However, if their amorous efforts appear timid, it is the task of the specialized messenger to arrange so that they sleep together.

52   The letter carrier [patrahārī] hawks only messages.

She only transmits what can be said in writing without moving oneself. She is a postwoman.
In this connection, it is said:

53   A devoted messenger studies the possibilities so as to indicate to them the most favorable meeting places and times.

She seeks the appropriate time and place, letting them know where they can go in order to meet.
This messenger decides the places where the heroes can meet and sleep together, once they have allowed themselves to be caught in love's snare and have already met together several times.

Some go-betweens, acting without a mandate, seek on the contrary to separate lovers out of duplicity, since they are at the service of someone else and are bound to another. They are called double agents [dvitīyātmārthā].

54 She may also be her own messenger [svayamdūtī]. Although sent by another woman, she acts on her own account, and strives to attract the boy herself. She tells him that she has made love with him in a dream. She claims that the married woman he lusts after is of low extraction and, out of deceit, she shows her jealousy. In giving him objects marked with scratches and bites, she claims "You ought to have offered them to me. In what way is that married woman prettier than I?" And, having succeeded in separating them, she ends by uniting with him. Such is one who becomes her own messenger.

Sent as a messenger by some other woman, she goes to the boy whom she desires for herself. She becomes her own emissary.

Seeking to make him unfaithful, she tells him, "Today I enjoyed myself a great deal with you, in a dream." She makes fun of his mistress's family and says, "I'm shocked that you should have fallen for such a woman. You should get together with a more beautiful girl than that." Thus, by mocking his lover's family, she shows her disdain. In order to indicate her state of mind to him, she brings him objects marked with scratches and bites, mixed with betel, to show her passion, so that he will understand that she is at his disposal.

In order to declare her affection, she says to him, "Formerly, my father swore that he would have married me to you. Am I not more beautiful than your mistress?" Thus, secretly, she manages to convince him.

55 She meets him in an isolated place, on the pretext of giving him a message.

56 Treacherously meeting him to whom she has been sent by another woman, on the pretext of a message, she conquers the boy and snatches him from the other. She is a go-between who works for herself.

Sent to take the girl's message to the hero and neglecting to let him hear it, she seeks to attract the boy to herself. Not letting him meet the heroine, the messenger is a go-between who works for herself.

57 In the same way, a man sent by another can act as his own messenger.

Similarly, a man who bears a message, in going to the heroine's house, takes the hero's place. He seduces her on his own account. He is known as his own go-between.

58 Messenger to an idiot (mūdhadūtī).
Having won the naive wife's trust without difficulty, she asks about the husband's amorous habits, what jewels he uses to adorn his person, whether he is irascible. She then reports to the heroine everything she has learned and shows the husband the scratches and bites with which she herself has marked the wife, so as to make him angry with her. In such a way, the messenger sent to the idiot woman wins the hero's trust.

The messenger then expresses her indignation to the husband. "Who wouldn't be angry in such a case and separate from his wife after what I have seen?" She knows, nevertheless, that he has no other mistresses. The confusion he feels serves her intention to possess him, which is the purpose of her enterprise. The messenger to the idiot woman has thus embroiled the wife, who has understood nothing, so as to make her cooperate in her aims.

59 She then unites him with her principal.

Meaning the heroine by whom she had been sent to the idiot woman. She arranges, out of vengeance, that he makes love with the heroine.

The messenger wife [bhāryādūtī].
If the hero is shy at receptions, when he dares not act as his own messenger, he sometimes charges his wife with it, making her his messenger to the other woman.

60   Utilizing his own wife, without her being aware of the fact, and getting her to establish confidential relations with the other, he makes use of her, thus showing his skill. The messenger wife is entrusted by him with snaring the other.

Out of stupidity, she does not understand.

He knows that she does not realize that through her, he is going to have intercourse with the other. Trustingly, she unites them. He catches the other by the intervention of his wife and thus demonstrates his skill. The messenger wife may also carry messages and the heroine's reply reaches him forthwith through the messenger wife.

If his wife is not successful in making contact, what will he do? He employs a mute messenger [mūkadūtī].

61   In order to send garlands of flowers, earrings wrapped in a secret message, marked with the print of his nails and teeth, he employs a very young maidservant, who sees nothing wrong in these dishonest enterprises. She is the mute messenger [mūkadūtī] through whose intervention he seeks to obtain an answer.

The hero utilizes a young maidservant who is favorable to him, innocent and without malice. Being innocent, she sees it only as a childish game. He sends her each day to the heroine's house and, when they have become familiar with each other, she carries secret messages, explaining, "My Master entrusted me with it." She brings her the necklaces and earrings that he has marked with his nails and teeth as an indication of his hope of amorous relations. This is the mute messenger, since she does not understand what it is about. She is like a letter-carrier, through whom the heroine can send a rapid reply. If the heroine accepts the earring marked by him, he needs no other answer.

In order to transmit a coded message by the girl, how does he go about it?

62   He utilizes a vātadūtī [a messenger as elusive as the wind].

She transmits the messages in an established, agreed-upon language, which they have prepared in advance and which cannot be understood by others, or else by using words with double meanings, or foreign words. She is known as the messenger as elusive as the wind. In the same way, she transmits the reply: that is her role.

The hero and heroine have previously established a secret language, which serves them as a means of contact, which others cannot understand, whose meaning they cannot grasp, thinking it must be a barbarian [mleccha] language, or else words with no meaning.

The girl to whom these messages are entrusted, without her understanding their meaning, is the messenger as elusive as the wind. She also strives to bring back a reply. The messenger faithfully repeats the message that has been entrusted to her and brings back the reply, if needed. According to the Bābhravyas, "picture face" means young girl, "parrot's game" making love, and so on. All the messages are transmitted in a secret language.

In connection with the messenger's role as intermediary, it is said:

63 On this subject, here is a verse:

"Widows, fortunetellers, slaves, beggars, worker women who frequent the house and whom one trusts, can easily carry out the messenger's task."

Because they have access to the house and inspire confidence, they can serve as intermediaries.

64 The messenger's role is briefly described:

She creates hostility toward the husband, she praises the woman's charms, and shows her and the other women obscene paintings.

By praising the hero's beauty, she earns the woman's liking. She describes the boy's character and his amorous qualities. She shows her drawings of sexual acts, describing the sixty-four positions, etc. This she does for the whole circle of girlfriends, not only for the heroine, and explains the same.

65 She describes the hero's passion, his skill in sexual practices. She exaggerates his successes with women and his wealth.

She describes the hero's passion, "*Listen to this, it's extraordinary!,*" and so on, then his amorous performances and exceptional talents. *He is much in demand by women. He is flattered by all those who desire him, whether or not they have previous experience. As far as the woman's security and fortune are concerned, she says of the husband, "Whether he is lying on your knees or in the cemetery, you will profit from his assets, even after his death!"*

First, the skill and other qualities of messengers were described. The overwhelming importance of their astuteness is now indicated.

66 When, through her mistakes, the desired result is not reached, the messenger lacking skill with words must be sent away.

Her mistakes have been the cause of failure, so she must be got rid of because she is incapable. Due to lack of reflection, the messenger attains the contrary of the goal desired and causes separation. The messenger's task requires skillful words and astuteness.

According to the authors of the *Kāma Sūtra* and Jayamangalā, the messenger's role consists of going to the heroine and talking to her about the hero. She describes practices that develop knowledge, beauty, and fertility. Her words are contrived to draw them together. When the heroine relies entirely on the messenger and has full trust in her, the latter incites her to meet the hero, embrace him, kiss him, and copulate with him.

In the *Koka Shāstra*, Pandit Koka says that the messenger must, first and foremost, establish a close relation with the heroine, paying her fulsome compliments, after which she gives an emphatic description of the boy.

"Having formed a truly intimate relation with the girl, she supplies her with highly advanced information. She explains to her the secrets of magic words and medicinal plants that procure knowledge, beauty and fertility. When her words have produced an effect, trust is born" (*Koka Shāstra*).

The messenger draws her inspiration mainly from the *Ananga Ranga*, *Kāma Sūtra*, and *Koka Shāstra*.

Following their opinions, the *Kāma Sūtra* recommends employing as the heroine's messengers vagrants, maidservants, widows, nurses, dancers, female building workers, female conjurers, cleaning women, waterbearers, slaves, kinswomen, young girls, nuns, beggars, sellers of dairy products, seamstresses, or complacent wives.

Sanskrit literature is full of tales of male and female messengers playing the role of go-betweens. Seeing the performance of these messengers in literature, it must be said that the descriptions given in the *Kāma Sūtra* are merely a suggestion or indication. The author of the *Sāhitya Darpana* (*History of Literature*) considers that male or female messengers, by exchanging letters, messages of love, and mutual expressions of feeling, are one of the main instruments in reciprocal experience and knowledge. Between lover and beloved, tender expressions, states of mind, and signs revealing feelings play a role of the highest importance.

"By loving words, rapidly transmitted in written messages brought by messengers, the feelings of libertines are made manifest."

The author of the *Kāma Sūtra*, in the second part dealing with special kinds of eroticism among the arts of love, has described the townsman's erotic desires toward village girls and peasant women. Vātsyāyana explains that country women are ignorant of sexual subtleties. However, it cannot be said that he is always right. It is true only as a general rule, and is not the case with certain peasant men and women. Throughout literature we find descriptions of the amorous skills of peasant women. At a signal from a peasant girl, a citizen went to her bamboo cabin. For some reason, the girl did not come to the rendezvous at the time established and arrived late, by which time the boy, weary of waiting, had already left. Seeing in this a sign of her beloved's displeasure, the girl was dismayed: her mouth became dry and she was deeply grieved at not having arrived on time. On this subject, the poet says:

"The young village girl and the young town girl are like flower buds. One takes advantage of them for a moment, then, in an instant, their image is blotted out."

What Vātsyāyana describes in the chapter on meetings, dealing with contacts between lovers by secret code, is familiar from poems and novels concerning famous women. Seeing a passerby, a village girl says to him, "Passerby! In this isolated village it is difficult to find shelter! But if you are happy with a sheep pen, stay here if you wish!" This description in the picturesque language of the village girl means that when she sees a young and handsome passerby, the beauty is attracted by this new young man. In her awkward language, she expresses her feelings, saying, "Here in this village of peasants, all refinements are lacking. If you, a young man of my own age, seeing my blossoming youth, wish to make use of it, stay here!"

In answering a townswoman who claimed to be civilized, a beautiful village girl, by her replies, dampened Vātsyāyana's convictions.

"It is true that I am a village girl, that I live in a village and do not know the customs and manners of townsfolk. But what I do know is that, whatever I am, I can steal the husbands of those townswomen who claim to know erotic science. I am a village girl. I live in a village and don't know town fashions, but seduce the townswomen's husbands we can and do!"

On the subject of special tastes, Vātsyāyana speaks "of the fascination that peasant women exercise on townsmen." He says that any relationship between a citizen expert in the art of love and peasant women, milkmaids, and female buffalo herder is considered a degrading coition (khalarata). In order to demonstrate that Vātsyāyana's opinions were without sense, a young Bhīl, speaking to his young and tender Bhīl girlfriend, said without ambiguity, "She thinks you are poor because you do not cover the cleft of your breasts. She feels she is superior for a matter of cloth over the cleft between the breasts."

The wonders performed by the charming little peasant, whose art of enhancing her value is not appreciated by Vātsyāyana, are described as follows in the *Sāhitya Darpana*:

"A traveler passes through a village. Reaching the fountain, he perceives a young peasant girl and is attracted by her youth and beauty. She speaks to him in rustic speech, "Why do you go further when you are thirsty? Nobody here will stop you from drinking. Come and drink the water, and not only once: no one here will stop you." Another country girl, acting as her own messenger, skillfully summoned her lover. "What shall I do? At home, my cruel parents-in-law torment me ceaselessly. Only in the evening do I have a moment's tranquility," meaning: "Come this evening: at that time there will be nothing to hinder us."

Another village girl, acting as her own messenger with a traveler who is lodging with her, leads him to his bed so that he finds himself next to her in the darkness. "My mother-in-law sleeps here, and here sleep I. Therefore, O traveler!, remember on which side of the bed you must not happen. The house is full, but, traveler, in the darkness of the night, do not mistake the wrong bed!"

In poetry and literature, the description of messengers is much more developed than in the *Kāma Sūtra*. In *Abhijñāna Shākuntalā*, *Mālatī Mādhava*, *Svapnavāsavadatta*, *Mrichakatikā*, and other plays, and in *Harsha Charita*, *Naishadīya Charita*, *Kādambarī*, *Sarasvatī Kanthābharana*, and other historical poems, important mention is made of messengers, as well as in many specialistic works, such as *Kuttinīmatam*, *Kuchumāra Tantra*, etc., dealing with the subject.

Besides female messengers, male messengers also play an important role in Sanskrit literature. In *Naishadīya Charita*, Nala, acting as his own messenger, goes to Damayanti. Numerous poems have been written on the messenger-cloud, the messenger wind and the messenger swan.

End of the Fourth Chapter
The Task of the Go-between
of the Fifth Part entitled Other Men's Wives

Chapter Five

THE
KING'S PLEASURES
[*Ishvarakāmita Prakarana*]

Not being able to introduce themselves into other men's dwellings, how do men in power manage? This restriction has its influence on the amorous adventures of kings, which will now be described.

1 Kings and ministers cannot enter other people's houses, since the conduct of the powerful is observed and imitated.

The masses constantly observe them as models. If they see them at fault, they imitate them. If their conduct is the highest, the same goes for others.

For kings, ministers, and important people, it is not possible to visit other men's houses, since the people observing them will imitate their behavior.

Of this point of view, it is said:

2 "When the sun rises, the three worlds, seeing the light, awake. When it sets, even if it is still light, they do the same."

The sun reigns over the worlds. When it rises, seeing its behavior, the people awake. When it sets, seeing that it has gone elsewhere, seeing its behavior, they go to sleep. They regulate their own actions by it.

3 This is why kings cannot behave in any blameworthy way.

They cannot go into a house to enjoy a woman, since the powerful are models. By entering a house, they would be imitated by others, and would be setting a bad example of behavior. This is why they cannot behave thus. Since they ought not to do so, it is difficult for them to practice the pleasure of seducing other men's wives.

4 If one of them is bent on a love affair, he must manage it while observing propriety.

If, under the impulse of passion, one of them wishes to enter another's house for lewd purposes, he must find a pretext.

Here there are two cases, according to whether things are done secretly or openly. There are therefore two ways of considering power, according to whether it is relative or absolute. In the latter case, dissimulation is imperative. It is said:

5 The unmarried sons of the head of the village with a dissolute frame of mind copulate with the village girls merely by request. The king's companions in pleasure call them "sex objects" (chārsha).

Serving for pleasure, utilized by the notables, the village women are at the disposal of licentious chiefs, at the slightest sign. This is why the village people call them "fields for ploughing" (karshana hālikā). Each of their sons takes one as a mistress. They are available simply at the prince's call. There is no need to wait for any of them. They are known as sex objects.

For the sexual amusement of their unmarried sons, the village worthies have peasant women, who accept to sleep with them at demand. The companions of the king's pleasures call them "utilizable."

6 They are employed without pay for various jobs, such as storing the harvest in the barns, going to seek provisions, cleaning the house, working in the fields, patching

garments, restitching bark garments, crushing or carrying materials.

He describes how these women-objects are used for unpaid work such as pulping, crushing, cooking food, and other ordinary jobs. Entering the palace, they do any job, storing wheat, etc., which they go to look for in the storerooms and put in order once it is garnered. They do housework, fieldwork, sowing and harvesting, cooking, restitching torn garments, and other needlework. They crush, pulp, and cook food. Being employed at these jobs, they are allowed to enter the royal palace.

These "sluttish" women are brought into the outbuildings or the house in order to crush and pulp the grain, do the cooking, carry burdens, do the housework, or else to work in the fields, spin cotton, wool, or hemp. When certain products are required, they are sent to the market or go to gather them. Thus, while doing all these jobs, they are utilized by minor officials.

7   The owners of herds do the same with the shepherdesses.

Cattle owners sleep with the cowgirls who come to milk the cows or make the butter.

8   The master builder [sūtradhāra] sleeps with widows, unattached women, or wandering nuns.

The contractor for the royal buildings copulates with widows.

9   During the night, the guards take advantage of the female thieves who roam about.

The town policemen, who check up on vagabonds during the night, sleep with female thieves and vagrant women.

10   The inspector of the bazaar, who controls the buying and selling, takes advantage of the pretty salesgirls.

The main opportunities for encounters are:

11   The amusements that take place at the festivals for the eighth day of the moon, for the full moon of the month of Ashvin [May], at the spring festival, and so on. On these

occasions, the women who come to the city market are invited as a group to visit the apartments of the royal palace.

At the festivals, the king's young companions come to inspect the markets of the capital and invite the women to the apartments within the royal palace, located outside the town.

12 There, during the course of an enjoyable drinking party, the town girls who have been chosen are taken, one after the other, into the pleasure rooms of the harem to be possessed. They are well treated and, after eating and drinking, they are sent back in the evening.

During the amusements, these women drink a great deal together with the inhabitants of the gynoecium. And then what happens? The market girls from the town and the townswomen of the capital [dronamukha] are taken into the chambers of love, the scene of amusement. There, pleasantly welcomed, they converse with the inhabitants of the harem, who treat them well. They make them drink to get them inebriated, and after having seduced them, when evening comes, they send them home so that they leave the palace while it is still light.

13 The king's maidservants are sent to speak to women selected for his use.

The king's envoys make contact with those women who are utilizable, those with whom he wishes to sleep. The one selected is informed that she has been chosen to sleep with the king that day. This is why she is invited to the palace. She is then skilfully chatted up.

14 She is invited to see the wonders of the palace.

Since the sight of these wonders will make her lose her head.

15 First of all, the king's messenger speaks to her in her own home: "I will show you all kinds of amusements and wonderful objects that are in the palace. I will let you see some magnificent carpets from outside. When the time comes, you will meet him."

Coming from the royal palace, the slave goes to her house, and speaks with her so as to stimulate her. She comes to see her at the right moment and, to attract her, tells her of wonderful things and precious carpets.

16 She lets her admire the floors of precious mosaic [manibhūmikā], shady gardens, bowers of flowering lianas, chambers formed like sea grottoes, mazes [gūdhabhitti sanchāra], rooms covered with fresco paintings, tame deer, chained falcons, caged lions and tigers, etc., of which she had only heard tell.

She shows her the mosaics made of tiny pieces of crystal and other stones, gardens planted with flowering and fruit-bearing trees, bowers covered with lianas, chambers in the form of marine grottoes with labyrinths in which springs run, and secret walks for strolling, astonishing live birds chained and others stuffed or artificial, animals for the hunt, birds such as swans, wild beasts in their cages that, even if they are stuffed, look as though they were alive.

17 Then, when they are alone, she speaks to her of the king's passion for her.

She explains that it is advisable to accept.

18 She describes the king's skill at making love.
19 Once intercourse has taken place, she advises her not to speak about it.

Once she has slept with the king, the slave explains to the woman that she must not speak to anyone about it.

20 If the messenger does not succeed in convincing her, the king himself comes to her politely and, having seduced her, then sends her away with kindly words.
21 If the husband of the woman the king desires seeks the king's benevolence, he will invite his various wives to the harem. Once there, the king's slave acts as above.

The one in whom he is interested, whom he wishes to use, is

respectfully invited by the slave for a love meeting. The slave respect-
fully introduces her to be enjoyed.

22   It may happen that one of the inhabitants of the harem
makes the acquaintance of a woman whom the king desires, and sends her a friendly message through a servant.
If the friendship grows, she will invite her to come and see
her, which she accepts. Once she has entered and been
welcomed, she is made drunk, after which the slave deliv-
ers her to the king, who acts as above.

Acquainted with one of the harem women, she is invited in a
friendly manner. Once confided in, the king, who desires her, invites
her using a slave as intermediary to come and see him since "I myself
cannot come."

23   When the king wishes to show off his well-known talents, he invites the harem women for an exhibition, during
which he gives them presents. When the one he desires has
entered, the king's maidservant acts as above.

If the king is an expert in singing and playing instruments, he
invites the women, making them gifts of garments or other favors, to
an exhibition. It is probable that the girl he wishes to utilize will also
come, mixed in among the harem women.
The king sends a maidservant to invite the girl to visit the palace
and bring her to him.

24   Finding himself in difficulty, or threatened, a man tells
his wife to find a mendicant nun who has access to the
harem. "If she speaks to the queen about my problems, the
latter will lend a favorable ear and will certainly be moved.
That way we can save our bacon. The nun will get you in
two or three times and you will be able to circulate among
the women. When the queen has been informed of the terrible difficulties of him who is your life, we shall be delivered from our anxiety." Once her fears have been calmed,
seizing the opportunity of conquering her, the king's maidservant acts as above.

A man with money problems or threatened by the royal officials speaks to a mendicant nun who is in the queen's good books. Following her advice, he takes her as an intermediary. Seeking some way to help him, the latter arranges to introduce his wife into the harem. "If you please the queen, she will listen to your words. What she says, the king does. He always listens to what she has to say. Your demands will be heard, since in this way she will show her benevolent nature."

Having pondered over her behavior, she will explain to her what she must do. "Knowing you are without resources, they will take away your fear." The woman returns to the palace two or three times. Later on, being known, she is free to enter, without any difficulties. Once she has been accepted, the nun says to her, "Don't make any difficulties about being possessed."

25   The case is similar for people who are persecuted by a minister in order to squeeze money from them, for those who are forcefully thrown out of their house, for those who are economically weak, or for those whose salary is insufficient and desire a raise, those who seek the king's favor, those who are victims of the royal officials or who want honorary posts in their caste, those who are persecuted by their family, and those who are looking for work. They arrange for their wives to be incited to sleep with the king, in the manner described.

Thus people who are frightened or in difficulty, who have no money, or are persecuted by the prime minister or other royal officials, who have been forcefully expelled by the government, have lost a lawsuit, are without income or find their salary insufficient and want a raise, who desire the king's favor or to attract his attention, who want to be respected by the king's men, but whose wife is pretty, should speak to a mendicant nun who will arrange a meeting and bring about the union of the king with their wife, who is otherwise inaccessible in their society.

Thus, those who hope for some means of livelihood from the king, who seek fame through royal edicts, who are ill-treated by the nobles, or are looking for employ, may be caught in the trap of seeing their wife sleep with the king in the manner described.

26 It may occur that the king has a woman living as someone's concubine seized, taking her for a slave, and makes her enter the harem in order to sleep with her.

She is friends with someone. He has her seized by order of the chief of police. Accusing her of immoral behavior in public, like a prostitute, then considering her as a slave, he makes her enter the gynoecium with the ordinary women so as to enjoy her, but not immediately, keeping her for further use.

27 The king's spies accuse the protector of a pretty woman of actions against the king, etc., so as to take possession of the woman and bring her secretly to the harem to be enjoyed. This is often practiced by princes.

Even if he is innocent, a man is accused of criminal behavior by the police. He is found guilty. His wife is arrested, but not accused. The couple is not defended by their family. This is often practiced by princes and their entourage, but not by the king himself.
Entering other men's dwellings for secret copulation is not allowed. If, in order to accomplish their purpose, the messengers enter secretly, such behavior is not approved by decent people. On this subject it is said:

28 The king never, under any pretext, penetrates into people's houses.

This is why he can only do it secretly.
It is also the case for respectable men, since Vātsyāyana considers it a serious offense.

29 In the city of Kotta, the King of the Abhīras, having entered someone's dwelling, was killed by a laundryman hired by his brother. Similarly, the King of Kāshī, Jayasena, was killed by the cavalry commander.

In a city of Gurjerat, called Kotta, the king of the Abhira tribe penetrated into the dwelling of the merchant prince Vasamitra, in order to make love with his wife. On entering the house, he was assassinated by a laundryman at the order of the merchant's brother.

Nevertheless, kings are often seen to have sexual adventures. He says:

30 The customs of certain countries facilitate amorous adventures.

Turning to behavior practiced since ancient times in certain countries, important men with an erotic temperament use it to their advantage, either publicly or otherwise, and kings in particular.

31 Among the republican tribes [janapada] of the Andhra country, a newlywed girl, in exchange for gifts, is led into the harem after the tenth day and, when the king has enjoyed her, she is released.

With gifts of garments, etc.

32 In the kingdoms of Vatsa and Gulma, the harem women belonging to ministers and high officials are sent to the king, at his disposal for the night.

The women who live in the gynoecium of the prime minister are at the king's disposal. This practice occurs in the south, in the kingdoms created by the two princes Vatsa and Gulma.

33 In Vidharbha, pretty country girls are made to reside in the gynoecium fifteen days a month, in order to learn to make love.

It is the custom in Vidarbha country that the queens, the girls who play the role of queens, are the most beautiful girls in the kingdom, and each month spend a fortnight in the royal gynoecium.

34 In Aparāntaka country, men offer their wives, if they are beautiful, for the pleasure of the king and ministers.

People send their beautiful wives as homage to the king and to the minister.

35 The custom in Saurāshtra is for women of the town

and those of the country to be sent, either singly or in a group, to the royal residence.

As a conclusion to what is said or is not said:

36 Here is a quotation: "Whether it is a question of these or other females, many are the ways used in various countries and practiced by kings for possessing other men's wives."

37 Being careful of their reputation in the world, kings do not give themselves over to such practices. The fairest victory of the great ones of this world is to overcome the six kinds of vice.

A great king is truly victorious if he is not the prisoner of the six defects, which are: lust, anger, covetousness, vanity, lack of judgment, and avarice.

In this chapter, Vātsyāyana explains how kings, ministers, high officials, and fortunate men make love with other men's wives, how they catch them, and what strategems and intrigues they employ in order to sleep with them. What means do sensual kings use to violate the virtue of their subjects' wives and daughters? What arguments do they bring to bear so that their subjects, considering it to be a tradition, make no opposition? And in royal families and kings' dwellings, in what way, by dissimulation, are natural or unnatural excesses practiced? When no women are available, they use mares, she-goats, bitches, with which they practice intercourse contrary to nature, and they give themselves over to masturbation. Thus, all forms of copulation have been described in detail.

Vātsyāyana condemns these tendencies and practices and declares that they are unworthy of man and should be avoided. He advises kings, nobles, and rich men to keep far from such practices, for the good of society and to avoid their spreading. Vātsyāyana depicts the morals of kings of his own time and in previous eras. He mentions certain primitive peoples among whom the newlywed wife was first sent to the king for him to enjoy her. He also speaks of kings to whose palace the wives of ministers and other officials were sent at night at the sovereign's disposal. While describing this behavior of kings, Vātsyāyana recalls that the king is the people's protector. He is not merely a respected personage. A king who desires riches, success, and glory must at all times abstain from such behavior and forbid the same wherever it takes place.

In Vātsyāyana's time and previously, the king had the right to be the first to enjoy newlywed wives. This is not surprising. Having once more found our independence, sovereigns of our own time have been discovered among whom amusements and the abduction of women are carried out in the name of tradition and custom. In order to satisfy their fantasy, they would sodomize boys in their harems and disguise their female companions, friends, and slaves as men, with whom they would exert themselves in erotic practices with the aid of artificial sex organs. For this purpose, they would use aubergines, turnips, etc.

Vātsyāyana mentions all kinds of ways, both artificial and not, of causing sexual enjoyment. It is astonishing, however, that he does not speak of secret relations for unsatisfied queens. It is probable that in Vātsyāyana's time such excesses were not revealed, or perhaps that such a prudent man would not wish to reveal these secrets. Nowadays, when it is the fashionable practice for girls to marry late, the employment of artificial instruments is much more widespread as a means of self-satisfaction.

Vātsyāyana had considerable power of intuition. In the chapter on other men's wives, he describes man's animal passions, but sometimes casts a veil over his penetrating gaze.

End of the Fifth Chapter
The King's Pleasures
of the Fifth Part entitled Other Men's Wives

Chapter Six

BEHAVIOR IN THE GYNOECIUM
[*Antahpurikā Vritta*]

Even a king is not entitled to enter a citizen's dwelling, yet in other respects, the ways in which a citizen can penetrate the gynoecium have been described. Relations between the gynoecium women and the outside world will now be expounded. It has already been said that:

1   As a protective measure, nobody may enter the inner apartments. There is only one husband, while the wives, who are often several, therefore remain unsatisfied. This is why, in practice, they have to obtain their satisfaction among themselves.

Given the fact that there is only one husband, how could he satisfy them? In practice, they mutually satisfy themselves sexually. In what way?

2   The nurse's daughter, female companions, and slaves, dressed as men, take the men's place and use carrots, fruits, and other objects to satisfy their desire.

Some disguise themselves as men to satisfy their fantasies. They use objects with the shape of the virile member: carrots, turnips, and fruit such as bananas, aubergines; roots like that of the sweet potato [āluka] or others, as well as wall pepper roots [tālaka]; fruits such as marrows [alābuka], cucumbers [kartika], etc. Having cleaned the fruit, they grasp it and insert it in the organ, so as to cause a pleasurable feeling. This is merely a question of erotic amusements and does not involve feelings of love.

The nurse's daughter, female companions, and servants dress up in male clothes with jewels and fabricate artificial male sexual organs with roots, carrots, aubergines. Then lying on the women, they satisfy them by means of this artificial copulation.

3 They also sleep with boys who do not appear to be men.

They have a man's body, but since their moustaches have not yet appeared, they look like girls.

The wives get boys without beard or moustache, whom they dress as women, to sleep with them.

In ancient times, how did the king, who was alone, manage out of goodness to appease so many women in heat?

4 Out of kindliness, the king, although he had absolutely no wish to copulate, would fix to himself an artificial sex organ, thanks to which he alone in a single night could sleep with many women. However, for the one that pleased him and whose period it was, he would change his way of doing things. This is an old trick.

Although he lacks any desire to make love, he puts on an artificial instrument, a false phallus. With this means of satisfying them, he can approach numerous women, have intercourse with them, and thus accomplish his aim: to sleep with all the women of the harem.

5 When men have no women to sleep with, they satisfy themselves with other kinds of vulvas, or with dolls, or else masturbate.

When a man does not find any woman to his taste, how does he satisfy himself? With men, or with the vaginas of other species, mares, she-goats, bitches, sheep, any animal of female gender, as he would with women.

Otherwise, he manages by simply "seizing the lion" [simhākrānta], meaning masturbation. In this connection, it is said:

In an upright position, seizing the lion means grasping one's sex with one's hand and thus scattering one's orgasm. Since spilling one's seed anywhere is a serious offense, a purification rite should then be performed.

On another subject:

6 Citizens dressed as women are sometimes introduced into the harem with the maidservants.

In the evening, dressed as maidservants, they are let into the harem.

7 They are assisted in their comings and goings by the nurses or other harem women, in the hope of a gift.

In order to be let in among the women of the gynoecium and allowed out again, citizens distribute tips to the women guarding the entrance, who thus derive a profit from their visits.

8 The maidservants explain to them that entry is easy and the exit assured; the palace is enormous, and the guards are not there all the time.

The way out is safe, the palace vast; no one knows where anyone is; the guards are careless and surveillance is not constant. The king and the princes are not always in the queens' apartment.

9 If the way in is not easy, men should renounce the task, since the matter is risky.

If entry is not easy, citizens should give it up due to the prohibition and risk of unpleasant situations.

From another point of view:

10 According to Vātsyāyana, however easy it may be for a citizen to get into the harem, he should not enter.

Because of the great risk to his life.
In this connection:

11 Knowing the secret entrance to the harem and having weighed his chances, he enters only if he knows the way out, if he is in the grip of violent passion, if the great inner apartments are separate and not well protected, if the king and his suite are absent, and if he has evaluated his chances of success in an adventure to which he has been several times invited.

He studies the harem entrance, through which he can go in and through which he will leave. Then, seizing the opportunity and disguising himself, he gets a servant to guide him.
The numerous great verandas stand open. The guards are few and inattentive. Someone shows him the way to enter the queens' dwelling.

12 If he is able to do so, he may go there every day.

Anyone who is in a position to enter without hindrance every day, should take advantage of it.
For his own safety, what should he do?

13 He should find some pretext to explain his presence to the guards outside.

With the outside guards, he should make mention of a family tie: "I am your brother, or the husband of your sister." He must strike up friendship with them so that they do not wish to drive him away.

14 If one of the harem maidservants shows a passion for him and obtains nothing in return, she will be saddened by it and risks becoming a spy.

She shows her passion by her behavior, so he should resolve to respond, since she would be very annoyed if she were not successful and would then risk denouncing him.

15 He must know how to recognize the king's spies.

In order to save his life.

16   If the messenger does not show up at the appointment, being disguised, he should stay quietly some way away, showing that he is available.

He waits for some time, having disguised himself and taken on another appearance, in a spot that is removed, but quite visible.
But if he cannot be seen to stay there, it has no point.

17   For safety's sake, he should get information from the maidservant.

Standing outside, he gets information from the maidservant about any risks for his safety, choosing the one who has shown her attachment to him.
Mixing with the guards, he contrives to see that maidservant.

18   When their glances meet, he gives her a sign.

When their eyes meet, arranging themselves so that they can look at each other many times, he signs to her to make his intentions clear.

19   Wherever she is able to meet him, he shows her his intentions by means of erotic drawings, songs, objects, actions, as well as material signs, offering her jewels for her nose, or rings.

At the spots where they meet or try to meet, he leaves the marks of his passion by writing on the walls. He chooses words with a double meaning, which, while saying something else, evoke his love, as well as the words of songs, scraps of poems, and so on, gifts such as balls, dolls marked with signs, wrapped in packages bearing the imprint of his nails or teeth, and rings on which her name is written.
At the spot where they can be seen by the maidservant who desires him, he draws images on the walls, writes obscene couplets, fragments of songs. He writes things that show his passion for the beloved, leaving balls, dolls, playthings marked with his nails and teeth, and also rings with her name engraved on them.

20   He awaits her reply, then strives to enter.

Once he has received her reply by letter or some other means, he waits a moment and enters.
After seeing her reply brought by a slave girl, he goes within.

21   Initially, he hides himself in the place where the slave is usually bustling about.

22   Disguising himself as a guard, he enters at the right moment, unperceived.

23   Or else, wearing a bed cover like a shawl, he enters without being noticed.

24   He may also make himself visible or invisible by the methods of Putāputa Yoga, and circulate without his shadow being seen.

By means of yoga practices, wrapped in a magic net or garment, his body no longer has a shadow. He takes on a form that disappears without having a shadow, so that he becomes invisible.

25   This is the procedure: without letting the steam escape, cook a mongoose's heart, long gourd fruits, snakes' eyes. Crush them all together to make eye salve. If applied to the eyes, one can move about without one's body or shadow being visible. Besides this method, there are also magic nets and exotic beverages prepared by the disciples of the Kshema Shiras sect, or Yoga Shiras.

26   As a general rule, access to the palace is easy on the days of full moon and during the festival of lights, or by way of the vaults.

On the nights of full moon, the nights of pleasure, or else during the festival of lights, when everybody roams here and there, one can tranquilly, torch in hand, enter the palace precinct, or the inner apartment, or else one can enter the palace through the vaults and leave in the same way.

27   It is also possible to enter and come out if one is bringing provisions or drinks, on the occasion of drinking par-

ties or strolls in the garden, when servants are running
right and left, during changes of domicile or changes of the
guard, during country excursions or departures for trips,
and also if the king leaves on a long journey leaving the
queens in the palace.

*Here are explained other ways of entering without difficulty: with
suppliers, carrying bundles or drinks in their hands, one can go in
without difficulty. Drinking parties are also an opportunity, by mixing
with the servants going ceaselessly hither and thither, as also when they
clean the house or garden, or when the king departs for a long journey.
But if the journey is a short one, the lover will not reach his goal.*

One can enter and leave carrying bundles on a cart, bringing or
unloading them. Among a crowd of guests for a drinking party, one can
enter and leave easily. When the servants, pressed by their work, are
running hither and thither; on moving one's business from one house
to another; by pretending to supervise the removers; or else if the
family goes out for a country walk, or the king leaves for a long trip.

*However, even in these various ways, entry into the harem is not
advised.*

28   The women living in the harem know each other's actions. If one of them acts on her own, if she gives herself
to a special adventure, she separates from the others and
risks being denounced. Hostility ceases when the others
share in the desired result.

*Knowing each other's secrets, harem women are bound together.
If one of them commits a forbidden act, all the others, even those
opposing her, are on the same side. For what reason?*

*If one is accused of bad behavior, it reflects on all those living with
her in the harem. Since they are bound together and have no differences of opinion, the secret is kept by the whole harem.*

In illustrating the customs of various countries, he says:

29   In Aparāntaka country, men with a feminine appearance freely enter the harem, which is not severely guarded.

*He alludes to women who let into the harem pretty, lively, girlish-
looking boys, who could pass as such and are for this reason kept by the
queens in the harem.*

30   Among the Abhīras, for their satisfaction, they let into the harem the soldiers on guard.

This involves soldiers belonging to the soldier caste [Kshatriya] and not others. The harem women let them enter the gynoecium and use them as they please.

31   In the countries of Vatsa and Gulma, the citizens, sons dress as maidservants, with whom they enter the harem.

Dressed up as maidservants, they go in as though they belonged to the royal family's household.

32   In Vidarbha, the queens sleep with all the princes, save those who are their own sons.

To the sovereign's knowledge, amorous frolics with family members are not forbidden, except with their own sons. Leaving their mothers aside, they enjoy them all.

33   The women in matriarchal countries only sleep with men of their own caste, even when they come from another state.

This is the case in the palace of Shrīpuri, "the City of Women."

34   In Gauda country, women make love with Brahmans, friends, servants, and slaves.

In Gauda country, the ancient Kāmarāja, they make love with whoever wants to take them, even servants or slaves.
And even untouchables.

35   In Sindha country, they make use of the guards, workers, and others to whom access to the harem is not forbidden.

They sleep and keep company with guards and workers, even with street sweepers [chamara], since entry to the palace is not forbidden to them. Sindha is a southern land.

36   The men of the land of the snows [Haimata] boldly

offer their services in the hope of obtaining recompense, but not otherwise.

In order to get money, in the hope of a tip, without any embarrassment, they offer themselves boldly, in the land of the snows, the Himalayas.

37 In the countries of Anga [Bhāgalpur], Vanga [Bengal], and Kalinga [Orissa], the Brahmans employed in bringing flowers for the domestic rites, with the king's approval, enter the inner apartments. They speak with the unveiled women and, on this pretext, seduce them.

When bringing flowers, town Brahmans enter the inner apartments with the king's permission and, according to the custom of the country, they speak with the women, either veiled or unveiled. Having come on the pretext of delivering flowers, they lead the women astray. In Vanga, they do it secretly, in Anga they are offered a good meal, in Kalinga they receive remuneration for their favors.

38 The people of the Eastern countries [Prāchya] hide one young man in the gynoecium for each group of nine or ten women. Such are the ways of having relations with other men's wives.

For each group of nine or ten women, a young man would be appointed, but in a secretive, hidden manner. Thus have been described the ways in which relations with other men's wives are practiced.

After describing the ways of frequenting other men's wives and of making love with them, he explains how one's wives may be protected.

39 It is for these reasons that one must protect one's wives.

Seeing what men get up to, however well the entrance is protected, the ways of getting acquainted, the role of go-betweens in establishing contact, the position of kings' favorites, and harem customs, the first means of defense therefore is to protect the house.

It is for these reasons that the women must be constantly under surveillance.

40 The masters explain that, as far as sexual matters are concerned, the harem must be protected.

The situation must be examined and a proper cleaning-up performed.

41 According to Gonikāputra, the guards can be influenced by fear, interest, or in other ways. Their honesty with regard to sex, fear, and money must be ascertained.

Although they may be irreproachable on a moral level, they may not be so under the influence of fear, the lure of gain, or other incitements. For this reason, these aspects must be examined.

According to Gonikāputra, even if the guards themselves are irreproachable, they may, under the effect of fear or the lure of gain, let someone enter the queens' dwelling. This is why they must be watched, not only for sexual reasons, but also for intimidation or desire for money.

42 According to Vātsyāyana, for guards, the defense of their master's interests must be a moral virtue that they fear to violate. He who watches over the purity of the harem must fear moral law.

A virtuous guard will not allow libertines to enter and, whatever the lure of money, he will not behave as his master's enemy. It is from fear of committing an evil deed that he will renounce it.

According to Vātsyāyana, it is a moral duty not to be one's master's enemy and this may act as a brake. Furthermore, to guard the queens' apartment, only virtuous and religious men must be chosen.

In connection with means envisaged for protecting wives, it is said:

43 According to the Bābhravyas, one must listen to the gossip of other women, especially those who dissimulate their behavior, so as to be able to judge the morality or immorality of one's wives.

Those involved in secret behavior may not know that their husband is aware of it. He examines their behavior secretly and finds out whether their conduct is pure or perverse.

44 According to Vātsyāyana, young women easily let themselves be seduced by bad men. This is why decent people should not be too hasty in accusing them of loose living.

Bad men are those who have no respect for virtue. Knowing this, the reasons for which a girl is deflowered or unfaithful must be considered. If she has gone wrong previously, one must not immediately punish a girl who is not guilty, or accuse her, without knowing the reasons for her losing her virtue. Thus it is said, the guilty must be punished if their behavior becomes a habit. Often, maltreatment is not the answer for an accidental sexual relation. It is only after studying the causes for her loss of virginity, therefore, that judgment can be made.

Vātsyāyana's opinion is that one should not, without reflecting, accuse those who are fundamentally honest.

45 On this subject, it is said: the causes for women's misconduct are too many parties, the husband's misconduct, uncontrolled relations with the husband's brothers, the husband's absences, his trips abroad, physical violence, contacts with lesbians, the husband's anger.

Too-free relationships with men, the husband's trips during which she remains alone, lack of money, contacts with lesbians of mannish behavior, the husband's anger, are circumstances that facilitate adultery.

Excessive gossip, the absence of authority, freedom of movement, are the causes of women's misconduct.

46 Being well informed by this book of the ways of having intercourse with other men's wives, a man who has understood the text properly cannot be deceived by his own wives.

Questions concerning the methods of seducing other men's wives have been briefly dealt with in this part. Let us see how other texts speak about it.

With regard to the ways in which dissolute men capture other men's wives, one who has thoroughly studied the parts of the *Kāma Sūtra* concerning other men's wives should, if he is intelligent, not be deceived by his own wives.

47 The ways to success in this field have been described, but those who seek virtue and prosperity do not attempt to possess other men's wives.

All this is seen from a theoretical point of view. If it is contemplated under other aspects, such as physical injury, one will take the opposite point of view, and avoid exerting oneself in trying to possess other men's wives.

Relations with other men's wives are detrimental in this world and the next. This is why an intelligent man must abstain from such evil deeds.

48 This is why men must avoid secret approaches. A wise man does not study this text to bring misfortune on mankind.

The main aim of this work is solely to assure that women are protected.

In this chapter dealing with persons who try to seduce other men's wives, mention is made of dangerous magic practices (shadyantra), go-betweens, the immoderate behavior of kings, the guilty amusements of the queens, so that being informed, people do not attempt to experiment with such practices by mistake. A husband's duty is to watch over and carefully protect his wives' virtue. In this chapter, Vātsyāyana clearly shows the causes for which women lose their virtue.

His suggestions are in conformity with the texts on morals. He says exactly the same thing as the *Dharma Shāstras*, which state:

"The six causes of corruption in women are drink, contact with corrupt men, absence of the husband on a trip abroad, dreams, changes of residence, and physical suffering inflicted."

Besides Vātsyāyana, other *Kāma Shāstra* authors have described the causes of women's misconduct. According to Master Padmashri, opportunities include walks in the garden, dance shows, festivals, pilgrimages, and temple visits. One must take care that, in visiting neighboring houses or in the fields, the women neither pronounce nor hear coarse language, because in the pride of her youth, a woman has no discernment. She is easily trapped by the words of go-betweens, and her good conduct, her faithfulness, her virginity, are all jeopardized.

According to the masters, a woman of great virtue is not affected at the sight of a handsome young boy and does not understand his signals.

According to the *Ananga Ranga*, a woman who lives too much with her fantasies, who is in contact with loose-living women, whose husband lives elsewhere, or whose husband is old or impotent, risks becoming a profligate.

In this chapter, it is necessary to realize that Vātsyāyana was a man of his time, bound by the prejudice of his caste, and that he did not write this treatise as a guide for misconduct. The fact of sleeping with another man's wife is a practice found in all periods, and Vātsyāyana's aim is to preserve women, their virtue, and their innocence from seducers, go-betweens, those who dishonor their family and attempt to divert them from their duty.

Here ends the Sixth Chapter
Concerning the Protection of Harem Women
and the Fifth Part entitled Other Men's Wives
of the Kāma Sūtra *by Vātsyāyana*

Part Six

About Courtesans

Chapter One

ADVICE OF THE ASSISTANTS ON THE CHOICE OF LOVERS

[Sahāya Gamya-āgamya Gamana Kārana]

In sexual relations, distinction must be made between women who will copulate at once, those who have to be courted, and those who prostitute themselves for some particular reason.

These three kinds of relationship are explained. For women who are easy, the reasons for which they copulate or do not copulate immediately are examined. Comparing the man and the prostitute during the sexual act itself, rather than being possessed, the prostitute is in charge of the game, not the man, due to the fact that, for her, it is her livelihood.

This is why it is said:

1 The prostitute who goes with a man gains pleasure and money.

391

What does she gain by sleeping with a man? She obtains pleasure from the act, and the means of subsistence. She lives on the money she receives. Pleasure is her livelihood. She sells pleasure for money.

2 In order to obtain money, erotic attraction may be real or simulated.

When these two aspects are in play and, in combining, desire predominates, the act of love is called spontaneous, and its pleasure is immediate. When relations take place for money, however, desire is feigned, and she does not experience pleasure.

3 In such a case, she should nevertheless pretend that she is enamored of her lover.

4 She must make the man believe that she is enamored.

She will not entrap him by talking only of money.

5 She traps him by showing her disinterestedness, by not speaking of money.

In order to trap him, she shows spontaneous desire. In such a way, the fact of receiving a gratification appears natural.
However, she must do nothing without a fee.

6 In order to maintain her prestige, she should never satisfy anyone without being paid for it.

So as to affirm her power, she must not neglect her interests.

7 She must always be elegantly attired so as to attract the attention of those who look at her while passing along the royal road. But she should not show herself off shamelessly, since it would diminish her market value by half.

She must always be well dressed. Otherwise, if she is without jewels, her value goes down. She must display herself to the people circulating on the royal road, but not in an immodest manner, since it would lower her price by half: that which is too much on display is not desirable.

She must sit in a place where she can be easily seen by the passers-by, but she should not display her breasts. A prostitute's value is similar to that of the products sold in the bazaar.

In connection with her pimp [sahāya], he says:

8 She must engage a pimp [sahāya], who knows how to recruit customers, draw them away from the other girls, is not coarse, and knows how to ward off trouble.

He attracts customers and leads them to her, breaking their attachment to others. He gets rid of people without money and knows how to keep accounts. Being a pimp means doing all these things.

9 This kind of occupation is suitable for an official, a man of law [lawyer, etc.], an astrologer. He should be enterprising, courageous, with an average education, and know the arts. Others may include administrators [pīthamarda], gigolos [vita], entertainers [vidūshaka], florists, liquor merchants, laundrymen, barbers, mendicant monks, unemployed men, or other such people.

A policeman, a man of law, whether lawyer or not, both being competent but unemployed; an astrologer, who advises her whether or not she should pursue a relationship, are suitable for this job. The man who earns his living by serving her as a bodyguard must be courageous, capable of warding off risks, understanding, skillful and gentle in bringing his enterprises to a successful outcome. If he knows the art of dancing, he may teach her and thus make her more desirable. Administrators and other men, under the pretext of their work, enter people's houses and arrange meetings. Sometimes, in order to make a profit, one of them may also serve another girl's interests. In betraying the girl he protects, he does not arrange encounters for her. He arranges matters in his own interest and not for her.

On the subject of acceptable lovers:

10 She should only sleep with a man if he is rich, independent, having inherited from his ancestors and with available goods, with access to hidden treasures, or having enriched himself by his own efforts, a financier, a vain man who loves flattery, someone attempting to appear virile

because he is impotent, a natural spendthrift, someone on good terms with the king and the ministers, a believer in the stars, not mean, free from parental control, belonging to one of the foremost families, ambitious, a rich only son, a religious playing an underhand game, a man renowned for his great deeds, a physician.

It is only for money and not for pleasure that she goes with customers who are independent, free from parental control, neither old nor poor, disposing of hidden riches. If the fortune is hidden for some reason, she makes enquiries to know how much he possesses. Men occupying important and highly remunerative posts are generous: they are not avaricious. The heir to a fortune and one who finds a treasure are difficult to part from their money. Ambitious men, out of a spirit of competition, pay a lot for intercourse. Financiers, tax controllers or usurers, people who believe in luck and do not wish it to be seen that they have been unlucky, since they would be spurned by the girls, spend freely. The vain give much in order to be flattered. The impotent pay to be believed virile. The envious, jealous of their equals for family, knowledge, riches, or other, spend more. Spendthrifts by nature give without counting the cost.

High-ranking people are taken at their word, if they themselves do not pay. Belonging to the king's entourage, "he will pay out of affection for me." Those who believe in destiny [in the stars], consider that luck will abandon them if they do not spend, paying freely. Those who depend on their parents spend a lot, because it is they who pay. The ambitious give with a view to the future. An only son, whom his parents do not try to check because they have no other, spends without taking count. A monk who, officially, has renounced pleasure and has no right to indulge in women, gives a lot. A courageous man who has rendered her a service in the past merits compensation. A medical man, even if he gives nothing, repays by taking care of her when she is sick.

Prostitutes have sexual relations for money with the following persons: those who are free from social or family obligations and are completely independent; who are young, with a fixed income and are free to spend; who have inherited a fortune from their ancestors and, themselves, have no expenses for other people's needs. She must attach herself to such persons, proud of their looks, youth, and riches.

11   She should also go with men famous for glory or money.

Wherever qualities are to be found, love and glory are also present.

12   A man's qualities are: to belong to an important family, to be wise, open, a poet, a skilled teller of tales, a good
singer, eloquent, expert in the arts, respectful of tradition,
ambitious, enthusiastic, faithful, constant, without slander,
generous, devoted to his friends, a lover of social life and
parties, appreciative of company and society games, in good
health, slim of body, sturdy, not an alcoholic, alert, compassionate, a defender and protector of women but without
falling into their power, financially independent, without
uncouthness, neither quick-tempered nor fearful.

*Learned in philosophy [ānvīkshikya] and other subjects, open, know-
ing heretical theories well, a poet, a good judge of poetical works in
Sanskrit and other languages, ambitious, fond of grandeur, eloquent,
lively in discussion, expert in the arts such as writing, a traditionalist,
with respect for the knowledge of his seniors, enthusiastic at meetings,
since he loves to shine—enthusiasm [utsāha] implies the qualities of
boldness, impatience, quick reaction—fond of dancing and other shows,
gatherings, drinking parties, society games, tall and well made, vigorous, not an alcoholic, sober as a Brahman, compassionate, forgiving
offences, faithful to his friends, a defender of women, giving them
prudent advice so that they stay on the right path, affectionate with
them, worrying about their health, without fear, going ahead without
hesitation: such are a man's qualities.*

*A man endowed with these qualities is qualified to be a partner
in love and to have relations with courtesans. If he possesses these and
other qualities, a hero is suited for seducing young girls, widows, other
men's wives, or prostitutes. Such a lover may enjoy the women of the
harem, if he manages to get in.*

13   Let us now see what are a woman's qualities:

Pretty, young-looking, gentle, devoted, appreciating a man's
qualities—and not only for money, making love lovingly,
constant, expert in love, saying what she thinks, knowing
what she wants, but always ready to adapt herself, fond of
parties and the arts: such are a woman's qualities.

As far as women are concerned, it is their aspect, color, and bear-

ing that make them beautiful, as well as those characteristics indicating fertility, their gentleness, their pleasant conversation, readiness for sexual relations, appreciation of a man's qualities, not only his money, making love with affection, fond of petting, with preference for long-lasting love affairs, doing what she has decided, not practicing magic, not fond of gossip, knowing what she wants, behaving according to her inclination and not only by chance, fond of parties and society games: such are a woman's qualities for sexual relations. Here, as previously, it is not merely the case of courtesans.

Explaining that these are general remarks concerning the two sexes:

14 The qualities shared by hero and heroine are intelligence; character; serious behavior; uprightness; gratitude; foresight; keeping promises; knowledge of local customs and ethics of the period; civilized conduct; lack of certain defects such as laughing without cause, intrigues, slander, anger, avidity, instability, unfaithfulness; not speaking first; and knowledge of the *Kāma Sūtra* and its various parts.

15 The contrary of these qualities are defects.

Habitually behaving in an abnormal manner, or adopting the behavior of the opposite sex, are defects. Behaving contrary to normal conduct is an error. On principle being of a different sex, with contrary nature and different mentality, if a boy adopts feminine attitudes and behavior, even his qualities become defects.

Which men should be avoided sexually?

16 With tuberculosis, sick, with worms in their excrement, with bad breath, in love with their wife, coarse in word, brutal, cruel, abandoned by their parents, a thief, idiot, practicing magic, insensitive to praise and insult, frequenting enemies for hope of gain, immodest: such men should be avoided.

By sickness, all usual sicknesses are meant, such as leprosy. If while cleaning the anus where there are worms, they come into contact with the sperm and then penetrate the vagina, the woman will rapidly decline. It is impossible for a man whose mouth is evil-smelling through lack of hygiene, who, without reflecting, approaches a woman, to possess her. A man in love with his wife is not attracted by anyone else, even for money. Brutal men, with a tendency to hit their wives or servants, should be avoided, or those in conflict with their parents, or who practice magic [mūlakarma]. Who would trust a man who, hungry for gain, will even make agreements with his enemies?

Some reflections are now indicated on good reasons for having sexual relations.

17 The masters of old considered as reasons for having sexual relations passion; fear; money; defiance; easy opportunity; desire to learn; protection; grief; virtue; fame; pity; loving words; shyness; resemblance to the beloved; the facts of being well endowed, handsome, and rich; excitation; congeniality; being of the same circle; cohabitation: such are the reasons for which sexual relations take place.

One has intercourse as a result of a sudden passion, from fear of ill-treatment, for money, out of the desire for property, etc. One sometimes seduces out of vengeance or to get back at an enemy; from a desire to know, in order to receive teaching; out of need for protection, in order to find shelter. Sexual relations conceived of as work are a means of assuring one's living. Intercourse can be practiced out of grief, when one is unhappy or does not courageously bear misfortune. In such cases, consolation is sought, whatever one's inclinations. A woman may seduce out of virtue, for example, by giving herself to a wise Brahman, or during certain ritual festivals, by practicing ritual marriage during a sacrifice, or out of pity, without desiring to, "I will do this favor for one who is about to die, if he requests it." "For loving words, I would right now sleep with the one who has loved me for so long."

Out of shyness, because he is in a higher position, she lets him do it. Because he resembles the man she loves, she accepts him as his image. A man who is well endowed, rich, and handsome deserves to be worshiped. Out of excitation, when the penis rises due to the pressure of the sperm, one will sate oneself with anyone. Easy relations can be had with women of one's own circle, since women of good family couple willingly only with men of their caste. By cohabitation, the fact of living in the same house incites people to sleep together.

18 According to Vātsyāyana, riches and poverty, hate and love, are the moving principles.

The author of the treatise enumerates the reasons for sleeping together, for example as a means of healing a sick person, out of friendship, in the case of sorrow, out of a taste for the arts and other similar subjects, due to physical aspect, during happy or unhappy events, because of a fondness shown by chosen words. He adds habitual contact, the desire for knowledge, the community of ideas, sorrow, virtue, fame, affectionate words, erotic excitation, fear, enmity, pity, in the event of catastrophe, as a result of love deceived, out of shyness.

19 **Interest and love are not opposed, but the search for the means of subsistence must be predominant.**

As far as money and love are concerned, when both coexist, money should be preferred to love.

20 **As far as fear and other similar factors are concerned, the partner's importance or insignificance should be considered prior to deciding whether to give in to him or not.**

People's importance or insignificance must be considered before deciding whether or not it is necessary to sleep with them.

If one accepts to go and visit an eventual partner, how can one refuse to sleep with him?

21 **When you are propositioned, you must never accept at once. Men have no esteem for easy women.**

When a boy approaches her with an invitation, she must not accept immediately. What is easy has no worth. One must accept after several requests.

22 **In order to know whether a suitor deserves her to sleep with him and to know his state of mind, she employs servants, the hairdresser who washes his hair, a musician, an entertainer.**

An entertainer is a vidūshaka, a buffoon. The others are devoted servants in her service, such as her masseur, or her musician.

23 **In their absence, she entrusts the task to her secretary**

or others, to find out whether the suitor is clean or dirty, passionate or not, amorous or indifferent, generous or not.

Speaking of her "pimp and others" means her usual companions, a gigolo, a maker of garlands, her perfumer, her hairdresser, etc. She charges them with gauging the suitor's mentality and, first and foremost, the intensity of his desire. In the event of her considering him as a possible sex partner, she wants to know whether he is particular about his appearance, or whether, on the contrary, he is dirty and she would be running risks to her health by contact with him. The intensity of his passion means the acuteness of his desire for sexual relations. The contrary is his indifference, whether he is sexually strong or weak, whether or not he has temperament, if he is generous or, on the contrary, mean.

24 If possible, she arranges for him to make love with a gigolo.

If possible, in order to get to know his nature, she sends a gigolo who sleeps with men who have the "citizen's vice," in order to couple with him, before accepting him herself.
The ways of arranging the meeting.

25 The pīthamarda, the courtesan's secretary, leads her to the candidate's house, on the pretext of seeing a fight between quails, cocks, or rams, to listen to mynahs or parrots talking, or to attend some artistic show.

Performances of dancing or music in the house are intended.

26 Or else he leads him to her house.

Or else he leads the suitor to the courtesan's dwelling.

27 When he arrives, he brings her, as a sign of affection, something charming or surprising that she would usually not have.

He must offer her things that are charming and also useful, or surprising, whose like has not been seen before, things that give her pleasure and not otherwise, things that are uncommon that she desires to possess and not otherwise, love gifts that will awaken her curiosity.

28 If she likes him, she welcomes him pleasantly and invites him to a party,

Such as dance shows or artistic exhibitions, treating him pleasantly, with drinks and betel, in attractive surroundings.

29 After an agreeable conversation, she orders a servant to send him back home.

A long and amusing conversation makes congeniality grow. In order to learn the hero's intentions, she sends him a gift, but she does not allow him to come inside the house.

30 Through the medium of the pīthamarda, explaining that she has to leave for a trip, she invites him to come back later.

Because she is leaving on a journey, the pīthamarda, who acts as her secretary, tells him to give up the idea of coming for the moment. If necessary, the courtesan herself goes to the suitor's house, accompanied by her bodyguard.

In this connection, here are some quotations:

31 When he comes to see her, he brings the girl he is courting betel nuts, garlands of flowers, and ultrarefined beauty products, and invites her to artistic meetings.

Always choose very refined things and arrange artistic evenings with spoken dramas.

32 As a mark of affection, she gives him various things in exchange for his gifts and indicates that she is disposed to have amorous relations, without restriction.

As a sign of affection, she offers in exchange unexpected things, such as parrots, rings, letting him understand her intentions in an indirect manner, which she will later declare openly.

33 By means of love gifts, messages, and special comportment, she lets it be seen that she is disposed to sleep with him. The rest will follow later on.

The small gifts of friendship, offered as a sign of affection, are transmitted through the pīthamarda or someone else. They show clearly and precisely that she is disposed, convinced, ready for the union. The continuation will be given in another chapter.

Three sorts of love partner are mentioned in this chapter: the wife, other men's wives, and the widow. Subsequently, the ways of gaining a courtesan's favors are indicated. Vātsyāyana explains the ways of starting relations with courtesans and why, before going ahead, one should consult the courtesan's assistants, verifying whether it is worthwhile meeting her, and what are the possibilities of sleeping with her, because if this is not decided, any idea of starting a relationship with her remains an idle speculation. Because of these uncertainties, he has chosen as the title for the chapter concerning them: "Preparations and Reasons for Sleeping with Her on Which Her Assistants Must Reflect."

When a man and woman sleep together, they both experience erotic enjoyment. What can be the reason, however, for which courtesans use so many artifices to trap a man with a view to sexual relations? They deploy all kinds of snares to subjugate him. Vātsyāyana claims that it is a characteristic they are born with, and that it must be so since it is the very nature of courtesans. They attract men for pleasure and for the means of livelihood. In this connection, a man should not let himself be impressed when a courtesan seems attracted by him. If the courtesan is only of a sensual nature, he should realize that it is her natural inclination, but if her inclination is the desire for money, the attraction is artificial. On seeing this false attraction, however, it is impossible to detect its lack of spontaneity. She charms the man in order to obtain money. From her behavior and her wiles, he cannot detect whether the love she shows for him is entirely fabricated. The courtesan who wishes to ensnare a man first uses the aid of her assistants. According to her assistants' evaluation, she establishes contact. After this, as a result of the flattering reports they make about her, the man gets interested. The prostitute, according to the rules of life she has observed since her childhood, has a double nature and makes love with two kinds of man. The first is a man possessing great wealth with whom the courtesan sleeps, pretending to love him, out of desire to squeeze money from him. The other kind of man is the one to whom the prostitute brings her real love, with the aim of obtaining sexual satisfaction, or for glory's sake.

Those who associate with courtesans who are only interested in money, and who seek them out because they are rich, run counter to family interests, caste taboos, and the rules of society, and live as they please. Such people, the victims of the courtesan's wiles, strive by every means to give her money, because they always want to see her satisfied. Individuals who do not understand the courtesan's wiles run to their ruin and, when the courtesan no longer finds any juice to squeeze, she breaks off immediately.

With the other man, the courtesan makes love not for money, but for pleasure. The satisfaction she shows in their relations is not feigned. Her love is due only to her lover's qualities. A courtesan is ready to give herself to a handsome young man who is expert in the arts, or even in a single art.

Vātsyāyana is of the opinion that if a man is affected by diseases such as tuberculosis, worms, or alcoholism, a courtesan should in no way frequent him, even if he possesses considerable means or is expert in the sixty-four arts. By making love with men affected by contagious diseases, there is a risk of catching them.

Besides the sick, Vātsyāyana indicates various categories of men with whom association should be avoided. The courtesan should avoid a man who is devoted to his wife, since he will consider other women as mothers or sisters. Nonetheless, if the courtesan deploys her snares in order to trap him and break his faithfulness, her efforts, apart from being contrary to ethics and society, are a form of violence.

The courtesan should also avoid malicious or cruel persons who beat their servants until they fall unconscious, who busy themselves with parrots and mynahs, or practice magic, since passion does not grow easily with them and if, for money, she shows she is amorous, it is like sowing in the desert, since it is useless to hope for money from such people.

Vātsyāyana considers that money, unhappiness, and pleasure are the main reasons for frequenting courtesans.

In this chapter, Vātsyāyana says two main things: one is that to seduce men and sleep with them are inborn tendencies of courtesans; the second is that courtesans are attracted by men for two reasons: a taste for money and a taste for pleasure.

Attracting men is an inborn aptitude of the courtesan. If one reflects on Vātsyāyana's contradictions on the subject, it appears that the human spirit contains spontaneous or preestablished tendencies, which are at the basis of our thoughts and actions. Through them, man's desires and passions develop. It is these energies that, either openly or secretly, determine our aims and our acts, through them that a man's actions are prepared and set in motion. These basic tendencies are sometimes such powerful impulses that all a man's efforts to control them are useless. These basic tendencies are called appetites. Hunger, love, food and drink, copulation, and hostility are the main appetites. According to certain authors, such appetites are multiple and the structures of the mind are so made that they are manifest in the same way among men, animals, and all living beings. These tendencies are transmitted by heredity. The final question is why prostitutes are born for copulation. Theory tells us that these instincts are hereditary. According to this principle, in the society of prostitutes, the search for copulation is considered as the very meaning of life. By family tradition, prostitutes' daughters acquire a whorish nature and their mother, father, and circle assist them in leading this way of life.

Another thing that Vātsyāyana says is that prostitutes, for lure of money or sexual pleasure, attract men to copulate with them. The basis of inborn appetites depends on four natural aspects: an impulse, a goal, an object, a domaine in which to develop. Impulse (vega) lies at the base of every tendency. The acuteness or mildness of this impulse should be measured prudently. The goal of any inclination is autonomous, and the inclination takes on all kinds of forms in order to reach its goal. Some inclinations must be satisfied in some way, while others may be curbed. The object (vishaya) is the thing by which the inclination can be satisfied.

Sometimes, an inclination abandons the path of its own satisfaction to attach itself to another object. The thing in contact with which a desire is fulfilled, however, remains the object of the inclination. For prostitutes, in their artificial eroticism, when a male sexual organ rises before them, they feel a desire for that member that they observe with attention and unite with, because the member is the object of their inborn instinct. The parts of the body subject to excitation, where desire is manifest, are called erogenous zones.

It is a commonplace occurrence that desire manifests itself at the sight of something exterior to itself. On seeing a woman, desire makes its appearance in a man's heart, and in a woman's heart the desire for copulation is manifest at the sight of a man. Vātsyāyana recognizes that the satisfaction felt by a prostitute in enjoyment and copulation depends on the man, but, in order to attract the man and lead him to copulation, the prostitute has to employ her wiles.

The essence of what Vātsyāyana says about the prostitute's trade is that the acquisition of money is its main aim and that this tendency must be inborn in her. As far as her nature and desires are concerned, however, it must be said that a prostitute is also a human being. On occasions she can experience pleasure and passion, but not all the time. She may also give herself totally to someone.

End of the First Chapter
Advice of the Assistants on the Choice of Lovers
of the Sixth Part entitled About Courtesans

Chapter Two

Looking for
a Steady Lover
[Kāntānuvritta]

1 In order to please the hero to whom she is attached, she behaves like a wife.

When a courtesan attaches herself to a lover, she becomes like his only wife. According to the ancient saying "The courtesan behaves like a faithful wife," even though she is not the wife of one man alone, she binds herself to a steady lover. Once they are attached, she only has amorous relations with this lover.

Considering her former conduct, he says:

2 She strives to please him and fence him in as though she were enamored of him.

She charms him by pretending she is enamored of him, that she is disinterested, repeating that it is the first time that she has been attached to someone.

But she fears the pernicious interference of her mother.

405

3   She is dependent on a mother whose behavior is cruel, who is attached to money.

Being dependent on her mother, she cannot disobey her.

4   In the absence of a mother, it will be an alleged mother.

5   The latter is not very pleased that she sleeps with him.

Whether it is a true or alleged mother, she will not be very happy, thinking that the lover is not in her best interests. If her daughter becomes attached to him, it will be harmful to her profits.

Whether it is her true mother or an alleged mother, neither the one nor the other will show much sympathy toward the individual who has fallen in love with her prostitute daughter, since to show sympathy would work against her interests.

Referring to this unpleasant behavior, he says:

6   When they are together, she comes to look for her daughter.

When they are ready to make love, she takes her off on the pretext of something that has to be done.

7   Consequently, the girl always appears unhappy, depressed, ashamed, and afraid.

Under such circumstances, so as to let her past be forgotten, even if she is happy, she pretends to be unhappy, depressed, ashamed: "What does he think of me?," scared, fearing that he will stop loving her.

8   Nevertheless, she does not attempt to escape from this tyranny.

Although she suffers and fears for her love, she cannot escape her mother's domination.

9   She suddenly pretends to be suffering from a particular, but not dangerous, illness, undetectable, but not long-lasting.

It is an invented illness, with the characteristic of being sudden, individual, not contagious, without visible cause, imposing no restrictions, undetectable since it cannot be detected by the eyes on examining her organs; it causes headaches, and stomach pains that are not lasting and disappear suddenly.

What advantage does she derive from her pretence?

10 It is a pretext for going elsewhere to sleep with other lovers.

She is called for by someone else.
She invents the excuse of a pretended sickness or pains so as not to sleep with him.

11 The girl may also send him a servant with betel and a flower garland that she has worn.

In order to be rid of him, since the girl is not in a position to have sexual relations, her mother sends a servant who brings him betel, telling him not to be worried.

12 When they sleep together, he expresses his appreciation of the quality of the things sent to make him welcome.

While copulating, the hero gives his thanks for the love offerings, the betel and cardamoms. He says he has never tasted any so good.

13 She wants him to teach her the sixty-four positions.

She pretends to be his pupil for the sixty-four positions and five techniques [pānchālikyā]: "I need to know them: teach me them!"
While making love, she plays the innocent, ignorant of erotic techniques. She says to the hero, "I will do what you want, I am very ignorant."

14 In order to please him, according to his instructions, she practices the various forms of copulation.

The hero is thus convinced that it is due to his efforts that she experiences pleasure.

15   When they are alone, she expresses her wish to belong to him always.

She tells him how happy she is to be with him.

16   She expresses her dearest desire.

Which would be to spend the whole night with him, to stay beside him laughing and making love.

17   She dissimulates the defects of her secret parts.

If she has some defect or deformity in the lower part of her body, her thighs or sex, she hides it, not letting it be seen or touched for fear of not pleasing him.

18   When they are in bed, she does not resist his touch.

In order to demonstrate her love, she puts her face close to his. When they make love, whatever their position may be, the courtesan turns her face toward his, to show the attraction he inspires in her.

19   When he touches her sex, she lets him do it.

If he touches her pubis or sex, she does not resist, nor does she stop him if he wishes to penetrate her.

20   Neither does she while he is sleeping, when he embraces her and clasps her unconsciously.

She has two kinds of behavior, one that she shows off and the other that is secret.

21   In public, she declares that showing herself on the street, staying in sight in front of the house, is scandalous behavior that destroys a reputation.

"When I see women who, in order to procure a man, show themselves on the public highway, or stay standing in front of their house, and have to pay the tax on prostitutes, I am ashamed for them. Those who do so dishonor themselves."

Winking at passersby, showing oneself at the window, walking in the street, nodding if a man looks at you, making amorous calls to him that he does not understand, are despicable acts.

22 She hates what he hates, loves what he loves. She lives according to his pleasure, showing sadness or gaiety with him. If he wants another woman, she is annoyed, but not for long.

23 She pretends that the tooth and nail marks are from another girl.

Although these marks are made by her, she assures him that they are the signs of another love affair, as a pretext for making him angry.

24. She is never the first to make advances.

She never says, "I am excited, I want to make love."
She shows her erotic desire only to overcome the boy's shyness, if it is necessary.

25 She then pretends that she wants sex.

So as to make him excited.
Then, in order to convince him,

26 She pretends to be nervy, unsatisfied, sick.

She pretends to be nervy, unsatisfied, ready to be sick, for lack of sexual satisfaction.
When her lover arrives, she pretends to be drowsy or faint, saying, "See what a condition I'm in when you don't fuck me."

27 She praises the hero's virtues.

She praises him, describing his piety, fame, and riches, his good deeds in favor of the temples and sacred pools.

28 Taking the meaning of these discourses seriously, flattered by her words praising him, he has intercourse with

her in response to her words, which he takes for an expression of her love.

Believing her words and unconscious of their limitations, the boy, not understanding the ubiquity of the gracious words flattering him, which he takes at face value, allows himself to be drawn to do what she wants without understanding the scope of her words. He becomes attached to her as a result of skillful words and insincere phrases, believing her admiration to be a part of true affection.

Being assured of the effect of her flattering words on the hero, she considers him definitively attached to her.

29   Without taking into account what her friends have to say, she pretends to behave as a wife.

Contrary to her companions' instructions, she neglects to follow their advice, since they consider that she is acting against her own interests by behaving as his wife. Even though her friends are furious at her wifely behavior, she does not obey them.

30   If he sighs, if he yawns, if he is depressed, if he falls, she shares his troubles.

If he sighs deeply, if he loses money, she shares his worries, even if she is not really affected by the reasons for his displeasure.

31   If he sneezes, or says or does something unexpected, she cries, "Bless you!"

She pronounces these exclamations as a mark of affection.

32   If he is worried or thinks he is sick, she consoles him.

If he is sad, because there is bad news, she asks him the reason. If it is a question of health, she comforts him saying, "I too have been suffering from this sickness for a long time."

33   She never praises anyone else in front of him.

She never mentions anyone else's qualities, not knowing whether he might detest him.

34 She does not criticize others' faults, since he may have the same.

And he would be afraid of displeasing her for this reason.

35 Gifts received must also be kept.

Objects given by the beloved must be made use of in his presence.

36 If she is unjustly accused, or if he has some misfortune, she takes off her jewels and refuses to eat.

To make him understand that she is not guilty, as a sign of protest, she makes her body thin by fasting, feigning physical suffering. At the same time, when he suffers some misfortune, such as the death of a son or a brother, a sickness or fever, she takes off her jewels.

37 At the same time, she bewails herself.

When he arrives, she throws herself onto the ground bewailing herself, proclaiming her sorrow so that he should see her unhappiness.

38 "I want to go away from here with you! Let us leave for another country!"

She wishes to leave the country with the hero, to go elsewhere, be separated from her mother. She whines, "If you can, take me somewhere where we can be free! If the king wishes to prevent my leaving the country and the government wants to arrest me, take me and let us fly away together!"

"Take me away to another country! Protect me without worrying about the law, or else let us fly secretly!" Thus she addresses the hero.

39 My life has a meaning since I know you.

She tells him, "If our meeting had not taken place, if I had not been adopted by you and if my life, thanks to you, had not been given a meaning, without doubt, I should be dead."

40 When money arrives for him, or he succeeds in some

enterprise, or his physical condition improves, before expressing his satisfaction, he must worship his guardian divinity.

When he has made a profit, or money has come in, or he has had success in some enterprise, or his health has improved after an illness, he must not express his satisfaction at once. He must consider that material wealth and the satisfaction of his desires are due to the benevolence of the gods, through whom desires are fulfilled. They must therefore be thanked by offerings brought to them.

41   A courtesan must always be well adorned and eat little.

"A woman must always be well adorned." This could be noted in times past. Eating too much and often is a defect for a courtesan. They must eat elegantly and without vulgarity. Coarse eating brings on fever.

42   When she sings, she must bring into the words her lover's name and patronym. If he is sick, she must lay her hand on his breast or brow. This calms him and he falls asleep.

When he is tired, staying beside him and holding his hand, she calms him down. The contact of her hand is pleasing to him.

43   Sitting on his knees, lying beside him, even when he is asleep, she does not leave him to go for a walk.

When he goes off to see his friends or visit a sanctuary, she follows him, without losing sight of him, so that she is never far from him.

44   She pretends to want to have a son by him and not to outlive him.

She desires a son. "I will sleep with you during my fertile periods, and not otherwise. And I think it better that my death should occur before yours."

45   Unknown to him, she keeps her own money and does not speak to him about it, even confidentially.

46 She refuses to share his fasting and abstinence, saying that it makes her ill. If he insists, however, she does as he does.

47 In the event of problems with someone, she refers them to him, saying, "I am not in a position to decide."

In case of litigation, she declares, "I can't do anything!" Even if she can, she pretends she cannot.

48 She considers her lover's money as her own property.

She takes her protector's money and assures her control over it.

49 Without him, she does not go to any party.

50 She considers it a privilege to put on the garlands of flowers he has worn and to eat his leftovers.

"Give me the flower garlands you have been wearing. Even if they invite me, I shall not accept. I only eat the leftovers from your meals."

51 She praises his gentleness, his family's merits, his character, his dexterity with his hands, his knowledge, his caste, his fortune, his country, his friends.

If his family performs the rites, she does not speak of them as unbelievers; if he is of pure blood, she does not treat him as a bastard; if he is deft and writes beautifully, she does not treat him as a clumsy person; if his house is ancient, she does not speak of an old hut. She does not call a golden cage "the yellow cage"; she does not call his honestly-earned money ill-gotten gains. If he is honored in his country, she does not treat him as an incapable. She speaks of his qualities, not his defects, to his friends; she shows him off to advantage and does not put herself forward. For her, he takes first place in everything, not second nor third. She says his voice is sweet, even if it is not. She deems it her duty to respect and praise him.

52 She encourages him to sing or play musical instruments, if he is able to do so.

If he sings badly, she will never make him sing out of fear of rendering him ridiculous.

53 Without worrying about danger, cold, heat, or rain, she follows him everywhere.

She draws her courage from his presence.

54 She says she will be with him in the flesh, when they live in another world.

"In our future life, when we leave this world, you will always be my lover," she says, in order to illustrate her feelings.

She tells her beloved, "When I die, I want you to be my husband in my future lives."

55 She comports herself according to his wishes, his feelings, his habits.

56 She puts him on his guard against spells.

Putting him on guard concerning the constant risk of falling victim to magic practices, she sows doubts about the evil intentions of his servants.

57 In order to stay and sleep with him, she is constantly quarreling with her mother.

Why does her mother make difficulties if she goes and sleeps with the hero? The reason is simply that, as soon as her daughter shows affection for someone, the mother creates difficulties.

58 When her mother tries by force to acquaint her with other men, she threatens to poison, stab, or hang herself.

If her mother wants to force her to sleep with another man, out of interest, she threatens to carry out the deeds in question, claiming that nothing would be more hateful to her. She declares that she wants to commit suicide, but does not carry it out.

59 When her lover learns of her infidelities, informed by his spies, she takes the customs of her guild as an excuse.

Denounced by his spies, she attributes the fault to her mother. She says that it is the way courtesans earn their living. Despite her desire to break free, her mother forces her to sleep with another man.

If he does not believe her in spite of her explanations, she herself will condemn the behavior of courtesans in front of him.

60 She never discusses money matters.

When she makes love with someone, she does not discuss this subject. Such questions are dealt with by her mother. She herself makes no effort to bargain on these matters.

If, besides her principal lover, she has sexual relations with another lover, her mother arranges matters with him, but she herself never speaks of money. She accepts the sum of money he gives her with pleasure.

61 She undertakes nothing without her mother's agreement.

In the end, if her mother advises her to sleep with another man, she does not refuse to do so. She conforms all her actions to her mother's instructions.

62 If he departs for a journey, she pronounces the wish "Come back quickly!"

If, for some reason, he has to go away, she pronounces a curse: "Cursed be my life should you not return soon!"

She tells him, "I formulate only one wish: that you come back soon!"

63 While he is absent, she stops looking after herself and putting on jewels, except the one that brings good luck, the shell attached around her arm.

As prescribed for women of good family when the husband is absent, she gives up looking after her body, which is useless if nobody sees it. The courtesan does the same, observing the prohibition, except for the lucky shell she wears on her arm. She keeps it only because it is the charm worn by women whose husband is absent.

She gives up soap, oil, and ointments and no longer adorns her person, or wears jewels.

64   Remembering times past, she goes to consult clairvoy-
ants, and questions the sun, moon, and stars.

She remembers times past, and the pleasure shared with the hero.
She goes to a clairvoyant's house to question her. She listens to the
voices of the night, so as to grasp the first signs of good or evil omen,
in order to know toward what crossroads he is directed. She invokes the
constellations and the stars to make them cast a benevolent glance on
the hero, so that nothing evil happens to him.

65   If she has a happy dream, it means "he will soon be
with me."

A good dream is considered a good omen. In the morning she tells
it to her circle, "So I am certain that his return is near." Even if it
is a question of pretended dreams that she has invented, she tells them
to show her interest and make the hero, who is far away, succeed in his
enterprise.

66   If the signs are unfavorable, she performs incantations.

Unfavorable signs and undesirable omens arise. If signs of evil
omen appear in her dreams, she calls a Brahman to perform ceremo-
nies of conjuration.
When he returns, this is how she behaves:

67   When he returns, she begins by worshiping Kāma, the
god of love.

When her beloved returns, safe and sound, she has a thanksgiving
ceremony performed for the god of love.

68   She also worships the other gods.

In sign of gratitude, she worships the protecting divinities of her
guild.

69   With her friends' assistance, she arranges a party.

Her wish having been granted, she invites her neighbors for a
great drinking party.

70 With the offering of first fruits to the ravens.

For the return of her beloved, she performs the rite of thanksgiving, which begins with an offering to the ravens.

71 The offering ceremony to the ravens takes place after their first copulation.

After the offering to the ravens, once she has made love with the hero, in order to celebrate his return, she goes with him to worship the god of love and the other divinities.

72 She vows not to survive him.

She speaks of dying with him. "I will not survive you: I am bound to you and to nobody else!" she repeats.
She speaks of committing suttee at his death.
What more does she say about her relationship?

73 The characteristics of love are the total gift of self, the fact of having mutual tastes, of doing what pleases the other, total trust, indifference to money.

A devoted wife does no work if not in accordance with instructions received, to the extent that she is able to do so. She shows indifference to money, "What I obtain from my family is yours."

74 Whatever there is to be known on this subject has been explained in Dattaka's treatise. What has not been explained, an experienced man learns from the behavior of people in real life.

The behavior of courtesans has been described, in an abridged version, after having studied the work of Dattaka. What has not been explained, a shrewd man, in honoring and observing courtesans, may understand from their behavior.
To get a good picture of courtesans, one must also learn the opinion of those who are against frequenting them.

75 According to them, here are two verses:
"They are mysterious and rapacious women, whose feelings

are unknowable. It is difficult to know whether they like making love."

In this passage, "women" means courtesans. Saying that their feelings are difficult to understand means that one cannot know whether their manifestations of pleasure or sorrow are spontaneous or simulated, and up to what point. They are mysterious, since their intentions are not evident. If one wishes to judge them according to their deeds, everything seems to come from their thirst for gain. But identifying their behavior with their rapacious nature means not knowing them. To men gripped by desire, they make believe what they want. To interpret their nature on the basis of impressions deriving from erotic experience is not a way of knowing them. It is difficult to know what is spontaneous or feigned in copulation, and what their true aims are.

Given the fact that moral concepts have nothing to do with the impulses of the senses, how can one understand whether a courtesan, who incarnates desire, is sincere or factitious, since for a prostitute, the illusion of love and the thirst for gain are equally important? Furthermore, their plan is often to ruin their lovers.

Indicating this result as the aim of eroticism, it is said:

76 "The courtesan arouses desire, brings pleasure, inspires love, then goes away after devouring all the money of those she seduces."

She inspires desire by her wiles; she likes to attract, but not to become attached, since it is said, "By her wiles, she lays hold of him; by erotic games she inspires love, but there too, without becoming attached. Why does she leave him after having drawn him? Because she has taken hold of all his goods. This is why one must not become attached to her, because the relationship is not permanent and lasts only as long as she can squeeze money."

In order to save the courtesans' female dignity, Vātsyāyana advises them to play the role of the single wife. A courtesan, who earns her living by singing and dancing, should belong to a single lover and behave like a wife in whom he places his trust and to whom he is attached. With regard to the courtesan who plays this wifely role, Vātsyāyana reminds her that it is not advisable for her to give herself entirely, since a courtesan is a woman who lives by her trade, and who, in deluding men, shows them as much love, as much affection, as she receives in the form of money. Seduction is her objective. Her declarations of love, her loving behavior are merely a display. She gives her lover her body, but not her heart, otherwise her working capital would be ruined. This is why she plays this game of love under her mother's domination.

If she were independent, she would not be able to stage this false love. For this reason, she plays the game of love, under the authority of her mother or of an alleged aunt. When the whore-mistress is with her beloved and another customer arrives, her mother—or aunt— takes her away. She pretends to obey her mother's or aunt's injunctions against her will, so that her lover believes she is wholly attached to him. However much she may oppose her mother or aunt in words, she does not oppose them on money matters. As far as other customers are concerned, she shows them enough love to squeeze more money from them than she should have.

Courtesans teach their daughters or the girls they bring up the duties of a prostitute, at an age when these girls have a woman's heart, when they dream of great love and of sacrificing themselves wholly for the beloved. Gradually, however, with constant incitement, their loving tendencies end by being expressed in terms of profit. Their love is no longer directed to a man, but to the goods he possesses. The courtesan's mother or aunt skillfully gives her an example of deceitful behavior. This is why an aunt is inevitably present in every house of prostitution. Out of fear of the aunt, the prostitutes dissemble their feelings, since they are protected and nourished.

Prostitutes' lovers also live in fear of the aunts' cruelty and hardness.

The result is that a courtesan never stays long with one lover: she measures out her time for him and goes with other customers.

Fearing ill-treatment from her mother or aunt, a prostitute has to frequent several lovers to exploit them. When she visits a regular lover, pregnant under her apron, she puts the blame on an ex-lover who is dead. The question of tying reponsibility on a current lover is very unusual and inconsiderate. When a courtesan is alone with a lover, lying beside him or speaking with him of love, and another customer intervenes, her mother or aunt knocks at the door and calls her. The courtesan then, giving as an excuse her fear of her mother and saying that she is cruel and diabolical, gets up sighing and leaves her lover unwillingly. The lover remains on the bed. In his mind, he is convinced that the mother or aunt is hateful, that his beloved does not want to leave him even for a moment. Happily, the new arrival is not aware of this secret.

When the lover arrives, if the girl does not wish to sleep with him or else if, after the preliminaries, she does not want to continue with this lover, from whom she has already received her fill of money, she pretends to have a headache or stomachache, which will be gone in an hour or half an hour, or else she says she has her period and leaves him.

Even if she is perfectly versed in the arts of love, she only shows interest for it at her lover's insistence, and only when they are sleeping together. She feigns complete ignorance about it: "I know nothing about it, but I will do what you ask me." Her stupid lover, believing that he has inspired unprecedented feelings in her, lets himself be robbed of everything he possesses and is unable to hide the pride he takes in his amorous talents.

When she is alone with her lover, the courtesan strives to keep him in suspense, by changes of mood and signs of tenderness. The description of the courtesan's seduction given in the *Kāma Sūtra* is similar to that found in the literature. "Unrivaled in singing, music, dancing, declamation, appearance, and eroticism, courtesans were set in the three worlds by the Creator." The courtesan, skilled in singing, music, dancing, speaking, presence, and eroticism, is a singular work of the Creator, in the three worlds.

"What can be said of the attraction, what can be said of the seductiveness, what can be said of the ways of embracing these heavenly courtesans, the mere sight of whom causes ejaculation!"

Vātsyāyana considers that a courtesan's conduct corresponds to her social duty, but the author of the *Kāma Sūtra* does not explain why men whose real wife is pretty, accomplished, young, run after prostitutes, even though in some verses he does emphasize the courtesan's erotic skill and seductiveness. In fact, courtesans are trained from childhood in the techniques of love and the ways of attracting men. The manner in which they subject them through the delights of pleasure is an art that exists among prostitutes and not among wives. The prostitute's superiority comes from the ignorance of eroticism among other women.

Vātsyāyana considers the courtesan's attitude to love as something essentially venal and mental. The prostitute's attitude to love is based on interest, which is why they are subtle, controlled by their intelligence. The prostitute's feelings of love and her interest form a whole. This is why, in appearance, a prostitute's love seems absolute, real, blameless, and totally devoted. As soon as any limits to her interest arise, it becomes a pure display. Since the change is very subtle, however, it is not perceived by her lover.

End of the Second Chapter
Looking for a Steady Lover
of the Sixth Part entitled About Courtesans

Chapter Three

WAYS OF
MAKING MONEY
[*Artha-āgama-upāya Prakarana*]

*Having taken control of her lover, she draws her livelihood from him.
The ways of doing it are now explained.*

*The means of squeezing money from him are of two kinds: normal
or otherwise. On this subject, it is said:*

1 Usually she assures her means of subsistence in exchange
for sexual practices.

*These are normal transactions, made without any special effort.
The wages of love go without saying.*

*In other cases, when relations have taken place, an effort is needed
to obtain one's due.*

2 According to the theoreticians, when, as is usual, she
obtains what she anticipates or more, she need not employ
special means to obtain it.

When, as goes without saying, she is given what she reckoned or more, she has no need to resort to tricks. She receives her due. This is done without asking for it.

3   According to Vātsyāyana, she can get him to give her double the normal price by using certain procedures.

By using certain procedures, she can get him to give her double the price foreseen.

4   In order to procure sweetmeats, things to eat and drink, garlands, clothes, perfumes, and other things, she says she has had to pawn her jewels and asks for money to recover them.

It is a matter of sweetmeats, pastries, or other things to eat, made of wheat, etc., whether prepared or not, clothes made of vegetable fiber, bark, silk [krimi], hair [roma], perfumes such as saffron [kunkuma] and others; garlands of flowers. The other things include pleasant appetizers such as betel, fruit, or areca nuts.
In order to procure them, she has had to buy on credit from the tradesmen. She needs money to recover her deposit, in fact, not merely to pay for the things she has bought.

5   She publicly praises the hero's fortune.

In the hero's presence, letting him see how elegant she is, she flatters him and gets him to show his generosity.

6   Under pretext of periods of fasting, planting trees, donations to temples, digging pools in the garden, festivities, she gets him to give her money as a sign of affection.

"For the next eighth day of the moon I have to fast, I shall need various things. One of my trees seems to be diseased at the top, I find the humming of the bees restful." An ear-piercing ceremony, the building or inauguration of a shrine, the digging or consecration of a pool that brings good luck, are all good pretexts. Under all such circumstances, she asks her lovers to contribute without fail, as proof of their affection. Likewise in order to buy whatever may be necessary to give a reception for her guests.

7   Or else, "while I was coming to see you, some policemen or thieves took all my jewels."

*She recounts how the cunning assistants of a magistrate, or else
experienced robbers, stole her jewelry while she was coming to visit the
hero. After having them evaluated, she asks him to give her some
more.*

8   Or else she claims that she is ruined because her house
has burned down and that, in the muddle arising from
checking the fire, her money disappeared.

*In the disorder caused by a fire, it seems that everything has been
destroyed. It was not she who started the fire, it was the fault of people
who want to ruin her. On the pretext of putting out the fire, some
thieves made everything vanish. "In the confusion, I was upset, like my
mother, and the money disappeared together with the house."*
It is because the house caught fire, or because burglars entered by
piercing the walls, or else due to lack of attention, that she claims to
have lost all her money.

9   Her jewelry, including what he had given her, as well
as the hero's own jewels and also the money he had dis-
bursed to sleep with her, have all disappeared. She asks
him to replace them.

*Together with what was destroyed by the fire she includes the
jewels he had given her, as well as the hero's jewels that she had
borrowed to adorn herself. Since they were destroyed in the fire, considering them lost, he will not ask for his own back. She sends a servant
as a spy to study the hero's reaction, charging him to inform him of
the loss. For her own part, in front of the hero, she asks him to pay
the expenses only for liquors and betel.*

10   Having taken money to pay an alleged debt, she quarrels with her mother, who does not want it.

*She takes her mother the money from her salary and that obtained
for paying the debt. They quarrel. "What is this debt? If he's paying
in order to get rid of you and end your relationship, you shouldn't*

accept it. It is a way for him to settle his accounts with you. This is certainly the reason why he gave it to you."

11   She does not go to the merrymaking, having nothing to gain thereby.

She refuses to go to the parties organized by the hero's friends, even if she is invited, even if the hero asks her to do so. The reason is that she has nothing to gain by going there.

12   "Before inviting me, they should have paid a fat fee that you have appropriated."

"My fee for attending the party is important. It should have been received by the hero. An invitation was not possible, without previously coming to an agreement. The organization is seen to after the invitation. If you don't give me that money, I shall certainly not go."

13   She breaks off for questions of expenses concerning her maintenance.

If his outlay for her maintenance is not sufficient, she breaks off.
She stops taking care of herself, being sociable, in order to make the hero understand that she is in such a position for lack of money.

14   She spends the hero's money with craftsmen.

She spends the hero's money by ordering works from craftsmen. "I have looked around a great deal to find a marvelous craftsman for this job that interests me, which cannot be carried out if you put it off."

15   The physician and police inspector ask for their fee for their work.

The physician gets the hero to pay his bill for consultation, as well as the chief of police, in recognition of his assistance in the case of theft.

16   She helps his friends and servants in trouble.

She takes care of the hero's friends and kin if they are deserving, but not otherwise. She helps them if they are sick, or have an accident, or are old. Once they have been delivered from their trouble, they will tell the hero of it.

17   She collaborates in housework. She pretends she wants to get pregnant, she busies herself with children's parties, and with his friends' sicknesses and sorrows.

She attends to the housework, as if it pleased her, taking part in the parties for his friends' children, making sure they are programmed for the right day. She takes part in the food offerings, tonsure ceremonies, she wishes to be pregnant like her companions, she assists in cases of sickness or unforeseen events. When a couple of friends lose a child, she shares their grief, she lets it be seen that she is concerned. In such ways, she participates in household interests.

In order to squeeze the hero's money, the courtesan pretends to busy herself with household organization, concerning herself with the rites of her companions' children. She pretends that she wants to be pregnant.

18   She sells part of her jewels to give the money to the hero in case of need.

Gathering her jewels, she sells some of them and gives him the money they fetch.

19   She shows the jeweler her worn jewels and sundry utensils, in order to sell them to him.

These are jewels the courtesan has worn, used utensils and objets d'art. She summons the jeweler in the hero's presence in order to show them to him and ask whether he wants to purchase them.

20   By exchanging them with similar things belonging to other hetairas, she gets a higher value attributed to them.

"By exchanging the objects, she has them estimated better." The meaning of this passage of Dattaka's is clear. In another verse, he says, "With other courtesans, their objects being similar, the objects are exchanged, their value being previously estimated so that they can then

be overvalued and a much higher price obtained from the jeweler's hands, in the hero's absence, than he himself had received for the operation. Used to such operations with courtesans, the jeweler gives back the authentic objects to other dancers."

Their weight is thus increased by several ounces.

21 She does not forget to have those valued that she has previously received as gifts.

If he remembers the objects he has given her and mentions them, what does she say? "For the sake of your reputation and so as not to appear without them, I have had copies made."

22 Through trustworthy persons, she lets him know the great profits made by the other courtesans.

Through trustworthy people, she lets him know that, as compared to her, the others have a better income, a much higher gain. Compared to what the hero gives her, their remuneration is two or three times higher.

23 As compared to the others, who earn much more, or as compared to her previous gains, she is ashamed of what she receives from her lover.

On comparing what she earns with the other courtesans' income, or with what she received from other lovers in the past, she says she feels ashamed at her current income and that he too should be ashamed of it.

If other courtesans come to visit the prostitute, they give an exaggerated estimate of their earnings in front of the hero. Even if they have not earned anything, they look at the hero in such a way as to shame him.

24 If a former lover seeks to renew intimacy with her, offering her a great deal of money, she sends him away.

A former lover, with whom relations have ended, seeks to re-establish relations, proposing a considerable remuneration. But looking at him as though he had poisoned her, she sends him away, making him understand that she is in love, and drives him out.

25 To arouse his competitive spirit, she tells him of the lovers she has abandoned.

In order to stimulate the hero, she speaks of former lovers whom she has left because they spied on her, or for their gossip.

26 For an occasional customer who will not return, the way of obtaining money for intercourse is by behaving like a child.

It is unlikely that he will come back. Like a child, she must beg shamelessly, "Give me that!"
Such ways of obtaining money for sexual relations are indicated, taking into account local customs and the times.

Having assured her means of subsistence through the gifts obtained in exchange for her sexual services, the ways of behavior with a view to separation are now described.

27 Separation becomes inevitable when one notes a change in feelings, and in ways of speaking.

It is inevitable because it is foretokened in every action. A change of attitude indicates that feelings have become different. All kinds of signs show that behavior is different, and it can also be understood from words and words of affection. Even if loving words can give an illusion according to the form they take, one must understand that the affection they betoken is, in reality, disaffection.
What is the way to proceed?
Desire to separate is shown by changes of attitude.

28 He gives her too little or too much money.

When the hero wishes to leave the courtesan, he either gives her too much or too little money.

29 As for her, she attaches herself to men of another social group.

The heroine takes a lover from an opposing group.

30 She does the opposite to what he tells her.

If he says, "Let us go and take a bath!," she does something else and goes and dresses. If he takes his toilet requisites, she goes to eat.

31 He does not do indispensable things.

He does not do what is expected and does not give what he had promised to give.
He postpones indispensable works.

32 He forgets his promises or else acts differently.

If he has promised to give something, he forgets. If she needs something, he says, "I didn't promise it" and brings something else.
A lover who is leaving is perfidious, even when he gives something. He insults her, saying, "When did I promise that?"

33 To the visitors she receives, he speaks only by signs.

To her friends or neighbors who come to see her, he only speaks by signs, without saying a word.

34 On the pretext of work, he makes his excuses to her friends and goes elsewhere to sleep.

He uses the excuse of a job with friends, "I've got something to do elsewhere." He goes to sleep in another house to that of the heroine.

35 He sends his own people to replace all the girl's staff.

He tells his own people secretly to replace all the heroine's personnel, and he sends all the heroine's former servants away.
When he has thus shown his detachment, the girl's way of proceeding is as follows:

36 Before he realizes it, since otherwise he would refuse, she gets her hand on everything.

Before he understands that she has realized his desire to separate from her, since otherwise he would take defensive measures and would stop her, she seizes whatever she can fraudulently.

She hastens to appropriate all the money on which she can lay her hands.

37   Or else she seizes by force whatever is in the hands of the bankers.

The courtesan seizes all his goods deposited with the bankers [sahukāra]. When the hero has a credit with the bankers and she is aware of it, she seizes it authoritatively.

38   Subsequently, if the bankers dispute with him, they will appear before the judge.

The hero accuses the banker before the judge, "Why did you allow my goods to be seized?" The latter replies that it was part of the agreement they had previously established. If there is no sentence, her attempt has succeeded.

The hero's dispute with the banker ends in legal proceedings.

When she is tired of him and wants him to leave, but due to his attachment he will not go of his own will, she must seize the first opportunity for sending him packing.

39   She treats with consideration a lover who has kept her for a long time, even modestly, even if he has behaved badly.

Even if he has given her little and behaved badly, out of affection for him, as one who has rendered her great service in the past, when she wants to be rid of him, she does not throw him out by force.

Ways of throwing out:
40   She throws out a lover who loves her but lacks money, with the help of a rich man who can keep her, but she does not do it herself.

He is without money, penniless, without a position, without a job.

Although she has told him, "I will always be yours," he is now without any means of livelihood, without a position. How can she therefore be rid of him, when she earns her living by means of sexual relations? She engages someone else to do it and makes the two of them rivals. The new one is favored, the other is humiliated and ends by leaving. Otherwise, without some means of action, she would not manage to throw him out.

In order to get rid of him, she may act either openly or discreetly. In connection with this latter manner, Vātsyāyana says:

41 How to go about it discreetly? It is necessary to be disagreeable to him, render him services that displease him, have recourse to forbidden habits, refuse contact with his lips, stamp one's foot on the floor, speak of things he does not know about, take no interest in what he says, reproach him for faults that are common to all.

Render the hero services that he does not want, services that he has previously said exasperate him, exerting herself in so doing either alone or with the servants' aid; practicing forbidden, vulgar habits, such as nibbling grass or leaves and doing it constantly in front of him, knowing that he considers it unclean; refusing the contact of his lips by clenching her own and turning away in horror and stamping on the ground with her feet—these two things always signify anger; speaking of things he knows nothing of, and discussing them in front of him, as if to make him shine, so that he appears stupid in front of other people; showing no admiration for what he says, in order to discourage him and make him look ignorant; humiliating his pride by attributing to another the deeds of courage of which he is proud, leaving him in embarrassment, especially when many people are present whose esteem he desires; without warning, appropriating things of value without his knowledge; complaining of trifling faults to let him know that he is unbearable: such are the ways described.

As far as sexual relations are concerned, these are the ways of detaching him from her.

42 Refusing erotic acts, not showing pleasure, covering the sexual area, pretending aversion to teeth and nail marks, showing opposition when he wants to put his arms around her, displaying a rigidity of the limbs, crossing her thighs,

wanting to sleep separately, being restless during moments of repose, accusing him of being impotent. When he is excited, she does not want to, or she has to go at that very moment to visit important people.

If he gets ready to make love, bringing accessories such as liquors, betel, etc., she does not reply to his invitation. If she accepts, she does it without pleasure. She refuses to give him her mouth, will not let herself be embraced, protects her sex and will not let it be touched. She makes opposition to the scratches and bites he wants to give her, since she detests such marks that she cannot remove. When he wants to put his arms around her to embrace her, she frees her shoulders and, freeing an arm, she shows her opposition to his hugs. She stiffens her body, and does not let herself be caressed. She crosses her thighs to prevent his instrument from entering. She sleeps apart and makes a point of staying alone while resting. If he wants to go anywhere, she declares she is tired and demands to return. She does not cooperate if he wishes to mount her. If he does not manage to have an erection, she laughs and treats him as a eunuch to make him lose all excitement. If he is in form, she says she does not want to and that she wants him to leave her in peace. Similarly, during the day, she says, "Some people are like asses, who copulate in full daylight, which is forbidden." When he shows a desire to sleep with her and begins his approaches, she leaves the house, pretending to have an important appointment, so as to destroy his desire.

If, somehow, the hero, being excited, ejaculates, she reproaches him, saying, "That's all you know how to do!"

If his sexual energy flags, she makes fun of him by applauding. If he is very ardent, she refuses to welcome him, pretending to feel ill. If he wants to make love during the day, she treats him as an erotic ass, insulting him.

43 She interprets his words wrongly; she laughs for no reason at ordinary words, giving them a different meaning. She laughs and winks at men present, in order to humiliate him. She says the contrary of what he says. She accuses him of faults and defects that he cannot get rid of. She reveals his secrets and accuses a servant of having revealed them.

She twists the meaning of his words. For no reason, for words that have nothing funny about them, she suddenly starts laughing. Even when he is not joking, she starts laughing. She laughs at the hero, as though he were really joking. She attributes a different meaning to what he says and points it out to those present, by winking, pointing the finger of scorn at him and laughing. When he speaks of subjects he knows, she shuts him up suddenly, in order to wound him. If he makes a joke, she interrupts him by speaking of other matters. She proclaims his defects or bad habits, such as cheating at games, etc., or else those that are inevitable and cannot be got rid of, so as to make enemies for him. She reveals his secrets in such a way as to put him in the wrong. She learns everything by bribing his servant.

If she does not manage to make him leave by these means, she continues without let, as follows:

44 When he arrives, she refuses to see him. If he asks for something, she refuses. In the end, she has him chased out by her servants, Dattaka explains.

When he comes to visit, she does not receive him. Every time he comes, she does not let herself be seen. If he comes without warning, she does not say a word, does not send him what he asks for. In the end, she throws him out of the house, or else leaves it herself. If these means are not sufficient, she has him thrown out by her servants. This way for the prostitute to have her lover thrown out by her servants is proposed by Dattaka, but is not recommended by Vātsyāyana.

Thus the ways have been indicated by which a courtesan can get rid of a lover.

Contrary to what has been said about being expelled by the servants, etc., it is considered preferable to reflect on what has been said by the Bābhravyas. If she has accepted money from him, what are his rights, and what are those of the prostitute?

45 In this connection, a quotation:
"It is only after taking their sexual relations into consideration, the pleasure they have experienced in intercourse, and the price paid for this amorous enjoyment, that the lover can be sent away by the prostitute."

She must take account of what she has received from her lover, the gains she has made by sleeping with him, the income from copulation, the pleasure she has felt in her relations with him, and the fact that gifts of money and love constitute her way of living, before contemplating the ways of throwing him out. All this only concerns the state of mind of a prostitute and would be unthinkable in a woman of good family. On this subject, Vātsyāyana says, "The wage is what characterizes the prostitute. It is the transaction that constitutes prostitution."

In connection with relations with prostitutes, he says:

46   In plying her trade, the prostitute earns her due. In sleeping with her, no close bond should be created, since she only seeks money.

Thus, in relations with prostitutes, a man is recommended not to bind himself too closely, not to be too familiar, since she is rapacious and only looks for money.

A prostitute who, in the manner described, meets, sleeps with, behaves correctly in her demands for money, and does not trick her lovers, ends by becoming rich.

This chapter on prostitution, composed by Dattaka at the request of the courtesan Vīrasenā, has been included by Vātsyāyana in his *Kāma Sūtra*. Master Dattaka was a great expert on the character, nature, and comportment of courtesans. The courtesans' way of life, as described in this chapter, even if in a somewhat summary form, is complete and covers every aspect. The essential of prostitutes' behavior described in this chapter is found in the dialogue between Muni Maricha and the courtesan Kāmamanjarī, on the subject of the fees mentioned in the *Dashakumāra Charita*. Kāmamanjarī describes the courtesan's state of mind, her mysterious character and comportment that is so difficult to understand, which she attributes to the prostitute's education. From birth, every effort is made to make her beautiful, seeking to improve every part of her body, for which purpose all the means taught in the treatises on beauty and in the *Kāma Sūtra* are employed.

From childhood, the food given to the girls is of a kind to improve their beauty and character during their developing years, and to enliven their spirit. As soon as they are five years old, they are kept under lock and key, without even being able to see a companion. It is at this age that they learn the sixty-four arts. They learn various languages and dialects; they study all the ways of playing, lying, and deceiving; copulation techniques are taught them by trustworthy men of assured discretion, so that they do not suffer too much. The little girls' birthdays are celebrated ostentatiously and, if they are taken to some party or festival, they are dressed in a very attractive manner.

As the little girl grows, her companions pay her compliments on her appearance, her qualities, character, nature, and beauty. According to treatises on beauty, treatises on the arts, and treatises on eroticism, such qualities are viewed from their remunerative aspect. By paying astrologers, they are made to say that the girl is governed by favorable signs, that she brings luck.

Gigolos, clowns, pimps, messengers, and mendicant monks propagandize the girl's beauty, her freshness and sweetness.

Hearing the young prostitute's qualities boasted of, enterprising young men commence buzzing like bees, ready to part with a large sum in order to be the first to enjoy her. All these anxious and agitated young men are examined and, when it is clear that a particular individual is suitable due to his age, money, courage, skill in the arts and professions, character, birth, and gentleness, and that he is ready to give everything to get the girl, he is granted the first copulation. Sometimes, in the case of a particularly rich person, taking money from him under the counter, he is allowed this first copulation in secret, after which they continue to say that the girl is a virgin. Or else, taking a considerable sum from some enterprising boy of a good family, he is trapped. Afterward, those who have trapped him claim damages and squeeze money from him. If he cannot pay, he is dragged before a court of law, and if he subsequently wishes to marry a beautiful, virtuous, and delicate young girl, the girl's mother, who wants her to be the only wife, will refuse his suit forcefully. The manner in which a prostitute, pretending to play the only wife, sucks all her lover's money, has been described in detail by the author of the *Kāma Sūtra*.

The author of the *Dashakumāra Charita* tells how a lover, enamored of the heroine but without the means of paying her, is brutally dismissed by her or by her mother. In order to throw him out, she calls in some bandits, who take everything that he possesses and, having reduced him to poverty, beat him and leave him lifeless.

On the subject of the prostitute's behavior, of her means of livelihood, and her guards armed with sticks, the *Dashakumāra Charita* quotes, from the mouth of a prostitute, the whole chapter of the *Kāma*

Sūtra on prostitution. The prostitute's character is the opposite of that of a well-brought-up woman of good family. A prostitute who adopts this contrary form of behavior is no longer a prostitute, but may become a virtuous wife. A courtesan like Vasantasenā, who fell in love with Chārudatta, was at all points a devoted wife. Such behavior, so contrary to that of the prostitute, is unacceptable to those who watch over her interests.

Seeing that Vasantasenā's behavior was contrary to a prostitute's rule of life or dharma, a libertine, reminding her of a courtesan's duties, says, quoting the *Mricchackatikā*, "You must decorate your dwelling, so that lovers, like young bees, come ceaselessly buzzing around. Your youth and your body must be like the goods for sale in a bazaar, which anyone who has the means can buy. Your only goal must be money. He who pays is the object of your love. He who does not pay must be rejected. You must consider yourself as a liana along the road, which the traveler who takes the road, whether noble or humble, may touch.

"Your body is made to be given for money, good for the use of all, whether you like them or not.

"Vasantasenā! You are the spring where both the wise Brahman and the barbarian draw water to wash themselves. You are that flowering liana made to bend by both the raven and the peacock. You are the boat on which Brahman or prince, merchant or workman may sit to cross the river. Vasantasenā! You are like the boat, the spring, or the liana, not knowing who is famous or insignificant. You yourself must also have this sense of equality, and take for a hero whoever brings you money."

The advice given to Vasantasenā by the libertine describes the prostitute's moral duty. As a result, it is clear that a prostitute belongs to nobody, and her love is given only to money. The reasons given in this chapter for leaving the prostitute, or for rejecting the hero, are based on poverty. "When a man suffers from poverty, his mentality and behavior are soiled. He becomes avaricious, and the prostitute, whose love is based on interest, abandons him." Referring to a classical text, Yashodhara describes the misfortune of the poor man: "He who suffers from poverty is soiled by it. Unable to practice the arts, he becomes coarse and primitive. He wears worn garments and, due to the defects attributed to him, he is kept at a distance. Badly fed, sad, he is rejected by women. He is overlooked, he is given no tokens of affection unless for charity, because he is suffering. He takes his pleasures alone. Nobody wants to have to do with him. In his pride and insolence, he gets angry and no one replies. Nobody will touch him and, when he wants to sleep, he finds no bed."

Such behavior, however, is not merely reserved to prostitutes. Apart from a few virtuous and devoted women, this kind of behavior can be found in all classes of society. Most women are attracted by someone for a special reason, whether it is a question of money, talents, or youth and beauty. This is not peculiar to a single country, but is found among women throughout the world. Basically, a prostitute is a woman like any other and although her profession is misconduct, she maintains a woman's heart and a woman's nature. Just as in noble families, not all the women are virtuous and devoted, nor all are corrupt, so, among courtesans, not all prostitutes are like Vasantasenā, nor are they all fond of money.

Nowadays, disagreements between husband and wife, household quarrels, and divorce are to be found everywhere, with all their consequences, of which the sole cause is that the wife does not seek to please her husband. Prostitutes try harder to be charming, at the slightest pretext weeping or laughing. "Conscious of their interest, they inspire confidence in all, but trust no one."

The defects and inconstancy to be found among courtesans is also seen among ordinary women. The lawgivers acknowledged this when they say that "A well-born and virtuous man should keep away from women, considering them as the urns in a cemetery."

The philosophers who are the worst enemies of women treat them as images of māyā (illusion) and say that "Woman is the only gate to hell," due to her instability and inconstancy.

Whether a prostitute or a wife of good family, because they are women, both are of the same seed. As a result of the influence of her surroundings, or circumstances, one woman becomes a whore and another a noble wife. Neither of them, however, loses her female nature. This is why the legislator (nītikāra), with great wisdom, explains that "A woman with large breasts distills neither ambrosia nor poison. She is, by turns, a liana of ambrosia if you like her, or a poisonous flower if you do not like her."

End of the Third Chapter
Ways of Making Money
of the Sixth Part entitled About Courtesans

Chapter Four

RENEWING FRIENDSHIP WITH A FORMER LOVER

[*Vishīrna Pratisandhāna*]

1   In order to free herself of the man with whom she is living at present and get rid of him painlessly, just as she removes the lacquer that adorns her feet, according to the principle that "one drives out the other," she reestablishes relations with someone who desires her, but with whom she had broken off because he was ruined.

In order to leave the man from whom she has squeezed all his money, the prostitute is reconciled with a former lover.
If she has left the one that was ruined, just as one removes lacquer, why does she take up with him again?

2   If a lover she has left has made money, lives well, and still loves her, she reestablishes their former intimacy.

He lives well, and no longer lacks money. He can therefore pay and he is fond of her. Without a doubt, she can be confident of what he will give her. "I was wrong to chase you out and leave you." Using this argument, she binds herself to him again.

If he is rich, he will certainly give her money. Consequently, since he is still in love with her, she immediately seeks to see him again.

First of all, however, she must learn whether he is attached to another.

3 In order to find out whether he is elsewhere attached, she must contemplate six kinds of situation.

As a rule, it is impossible to appreciate a situation on the strength of what is talked about. If he has formed an attachment elsewhere after their separation, six kinds of situation can be contemplated, according to his way of acting.

4 He left here because he wanted to do so. He has another mistress at present. Will he willingly leave the place he has gone to? This is one of the situations.

5 He departed from both here and there, because he was thrown out.

He has not lost the defects he had here. He will therefore be sent away just the same. This is the second situation.

6 He left here of his own will, while from there he was thrown out.

From here, he departed of his own will; from there, he left because he was thrown out. Such is the third situation.

7 From here he left of his own free will, but there he has settled down.

He departed of his own will because cohabitation was not working. He has settled down there, however, and is cohabiting, which he did not do in the first case. This is the fourth situation.

8 He was sent away from here, whereas he left from there of his own accord.

He departed from here because he was thrown out, since cohabitation was not working. Will he leave there of his own accord, now that he is cohabiting with no problems? This is the fifth case.

9   From here, he was thrown out, while there he has remained.

Cohabitation was not working. Being thrown out of here, he did not leave of his own accord. There he has remained, although he did not do so in other cases. This is the sixth situation.

10   If he went away from here and there in an underhand way, without warning, without taking any account of the qualities of the one or the other woman, he must be considered unstable and untrustworthy.

Having established a relationship, he left without warning, and she learned of his departure from the mouth of her pithamarda (manager). It is not certain that his behavior with the other woman will be different. It is a matter for discussion in one case, as it is in the other. It has nothing to do with the merits of either woman. Neither of them sent him away. He put himself in the wrong by leaving in such a way, showing his instability. He does not settle down, he is not reliable. This is why, even if he is interesting, he must not be trusted.

11   He has left, sent away both here and there, against his will. She threw him out because she could earn much more with another. But now he once more has money. By arousing his jealousy, he will probably give her a great deal.

At present, he is negotiating in secret. Being of a persevering nature, he never broke off completely. In such a case, she has no reason to hesitate. It is merely a matter of money. She sent him away because she could obtain much more money from another. Knowing, however, that by arousing his jealousy he will give more, she decides to sleep with him again.
The prostitute considers that, because he is furious at the man for whom she left him, he will give more. She must therefore reestablish relations without doubt.

12   If she left him because he had no money or was mean, he is not recommendable.

She sent him away because he lacked money or because, even having money, he was mean and gave nothing. A renewed relationship would be just the same.

13   He left here of his own accord and left there because he was sent away: he should not be accepted unless he gives a considerable sum in advance.

He abandoned one prostitute of his own accord, and was sent away by another. It is better not to have relations with him immediately, because, sooner or later, he will probably go away. He must only be accepted under conditions, or else, according to another opinion, accepted for want of a better.

14   He left here of his own accord, but he has settled there: his bad faith is debatable.

The debatable point is to know toward whom he is in bad faith. Before judging him, reflection is necessary.
Why is it debatable?

15   Seeking new sensations, he has installed himself in another woman's house, but not having found what he was looking for, he now realizes that he can find them with me, and thus he returns. Having judged the other's limitations, from an erotic point of view, and having realized her defects, he now sees the superiority of my qualities. He is ready to pay more.

There are some uncertain cases.

16   Or else he is as thoughtless as a child, or cunning, or an adventurer, or irresponsible: considering this, she does not know whether she must sleep with him or not.

He is an adventurer, his loves are not lasting, he desires her, but wherever he goes he captures affections. He wants to make love immediately. What can he give? He is irresponsible, he could do her wrong. It is only after considering all this that she decides whether or not to give herself to him.

17   He left here sent away; there, he left of his own accord. His honesty is open to question.

His good and bad sides must both be seen, whether he should be taken up or rejected.

18   "He is enamored of me and desires me. He will therefore give a lot. He is so impressed by my qualities that he desires no other woman."

He wants to make love with her because he is enamored, beside himself with desire. He is absorbed, enchanted by my qualities. The other woman, whom he is leaving, does not please him.

19   Or else, "I previously rejected him without consideration. Lusting for revenge, he seeks to persuade me, or else he wants to get back the money he gave me. He is attempting to give himself the aspect of a trustworthy person, but what he wants is to recover what he had paid me. He wants to take me away from my current lover and make me leave him. I must therefore be on my guard against his evil intentions."

They had previously separated in an unpleasant fashion and he was sent away. He is now trying to persuade her by pretending to be in love, so as to worm his way into her house to carry out his revenge, forcing her to give up her current lover and making her leave him. His aim is to appropriate the money she obtained as the price of their union, as well as what she has earned with others. He is attracted by the abundance of this money and will do anything to get hold of it. On the pretext of love, he seeks to inspire confidence in her, with the intent of taking back what he had given, desiring to appropriate the fruit of her work. He wishes to enrich himself with the earnings she has saved. He desires to recover what he gave and not to give any more. He wants to separate her from her current lover, who is her livelihood, and being in contact with him who finances her, he is striving to separate her from him in order to unite himself with her. He wants to make her break off with the man who pays her.

Someone who wishes you ill, and is bent on vengeance, should not be frequented.

20 If his state of mind is now different, one may benefit by it after a certain time.

If his mentality has really changed and he now wants to return out of love, he should be kept at a distance for some time in order to judge this change. "It is possible to take advantage of it, if I decide to take him back, but not immediately, and in all cases while maintaining my independence."

21 Sent away from here, he has settled down somewhere else, but is now making discreet overtures through intermediaries.

Given the former relationship and the unpleasant words exchanged previously with him, if his bad character has now become sweeter and he has changed his attitude, advantage can be taken of it after a certain time. Sent away from here and having settled down elsewhere, he is making discreet approaches. It is a matter for discussion.

22 Now established elsewhere, he sends messages through intermediaries. He must present his suit himself.

He is settled elsewhere. His suit, presented either through the offices of the people with whom he lives or through his kinsmen, must be considered with prudence. The possibilities are two: either he has left there already, or else he is seeking an excuse for leaving. He should make his suit himself.
In connection with other situations, Vātsyāyana says:

23 "I threw him out because he committed an offense. After having obtained me, he went away. I must strive to get him back."

He behaved badly, had committed an offense: it was I who sent him away. If I manage to get him back, I can once more take advantage of him and derive new benefits from our relation.

24 If he went away from here after a quarrel, it is now for me to separate him from the other woman.

He left here following a quarrel, a quarrel caused by my words. I must apologize for it and it may be that he will separate from the woman to whom he has gone.

25   I can still squeeze money out of him.

Why should he give it to another? Taking advantage of his vanity, I will make him come back and, through my astuteness, will lay my hands on everything he possesses.

Once he has come to me, his ruin is assured.

26   He has made money by trading, by extending his properties, by winning lawsuits. Financially independent, he is separated from his wife, his father, and his brothers.

He is adept at making money by trade or through the civil service. He has increased his property by purchasing new land. He has also won in legal proceedings. He is separated from his wife, and his father, even if the latter is alive. His grandfather and his brothers are dead. He is therefore independent, free in his work and at home. He can spend freely. This is my chance!

He is wholly independent. This is therefore the right moment to obtain money from him.

27   It happens that the man with whom I live has made friends with this rich man, whom I am going to lay hands on.

The man I am living with has become friends with this man. By sleeping with him, I shall draw the other man to me.

28   Because I have been humiliated by his wife, I will separate him from her.

She was offended because her former lover has gone back to his wife. Wounded in her pride, she decides to separate them, stirring up conflict. For revenge, she stirs up quarrels.

29   A friend of my lover has fallen in love with the latter's legitimate wife. She hates me: I will separate her from him.

A rich elderly man, a friend of my lover's, wants to have relations with his other wife, who is my enemy and wishes me ill. I will separate them, thanks to this old man, so that she will no longer draw any advantage. My mother will take care of it.

30 He is changeable: I shall not keep him for long.

He is an adventurer: here, there, and then somewhere else. He gads about because he is unstable. I shall not keep him for long.

He is known for his instability. He will fall for the wiles of other prostitutes.

A description is now given of one who intrigues on his own.

31 He is truly in love with the heroine and has explained it to the pīthamarda and the others, but her mother, out of malice, has ousted him. He is desperate: she has warned him to leave the place.

Out of spite and the lure of gain, her mother has sent away this former lover. The girl loves him, nonetheless, but she is dependent.

Going to see the pīthamarda and the other confidential servants of the prostitute, he has explained that he is in love with her. He was discouraged, however, by the mother's intrigues and was rejected by her.

32 Her current lover does not please her and she hates having relations with him.

Contacts and sexual relations with her current lover do not please the heroine, because he takes drugs. She is hostile to him as soon as he appears on the path. She does not manage to dissimulate.

She has to sleep with him against her will, but she has a horror of him. The occasion is therefore favorable.

33 Recalling their past love, her former lover wishes to reestablish relations with her.

Noting their former amorous pleasures which are over, the hero calls them to mind in order to renew them.

Seeking to regain her trust, the hero recalls to the heroine their love prior to his expulsion by the pīthamarda and the other servants.

34 Having acknowledged his errors during their first relationship, he convinces her to renew their intimacy.

Having acknowledged the faults he committed and having apologized for his failings in terms of money, the union becomes acceptable since he will pay willingly.

In the absence of a new one, a relationship with a former lover is advised. When the possibility of a new lover arises while the former one is making advances, which of them is it better to accept? He says:

35 The masters say that between a new one and someone with whom she has already had relations, the latter is to be preferred. His character is known, his desires are evident, and it is easy to satisfy him.

His character is clear: by sleeping with someone, one knows his mind. His sexual desires are known, due to their former relations. To the benefit of their mutual rules of life, their relations are easy.

36 With a former connection, there are, as a general rule, no money difficulties, although he does not give much. It is difficult to reestablish former trust. Vātsyāyana says that a new one is easier to manipulate.

He used not to give much money: now one sleeps with someone for money. If he is not suitable, why join up with him again? It is difficult to reestablish mutual trust. Considering his character and seeing his attitude during the affair, his attachment changed from the moment he was sent away. It is easier to satisfy someone who does not know your defects, and money can be obtained from him without difficulty. The money that counts is the money that is actually received. A former lover is of two kinds, one who has had relations with other prostitutes, or one who has not; if he has had, there are again two types according to whether he was rejected or not. The reestablishment of the relationship should be contemplated on the basis of such relations.

According to Vātsyāyana, intercourse takes place in order to obtain money. If the hero had formerly been sent away because he had become avaricious, what would be obtained by reestablishing relations? Apart from this, recovering a trusting intimacy will be difficult, while it is easy to attach oneself to a new lover.

37 Nevertheless, man's nature is unpredictable.

Man's nature means his behavior. It is possible to reestablish a confidential relationship after a break with someone who formerly behaved badly and showed little generosity.

Men are different according to their nature. There are young men who behave like old men. A new lover can show a mean side, giving nothing and, once he has been satisfied, demonstrate no attachment. Others are so made that, after having been exploited, even if they have been thrown out, they conserve their trust and their attraction for the heroine.

Three situations may arise when the hero is bound to another woman, whether it is an old or a new relationship. In explaining this, Vātsyāyana says:

38 In this connection, a quotation:

"She sleeps with him in order to separate him from another woman. She seeks to establish a relationship in order to break up an affair."

"I shall succeed in separating them because their relationship is deteriorating," or else "Because he despises her, I will separate him from his wife," or else "Because he is in love with my enemy, I will separate him from her." On the basis on these intentions, she establishes a loving relationship in order to break up the existing intimacies. Thus she seeks to separate other girls from their weary lovers in order to get them for herself.

39 A fearful man, who is afraid of others and is attracted by her, will not see her defects and will give much.

When a timorous man finds himself in the presence of an enterprising girl, he sets his face against any kind of relation and is some-

times insulting. He takes no account of the heroine's defects, nor of her misconduct. He is impolite with people who approach him. In order to overcome his anxiety, however, he gives a lot.

A lover who is greatly enamored and who is afraid to sleep with another woman, will not see the heroine's defects. He will give a lot because he is fearful.

40   She finds satisfaction in novelty. By utilizing a skillful messenger, she can be possessed.

Her former lover remains greatly enamored of her, and her current lover is also very attached to her. She is only interested, however, in someone with whom she has no bonds. Knowing her state of mind, her desire to conquer an indifferent man, the messenger contrives to detach her from those with whom she is intimate, in order to attract her to his principal. By giving her mother money, a skillful messenger arranges their union.

41   It is not possible to set up a durable relationship with a woman with whom one has slept previously. If she now has a permanent relationship, it is difficult for her to give it up.

It is a question of a former relationship. Given the subject of the chapter, it refers to a prostitute, not to women in general. If her relationship with her current lover is a lasting one, the risk is that she will have trouble with him. A former lover, even if he is very much in love, can wait. She cannot leave her current lover because he is useful to her.

When two lovers present themselves, one rich and the other less fortunate, in her own interest it is advisable for a woman to sleep first with the rich one, since the penniless hero can wait. He must not make a fuss and force her to leave her rich suitor, just because he has been put in second place for copulation.

If, compared to her actual profit, it would be greater with the other, how could she refuse?

42   A woman in the power of a lover may, with his consent, go and pleasure another. Having earned money in this way, she may let her lover profit by it.

Being in the power of the man to whom she is tied, invited by another, she satisfies him and, after this adventure, she makes her lover happy. Having gratified her customer, she returns to base, and does not make friends with the other.

By bringing money home, she makes her man happy.

43 A woman with foresight first examines the income, profits, and solidity of the affair, and the man's constancy, after which she can renew intimacy with a former lover.

Considering her revenues, way of life, the possibilities of making a profit, is it in her interest to reestablish relations? She examines it carefully and ponders the matter with skill.

An adroit woman must, first of all, consider fortune, profit, the strength of the affair, and constancy, prior to reestablishing relations with a former lover.

Having sucked all her lover's money by various means, a prostitute leaves him without resources and then throws him out, either with grace or else without ceremony.

With such lovers, bereft of common sense, in what situations or under what conditions can the prostitute renew relations?

The whole chapter on prostitution was written by Master Dattaka. He has described in detail the states of mind of prostitutes and their lovers from the scientific point of view. Vātsyāyana has, however, briefly introduced his point of view in this detailed description, in such a way that as a whole, the description reflects the essential, i.e., all the aspects of prostitution.

In describing the state of mind of the amorous candidates, Vātsyāyana says that, in questions of meetings or separations, the prostitute accepts or rejects a man after analyzing his intimate nature. Some persons take up a prostitute after she has sent her former lover away. If, however, one contemplates all the prostitute's ways of behaving from the point of view of vice and her greed for gain, one risks making a mistake, since there are also persons who, having been insulted and thrown out by a prostitute, gather all their goods and money to give them to her. They remain attached to her and desirous of having relations with her again. After having given her all their money, they continue to run after her and, even after being insulted and deceived, continue to trust her. This is why a prostitute appreciates the idea of renewing intimacy with a former lover who sends her messages, out of a question of feelings. Often, however, if she gives way and decides to do so, she is deceived.

In this chapter, prostitutes are described as being changeable, undecided, completely selfish. On taking a closer look, a prostitutes' moods effectively appear as shifting as the waves of the sea.

In a prostitute's dwelling, her lover's presence lasts no longer than the reddening of the sky when the sun sets. Just as the henna leaves crushed to color one's feet are thrown away, so a prostitute, having extracted money and success from her lover, throws him aside.

In this chapter, by studying the prostitute's ways of behaving and her lover's position, the difference between men and women becomes evident. In one of the last verses, the prostitute is called "the woman" (nārī), while in another passage it appears that, from the point of view of the wise author, one should see no difference between a prostitute and an ordinary woman, since it is a matter of women in general. In such conditions, it is not a mistake to consider the prostitute and her lover as an ordinary man and woman and treat their psychological traits on the same level.

It seems that, in a man's life, satisfying his love, his excitation, and his erotic desires is an everyday activity, having nothing to do with his inner being. For a woman, on the other hand, love and erotic satisfaction are the mainspring of her existence and are strictly tied to her state. A man makes love with the woman he loves, after which, considering that he must have been mad, he ends there but, according to the differences of mentality, it is evident that for the lover, it is only with his body, his substance, that he makes love with the body and substance of his mistress. His love has nothing to do with his soul or mind. Nevertheless, it is curious that he believes that the woman loves him with her soul.

Contrariwise, when a woman is in love with a man, she loves him with her whole body, soul, mind, and substance, and thus the closer she is to nature the more primitive she is. When she is educated, she easily becomes more calculating. The fact must not be overlooked that a woman knows much more than a man about procreation and other realities. This is why wise, scholarly, important men are like ignorant street urchins in front of women. Woman is intuitive. By her intuition, she sees more or less that mind and matter, the one without the other, lead to nothing. This is why she uses her body and soul in love. But when does a man ever give himself in such a manner? The result of this mistake on the man's side means that most relations between married couples, as well as most amorous relations with prostitutes, remain without hope and without peace. The way to find a remedy would be for the man to realize, starting from the wedding night, from the first relations with a prostitute, that it is a question of two souls, two hearts, and not merely an opportunity for intercourse, rubbing against each other.

End of the Fourth Chapter
Renewing Friendship with a Former Lover
of the Sixth Part entitled About Courtesans

Chapter Five

OCCASIONAL PROFITS
[*Lābha Vishesha*]

There are three kinds of prostitutes.

The one who lives with one man, the one who is tied to several, and the one who is tied to nobody. The profits of the first category have already been described; those of the second category will be spoken of. With regard to the third, which is without attachments, the profits she makes from each customer are called occasional profits. The income of the one who is independent will now be described.

1   Sleeping with different individuals, her daily earnings come from various persons, since she does not settle on a single one.

When she sleeps a single time with each of her numerous custom-ers, she makes them competitors. Each of them gives little. Her daily profits are therefore uncertain, and often very meager. If she happens to have only one customer, she must be content with what he gives her.

2   Considering the country, the period, her own condition,

her qualities and chances, her advantages, whether greater
or lesser than those of the others, she establishes her price
for the night.

*In order to evaluate the price of a night, a man considers the
relative advantages of the prostitute with whom he wishes to sleep,
which vary according to country, region, period, and customs, in particular the value relative to practices concerning the upper or lower
parts of the body, and the girl's qualities, beauty, skill, and superiority
as compared to the others.*

*If he wishes to stay the whole night, it is better not to argue over
the agreed price.*

*If it is worthwhile sleeping with him, once the price has been fixed
and following the information furnished by her messenger, she calls
him and the business is settled.*

3   She uses a messenger for her amorous relations. If he
encounters difficulties, she gives up the enterprise.

*If the messenger finds difficulties, if it is difficult to discover the
customer's intentions, she gives it up, after examining his proposals, if
her profit is uncertain.*

*Following the messenger's instructions, she fixes the price for half
a night, for a single copulation. She thus earns more, but it is not
honest.*

4   If, by chance, she manages to obtain from a single customer the price of two or three or four nights, she stays
with him, behaving like a wife.

*During the following days, dropping the others, she makes him
welcome.*

*On what grounds does she choose the man with whom it is advis-
able to sleep?*

5   According to the masters of old, when two customers present
themselves to enjoy her and propose the same fee, she must
clearly go with the one from whom she can obtain an extra.

Financial possibilities are the same and both are anxious to fuck

*her. In order to obtain more money from one than from the other, she
goes with the one who gives more than the price, thus obtaining an
extra profit.*

**6 According to Vātsyāyana, anything may be obtained by
giving something in exchange: the coin is the basis of every
transaction.**

*The coin referred to is the kapardaka, the shell that serves as
money, known all over the world. Even if copulation does not take
place, once given, the coin is not returned. If one sells clothes, etc., one
receives something in exchange. It is the same for every transaction.
Every activity from which a profit is made is based on money. This case
too is a commercial transaction.*

Jewels, precious objects, etc., can be bought for coin. This is why
a prostitute must squeeze as many coins from her lover as she can.

What are the things that one buys?

**7 They are, as the case may be, objects of gold or silver;
copper, bronze, or iron utensils; hangings; shawls; garments;
perfumes; spices; accessories; ghee; oil; wheat; cattle.**

*Gold and silver may be worked or not. The utensils are vessels of
copper, bronze, or iron. Hangings also include cushions, shawls, rugs,
luxurious garments of silk, etc. Perfumes mean sandalwood, etc., spices
(pepper, etc.), accessories (plates, seats, etc.), consumer products, flour,
ghee, oil, meat, and others. Before purchasing, the prostitute must
choose things of the best quality.*

**8 When two candidates are similar, if she likes them both
equally and they are equally rich, she refuses or accepts to sleep
with one of them according to the advice of her household.**

*When she has two similar suitors and likes neither more than the
other, if they are equally rich, equally generous, equally handsome and
important, she consults her household and follows their advice. Or else,
when one of them makes advances, she chooses him because he loves her
or because she is attracted to him.*

Which are the ones most deserving of her to sleep with them?

9   According to the masters of old, she should prefer the one that pays well rather than a passionate lover, because it is to her advantage.

Material realities must always be considered. It is thus that money is obtained.

10   She must be capable of leaving a lover for someone who pays.

She must find the means of ridding herself of someone who is greatly enamored, but who does not pay.
Vātsyāyana's opinion is that:

11   "He who is in love parts easily with his money, even if he is mean; but he who wants to go away cannot be recovered."

Parting with something means giving. It is useless to try to please someone who is ready to break off relations.

12   According to the masters of old, between a rich man and one who is not rich, it is the rich man who is interesting, and between one who spends willingly and one who tries to render services, the useful one is often preferable.

Between the rich and the poor, the rich man is preferable. However, the one who arranges her encounters, who assists her in her work, is preferable to someone who spends freely, since the former makes himself useful, and it is not certain that the spender will give money.

13   "He who renders services and acts immediately is useful in any enterprise, while the spender will end by going away," says Vātsyāyana.

One who renders services does what she asks of him immediately. "What would I do without him? The other will go away. Even if he pays me, I must not expect that he will give me money later on, since he is a spender by nature. There is no continuity in his acts of generosity."

14   There too, of the two of them, one must consider whose absence will cause the most inconvenience.

The one whose services I shall miss is therefore the more important. Although both are useful, according to the circumstances.

15   According to the masters, between a serious, faithful man [kritajña] and a fickle man, it is advisable to favor the fickle one.

16   The past attentions of the fickle man [tyāgī] who has been courting her for a long time, even if he has once behaved badly and has betrayed her with other courtesans, must be taken into consideration.

For a very long time, the heroine has been courted, overwhelmed with attentions, by a guilty lover who, lacking in respect for her, was openly caught betraying her. Despite his offense, his efforts and the trouble he has taken to serve her must not be forgotten.
What has he done?

17   Fickle people are often impulsive, changeable, distant.

Being impetuous, they are unstable by nature. No attention should be paid to their misconduct, due to their ardent nature. Their vanity may cause one to mistake their real uprightness. One must not bear them a grudge.
How does the faithful lover behave?

18   He who is faithful is conscious of what he has acquired and will not let himself be easily seduced. Careful in his behavior, he does not commit the offense of deceiving her, Vātsyāyana explains.

Aware of his former experience, the conscientious man, because he is faithful, does not allow himself to be seduced by another, even if he is ill-treated. Being of a reasonable nature, he does not make the mistake of deceiving her, since he knows her temperament.
Neither does he go frolicking around with other prostitutes.

19   Here too, it is the yield that counts.

In the choice between an influential person, but with whom, according to her friends' opinion, she risks a financial loss, and someone who is rich, it is the second that counts, without any hesitation.

Between two influential persons, she must prefer the one from whom she will obtain most.

On what basis?

20 She must follow her assistants' advice in sleeping with the one from whom she will obtain the most money. She must always prefer a relationship that pays, say the masters.

According to the advice of her kin, she chooses the most advantageous one. With the other, she only has social relations.

21 According to Vātsyāyana, if she chooses to sleep with one for a matter of money, without following the counsel of her assistants, they will make difficulties.

When she could receive money, but refuses to and does not follow the advice of her kin, the latter will be furious and foment difficulties which will do her harm.

22 She may not neglect her assistants' advice.

If she neglects their interests, she must compensate them.

They must, without fail, receive their share of the money she obtains.

In connection with discontented collaborators, it is said:

23 In such a case, she summons the assistant who organizes her work, saying, "Tomorrow I will do what you advise, and you will recoup the money for my transgression."

The one who organizes her work supervises her relations with people, and does not tolerate her acting without his consent. She says to him, "Tomorrow I will do what you ordered and you will receive your share."

24 According to the masters, when there are several pos-

sibilities, the collection of money is always preferred by prudent persons.

25   According to Vātsyāyana, earnings may be meager, but if no money is produced by what one does, one will not know what to live on.

When money is scarce, someone who has never had much can make do. Once the constant flow has stopped, however, one no longer knows who to turn to. In this connection, one calls to mind the example of the drip of honey, that little by little empties the honeycomb.

26   There is also a difference to establish between the fat and the thin.

When compared to the thin ones' lack of money, the lack of money of the fat ones seems to be prosperity. It is necessary to understand the meaning of plus and minus.

27   When one fears that money may be lacking, the different levels concerning the lack of money must be considered.

Everything depends on what is meant by lack of money. It is clear that people's behavior is based on this doubt. To have limits to what one can spend is to lack money. As far as current needs are concerned, one must try to define what they are based on. In this case too, there are differences. According to the saying, "What can be extracted from a fat man who lacks money passes for abundance compared to the thin man's lack of money."

For half a night, by specifying a suitable price, she earns more. In order to obtain a greater income, she should make the others wait at the door.

28   Having temples and reservoirs built, setting up altars on raised platforms to Agni, the fire god, giving Brahmans herds of cows and covered vessels, arranging pūjās and offerings to the gods, bearing the expenses involved with the money they earn, this is the concern of high-ranking courtesans who reap large profits.

There are three kinds of prostitute: courtesans [ganikā], girls who live on their charms [rūpājīvā], and slave water carriers [kumbhadāsī]. These three categories correspond to three levels: upper, middle, and lower.

In order to procure what is destined for the gods, what counts is money.

This is why only the top-ranking courtesans can take on the expense of digging pools of flowering lotus, or building fire altars in high places and, in order to reach them, build bridges, have shelters made of earth to house the oil, perfumes, and choice grain for the fire offerings. For this purpose, she must use covered vessels. A prostitute's offerings may not be received from her hand and must be brought by someone else. Things intended for the gods' pūjās are therefore placed in covered vessels, mostly for food offerings.

Seductive girls of middling and lower status may not take part, even if they have the means, since they are only half-qualified.

By supplying all the accessories required for the rites performed daily for the Agnihotra ceremony (fire worship) through the offices of a ritually acceptable person, she assures the outlay for meritorious and charitable works.

29 Covering all her limbs with jewels and carefully decorating her home with priceless vases, utilizing her servants to polish all the openings of her house, those who live on their charms succeed in improving their status.

They cover their limbs with jewels, wherever they can put them. They decorate their dwellings with expensive vases of copper and iron, with the assistance of the servants they employ when they earn well. Of the seductive girls, the richest, the most beautiful and expert in the arts, although they only enjoy middling or lower status, are put on the same footing as courtesans.

They employ servants to keep clean their windows, doors, hangings, curtains, and garments, which must be as white as milk.

30 A slave water carrier who wishes to make considerable gains must always wear spotless clothes and feed well, always have scented betel, and wear silver-gilt ornaments.

Her underclothes, like her top garments, must always be white. She must not appear famished, eat sugarcane, oil, or ghee. Her perfumed mouth must smell good, and always contain betel. She must always imitate the courtesans and girls of charm. She is advised to wear gold-plated jewelry. In order to have good earnings, she must raise herself above her slave status. She is considered as a water carrier. She does this work in order to be able to stop carrying jars. She has clearly left an overhumble job for a superior occupation.

31 According to the masters, prostitutes of middle and low class also make considerable profits.

Compared to the courtesans, girls of charm and water carriers have an income proportional to their status. After her essentials and setting-up expenses, whatever the prostitute has left over is considered a gain, which may be considerable.

32 Vātsyāyana explains that the profits and remuneration given are determined according to place, times, living standards, ability, eroticism, and customs.

According to whether the country is rich or poor, the period prosperous or poverty-stricken, whether living conditions for the individual are abundant or limited, profit-making capacity may be wide or restricted. The remunerations indicated here as an example correspond to a favorable financial situation, but they may be higher or lower.
On the other hand, in relation to the job performed, her earnings are sometimes scarce. Sometimes she receives nothing, sometimes she is given much.
Thus, it is said:

33 A courtesan may even accept to have intercourse for very little money, if it is a question of taking another girl's lover, preventing him from setting up house with her, stealing the permanent lover of another or appropriating another's profits, separating her from a potential lover by appropriating him, widening her relations through her amorous contacts, or else, to have his assistance in the spiteful actions she has in mind, to induce another's steady lover to behave

badly: considering everything he has done for her in the past, the courtesan willingly accepts him for a small sum.

Desirous of separating another courtesan from her lover, of preventing him from cohabiting with another girl, wishing to seize a man who is attached to another and make him leave her, wanting to appropriate what another girl has earned, she wishes to take advantage of the man to whom she is tied. Anxious to separate them, she organizes a breach between them. For this purpose, she makes amorous advances and, by sleeping with him, she establishes a bond.

She wishes to enlarge her property, her home, her reception rooms. Having won a position of influence, thanks to her earnings, she wishes to dominate the other courtesans and, to this end, she needs means. Seeing that someone is attached to another girl, she exerts herself to seduce him, even if she already has a lover. She looks for one who has rendered her services in the past, even if at that time she was only making a small profit. She accepts to take back someone who, in the past, was not correct in his financial dealings and from whom she earned little at the time, but who has apologized for his offense.

She accepts him only because she is seeking affection. She accepts him for love and not for money, welcoming him with pleasure.

According to the occasion and necessity, one must sometimes be content with a modest profit.

She must foresee the possibilities of profit or loss.

34   Her protector has no money, but is expecting considerable funds. To safeguard the future, she takes nothing from him.

He is expecting a considerable sum, but it has not arrived and he is without money. She takes nothing from him in the expectation of future profits.

35   On leaving this man, I shall find another with whom I can have a serious attachment; going back to his wife, that man will leave me in poverty; another is under the thumb of his master, or father, etc.; or his position is threatened; or he is unstable: in all these cases, she must take in advance the remuneration given on account.

On leaving this man after taking his money, I shall attach myself to another who will give me more. If he goes back to his wife, how will he be able to pay me? I shall be ruined and without resources.

If he is in someone else's power, held like an elephant by the goad, he must obey. If he is not independent, how will he be able to pay for his amorous relations, being under the rule of his master or his father? His position is in jeopardy. He risks having to leave the position he occupies. Since his future is uncertain, how will he be able to pay? In all these cases, one must make sure to be paid at once.

If the prostitute sees that things are going thus, she must squeeze all she can immediately from the hero.

36   He is certain to receive considerable goods from the king, or he will be given an important post. He will soon be able to enjoy his revenues. His ship is about to come in. The revenue from his estates and houses is due. He does not forget what has gone by. He knows that she desires a constant income, without arguments. This is why she decides to stay attached to him.

She does not leave him in the knowledge that, if she takes him as her lover, he will give her whatever she needs, without difficulty; that he is expecting an important post to be given him by the government, that the time is ripe to draw the revenue for his services, that the moment has come when his means will be assured, even if for the time being delays are being made by the court or the king, that ships full of goods are about to arrive, from which he will make a profit by trading, that he is waiting for the harvest from his estates. He does not forget past deeds, and having slept together will not be fruitless, since he is not ungrateful and does not go back on his commitments; when he is able to enjoy an unlimited income, he will honor the promises he made during their relationship and will give the money he promised.

He is not a chatterbox or falsehearted. He will do what he promised. Thus, by choosing from among all the others her hero, from whom she expects important profits in the future, a courtesan may, with this end in sight, devote herself to him like a wife.

On this subject, a quotation:

37   "She must stay away from anyone from whom she can

only just obtain her livelihood or from anyone who performs dirty work in the king's service, even if she can make a profit thereby."

Someone from whom she only just makes a living, from whom she has difficulty in squeezing the means of existence, or someone who does dirty work for the king, who performs unpleasant and cruel business for the state that one should avoid doing, even if she counts on making a considerable or modest profit thereby, she should hurl him far away from her. She must neither see nor speak to such men, since she thereby risks serious trouble. For what reason?

38   To avoid the misfortune due to them. In order to get free, she strives to attach herself to someone else.

In order to leave the man to whom she is tied without profit, or to free herself from another, she strives to grab someone by sleeping with him. This expedient serves her as a pretext, even if she gets nothing out of it. She does not go with this new lover with the intention of becoming tied to him inasmuch as, since he is without resources, it would not improve her position.

With regard to those whose resources she may use, it is said:

39   The rich man, who gives without counting and is satisfied with little, is a magnificent character. She must go with him to assure her expenses.

An important man, whose prestige is seen from his splendor, who is satisfied with little and is ready to spend a lot on the prostitute: she must attach herself to him, considering that her expenses will be assured.

This chapter deals with the occasional earnings of prostitutes, which they obtain from their lovers by all kinds of expedients. To begin with, the three types of prostitute are described, those who have only one steady lover, those who have several lovers, and those who have nobody permanent. The one who sets up with the hero, playing the role of the single wife, has relations with only one man.

The one who makes money by sleeping with several lovers is the girl of several.

She who is attached to no one and sleeps with anyone that comes to her, receiving money for it, is called an unattached prostitute.

The author of the *Kama Sutra* describes the ways of going about things of those that have several lovers and of the independent ones who, by easily satisfying their lovers, obtain money from all of them.

As regards prostitutes who have several lovers, the author of the *Kama Sutra* describes their art of proceeding secretly and discreetly in their amorous relationships. Their behavior is such that, even if they have contacts with several lovers during the same night, none of the lovers realizes the existence of the others, neither their arrival nor their departure. The kind of joke practiced by prostitutes is charmingly described in the *Bhoja Prabandha*.

Bhoja, the king of Dhārā, and the great poet Kālidāsa were both in love with a courtesan of the city, who had amorous relations with each of them. One day, King Bhoja learned that Kālidāsa was going to visit her. He told the prostitute that, in order to have proof of Kālidāsa's love, she must ask him to shave his head. Following Bhoja's suggestion, the prostitute said to Kālidāsa, "I have had proof that you are not very much in love with me." Kālidāsa said to her, "Yet I do whatever you ask of me." The prostitute replied that "The coils of your hair are better loved by you and by the public than I am. And I am jealous. If I were to tell you to do so, would you be capable of cutting them off?" "Certainly," said Kālidāsa, who lowered his head and let his hair be cut. Touched, the prostitute then said to him, "It is King Bhoja who claims that you would leave me rather than give up your coils of hair. I now see that your love for me is boundless." Kālidāsa realized that King Bhoja was greatly in love with the courtesan and had invented this stratagem to detach him from her and humiliate him. The poet, however, did not consider all was lost. He said to the girl, "If you believe that the king is more in love with you than I am, you must put him to the test too." The courtesan asked how. Kālidāsa replied, "Tell him to go into the garden and bray like an ass." She accepted to do so and, when King Bhoja arrived, she told him that as proof of his love, he must go into the garden and bray like an ass. The king did not refuse and, standing in the garden, started to bray: "Hee-haw, hee-haw!" He thought that no one besides the prostitute knew the story of his braying.

This is why, the following day in the audience hall, in order to ridicule Kālidāsa, he asked him, "Kālidāsa! Sublime poet! What was the occasion that made you shave your head?" Kālidāsa immediately retorted,

"Sire! Under the same circumstances that make kings bray like asses!"

On hearing Kālidāsa's words with their hidden meaning, the king was abashed and said nothing.

In the *Kāma Sūtra*, suggestions are given with regard to the prostitute's remuneration according to the region, period, situation, her qualities, beauty, etc., in order to enjoy her for a night.

According to the *Artha Shāstra* by Kautilya, however, it is not the prostitute who decides: the price is fixed by the government. Kautilya studied the prostitute's trade. In order to have a look at their condition and morality, an intendant of prostitution was appointed, who fixed the courtesans' remuneration, taking into account the people who frequent them, their income, and expenses. The independence enjoyed by prostitutes at the time of the author of the *Kāma Sūtra* did not exist at the time of the author of the *Artha Shāstra*. At that time, prostitutes were controlled by the government. They could not demand an excessive price from anyone, nor steal his money, nor insult him. They could not earn more than necessary, nor spend more than foreseen. Since their adolescence, they had to learn the prostitute's business. Their income was fixed by the government and, if they acted contrary to the laws, they were severely punished.

But it does not appear that the prostitutes of the *Kāma Sūtra* were under any restriction. The chapter on prostitution describes lovers, customers of all kinds, and the ways of exploiting them or getting rid of them after despoiling them and accusing them of faults, spreading hostile rumors about them. They had every freedom. The king's and government's supervision of prostitutes was relative. If somebody did not pay them properly, they went before the judge and obtained justice. By studying and comparing the chapter on courtesans in the *Artha Shāstra* and the chapter on prostitutes in the *Kāma Sūtra*, certain authors have concluded that Kautilya and Vātsyāyana were the same person. It is true that the type of composition of the two works is similar, but if they had been composed by the same author, in the same period, such differences in the laws, ways of behaving, social traditions, and government practice would not have existed.

Like Vātsyāyana, Kautilya considers three kinds of prostitute: upper, middle, and lower. Principles and aims, however, are different. For Kautilya, the differences concern the tax office, whether to levy more or less tax, while for the *Kāma Sūtra*, the differences concern demands for money and services rendered to customers.

There is such a difference in rules and behavior that it is evident that the *Kāma Sūtra* belongs to a later period than Kautilya's *Artha Shāstra*. With regard to rates, Vātsyāyana mentions a gold piece for the highest category. During the Gupta period, gold and silver pieces were used. During the Maurya period, the highest piece was the pana.

Concerning prostitutes' remuneration, earnings, and savings, Kautilya speaks of the pana, whereas Vātsyāyana does not even use the word. In speaking of the prostitute's wage, he talks of the gold piece (suvarna mudrā) and even of the rudra vrati (the one of Shiva's fast), which clearly indicates the Gupta period (fourth century). The courtesan Sugandhā of Ujjaina asked for one gold piece for a single time, a price that few young people could pay. Because of her unrivalled beauty, famous and scholarly Brahmans lost their goods, kings and princes gave her everything and were thrown out of her dwelling. Stripping them naked and insulting them, she had them forcefully thrown outside.

A courtesan spends her assets on religious, cultural, or social enterprises. Being a high-class heroine, a courtesan has relations with heroes belonging to high society. She behaves like a woman of good family, without making a show of eroticism or rapacity.

Pingalā, from the *Sānkhya* treatise, Indumatī, the courtesan of King Sāgara, Vilāsinī and Sugandhā of Avantī, Lakshmanā and Karnātakī from the south, and Āmrapālī of Vaishālī were courtesans who have remained famous in the *Purānas* and epic poems for their incomparable beauty as well as for their merits and behavior. They were predestined creatures and, as soon as their destiny was revealed by circumstances, they renounced their profession and devoted themselves to the gods, acquiring the ability to attain liberation. These are the kind of prostitutes whom Vātsyāyana calls upper (uttamā) or courtesans (ganikā).

The rūpājīvā, one who lives on her charms, is a prostitute endowed with beauty, talent, and merit, who spends her life practicing the arts. She attracts men who love and practice the arts. In all their activities and relations, the arts have a predominant place. Because of their talents, they are a kind of fiancée for the whole town.

The third category of prostitute, the slave water carriers, recall those seen today by the thousand, who sell their youth. They are considered inferior due to their character, behavior, and incompetence. Their only resource is sex.

Subsequently evoking relations with former lovers, ancient verses are quoted as examples. Among these, in the twenty-second verse, the whore is called a woman like the others (nārī) and in the forty-third, she is called a female being (shrī). In this connection, the author does not consider them as a separate category among women and, according to this principle, he speaks of prostitutes at the same time as women in general and their virtues.

In describing womankind, the *Brahmavaivarta Purāna* (I-31) says: "A woman who has only one husband is a model wife (pativratā). She who has two husbands is called kulatā (stray). She who has three husbands, vrishalī (broad view), she who has four husbands, punchālī (shameless). Those who have five, six, or more husbands are called prostitutes (veshyā). Those who have seven or eight husbands are known as yunmi (public women), and those who have even more husbands are the superwhores (mahāveshyā) for the satisfaction of all castes."

As in the *Kāma Sūtra*, according to the *Brahmavaivarta Purāna*, the nature of all women is the same.

It is according to her behavior, her character, that a woman belongs to different categories. In the opinion of the author of the *Purāna*, a woman, according to whether she has one, two, or three husbands, is called virtuous, stray, etc. In the *Kāma Sūtra*, only prostitutes are concerned. This is a basic difference. For the *Kāma Sūtra*, a prostitute is born into this class, while for the author of the *Purāna*, it is a question of behavior. For the *Kāma Sūtra*, a prostitute's daughter is a prostitute by heredity, so that it is right to say that she is a prostitute by nature. Contrary to the *Kāma Sūtra*, however, poets, historians and playwrights consider that the heroine belongs to the prostitutes' class on the one hand, and to the class of women on the other.

At the same time, the apsaras, Rambhā, Menakā, and Urvashī, and the other heavenly nymphs form a separate category. In the *Purānas*, the legendary accounts, and works on ethics, the nymphs are considered as a kind of courtesan.

It may be considered that, just as among the gods the yakshas and gandharvas form lower categories, in the same way the apsaras, who are superhuman beings, are nevertheless women. To consider courtesans and prostitutes as forming a separate category of women is an indefensible argument for human intelligence and science. It can be said that by birth one belongs to the Brahman, Kshatriya, Vaishya, or Shūdra caste and that, for each person, this is considered as forming part of his nature. But it cannot be said, in the same manner, that certain women are prostitutes by nature. This is not acceptable either in principle or in practice. In reality, a courtesan is a woman like others, included in the prostitutes' category. She has debased herself by her activities. If a woman who was irreproachable misbehaves, she too becomes kulatā, vrishalī, punchālī, or veshyā. When she falls increasingly lower, she is called mahāveshyā, superwhore, and is considered untouchable and despicable. The author of the *Purāna* adopts the point of view of the *Kāma Sūtra* that a high-class prostitute, being unable to accept an object from the hand of any prostitute of another category, would use an intermediary's hand to take it. The author of the *Purāna* says that a prostitute's gifts are unacceptable. The twice-born who accept money from a prostitute end up in a hell called kāla sūtra.

End of the Fifth Chapter
Occasional Profits
of the Sixth Part entitled About Courtesans

Chapter Six

Profits and Losses

Reflections on Doubts Concerning the Advantages and Disadvantages of Relations
[*Artha-anartha Anubandha Vichāra*]

1   It can happen that in pursuing profit, one ends with a loss. A relationship must therefore be considered prudently.

Profits include the occasional earnings that the prostitute may make. If a steady relationship offers the possibility of gain and the risk of loss, it is better to renounce it, if she has the means of getting along. What can the losses be due to?

2   They can be due to lack of intelligence, to excessive love, to vanity, dishonesty, cupidity, excessive trust, anger, pride, brutality, belief in luck.

Losses come from a lack of intelligence, meaning discernment in appraising would-be lovers, from the violence of feelings of love, from vanity or egoism, cunning and deceit, from cupidity, excessive trust given to someone, from anger, from crises of wrath. When such defects interfere in a relationship, even if they are slight, it is better to renounce it. Pride separates you from other people, brutality provokes fear. Such are the defects concerning a man. The prostitute's loss often consists of attributing the difficulties she encounters to the stars.

3 The results of such defects are that, once the relationship is established, the promise of money as an income from the sexual relation does not materialize. Her earnings do not cover her expenses. He leaves her for another. The sexual relationship is a brutal one, injuring her body. He tears out her hair, throws her to the ground, breaks her limbs. These are the possible risks.

All these misfortunes, caused by stupidity and other defects, are the result of a lack of prudence in establishing a relationship that will not give the expected results. Financial questions must be dealt with prudently, otherwise any profit is in jeopardy. The expenses are those made to arrange love meetings that, for lack of income, lead to a deficit. It must be seen that expenses do not exceed income, since otherwise the verbal contract is reversed. He may go away because he has some other attachment. Cruelty manifests itself in hostile words, overly numerous copulations, physical brutality to the point of killing her, tearing out her hair, throwing her to the ground, attacking her, beating her, breaking her limbs, cutting off her nose or ears.

Possible misadventures are as follows:

The money spent for his welcome is lost. Her influence over the hero is not lasting. The money expected is not received and what has been saved up goes. In the case of repeated quarrels, when the hero gets angry, he seizes the prostitute by her hair, throws her to the ground, beats her, breaks her limbs: she may even die of it.

4 In order to avoid such risks, even if she could obtain a lot of money, she must give it up.

She must learn to overcome her stupidity and other defects since, if her monetary earnings are tied to perverse practices, instead of prof-

its she may find misfortune. In the eventuality of ill-treatment, even if her money is certain, but, in order to earn a lot of money she must expect brutality, she must look for other sources of earning.

Concerning relationships to be avoided, he says:

5 Money, virtue, and love are the three goals to be attained.

6 Lack of money, lack of virtue, and hate are the three sources of sorrow.

The goal to be attained is of three kinds, whose opposites, the sources of sorrow, are also of three kinds. This is why these two aspects must be pondered since, besides the question of profit and loss, this verse simultaneously contemplates moral/immoral and love/hate aspects, although some opinions do not consider this aspect.

7 In practice, the other kinds of misfortune depend on these.

Apart from these six possibilities of success or failure, five other troubles may also be experienced, some of which are of the same nature, while others are of a different nature.

8 If the expected profit is not certain to be obtained without difficulty, it is proper to have some hesitation.

9 It is difficult to foresee the outcome right at the start.

This dilemma makes any decision uncertain, the mind remains confused.

10 It is only in practice that one or other of these eventualities may occur.

Only when the deed has been accomplished is it possible to know whether the relationship is profitable or not. Uncertainty, in this case concerning money, is found in other aspects, whether they are of the same or of a different nature. There is always a dilemma.

When the result of a deed is not as expected, it is called an ambiguous relationship.

11 A relationship may also have a multiple outcome, of which examples will be given.

An action may have a multiple effect. If the result is uncertain to start with, it is better to avoid the relationship. Some examples will be given.

Since the form of the three kinds of failure are unknown, what examples can be given?

12   The form of the three kinds of success has been contemplated. Their opposites are the three kinds of failure.

They are success in the three aims of life: love, money, and virtue.

13   Having had an excellent sexual relationship with someone, she expects that her monetary earnings, when she receives them, will show a tidy profit. If it is not so, it is a failure connected with money.

Lovers are of three kinds. She has slept with the lover of her first choice, who is endowed with every quality. Her earnings are assured with him. It is obvious that she will receive her due, the amount generally agreed upon. She is enhanced by it and other suitors immediately press her, desirous of sleeping with her. The money earned from them is the result of her earnings with the first one. The money she receives is connected with the money already received. Thus, there is a relationship between things of the same nature.

14   If she sleeps with just anyone solely for gain, the relationship is a purely commercial one.

When, solely for gain, she sleeps with just anyone whose qualities or defects are unknown to her, she does it without reflecting.

15   By accepting money from someone else, she risks losing the affection of her faithful lover, who will cut off her allowance, so that there will be a money loss. Furthermore, she incurs everybody's contempt. Or else, by sleeping with men of lowly status, she risks losing his esteem. In this case, the gain is accompanied by a loss.

Because her lover lacks money, he gives her money stolen from someone else. By accepting this money, she loses her reputation and is compared to a thief. She is condemned because of this money stolen from a citizen, since what is acquired by stealing is detested by the people.

Or else, by going with men of low extraction, she loses everyone's esteem and destroys her reputation. Here the profit is accompanied by a loss, since they are incompatible.

16 Wishing to acquire notoriety by frequenting famous men or ministers at her own expense, sleeping with them will win her nothing, since her outlay is exaggerated. Although her lack of earnings is considerable, she gains in security. This is because there is a relation between advantages and disadvantages.

When, out of ambition, she herself goes to some expense to receive a famous warrior, an influential personage, or one of the king's ministers, she does not make a profit from it. However, in the event of difficulties, in order to remedy some disaster or acquire social notoriety, such meetings are profitable. One of the aims is not attained, but another aim is attained.

17 A girl who, believing herself to be beautiful, is authoritarian, vain, or else very keen on sex, receives her lovers at her own expense, gaining nothing thereby. The absence of profit is not considered as a loss.

Being authoritarian, she beats her servants. She thinks she is beautiful because she has amassed money. Not being beautiful, she pays her lovers. She who is ugly but believes herself to be beautiful pays to be slept with.

Such relationships are different to the former. Being very inclined to sexual relations, she manages it by her intrigues.

If she likes someone, she sleeps with him at her own expense, without a profit. The pleasure she finds in it is her profit. The outlay incurred is not considered a loss.

On the subject of mean men, he says:

18 If she is courted by an upper civil servant with a particularly cruel character who, after being generously welcomed by her, leaves her with threats, without giving her anything, in this case, inconveniences are piled upon inconveniences.

With such a cruel-tempered person, she has to put up with three inconveniences: she must face the expense of receiving him; she earns nothing for having slept with him, since avaricious men give nothing; and to send him away after having received him would be risky. Moreover, his violence and ill-treatment cause her injury. Here, the inconveniences are accompanied by other inconveniences: it is a relationship between things of the same nature.

Thus, sleeping with a royal personage or a member of the government who is cruel brings her nothing, but it would be a serious mistake to send him away. In such a way, the loss suffered is accompanied by other inconveniences.

19 From now on, the questions will be connected with virtue and pleasure.

Besides the above, there are deeds connected with virtue and pleasure. Such is the case of a married Brahman, so in love with her that he risks dying of it, whose life she saves. She thus preserves his family and allows him to perform his duties as the head of the family. Meritorious deeds of this kind are connected with virtue. Those who have intercourse only to procure shelter and nourishment practice a loveless eroticism. There are thus six kinds of relation between values of different nature, becoming twelve with their opposites.

20 Besides simple contrasts, there are also complex contrasts.

Apart from simple contrasts, there are contrasts between values of different natures, as, for example, when profit is in contrast with pleasure, virtue, and another profit, or a loss is in contrast with virtue and pleasure, a profit and another loss; or else immorality is in contrast with profit, loss, pleasure, and virtue; the same goes for enmity [dvesha], forming a total of twenty-four cases.

These relations must be studied with discrimination.

In describing situations in which choice is simple, he says:

21 Even if he is satisfied, one does not know whether he will pay or not. The profit is doubtful [artha sanshaya].

Although he may be perfectly satisfied with the girl's sexual behavior, he does not pay what he should. Not knowing his character in advance, she does not know whether he will pay or not: this is financial doubt.

22 Having sqeezed his money from him without violence, she throws him out, seeking only her own advantage, and does not consider that it is unethical: her morality is doubtful [dharma sanshaya].

She resists and throws him out, after he has paid his due: is this unethical?

Giving her body is the prostitute's duty [dharma] and "duty is to act according to one's status," say the Masters. She throws him out after having taken his money. Is this a question of ethics, of dharma?

This is moral doubt (dharma sanshaya).

23 Having found someone she likes, she makes inquiries, through one of her assistants or some other low person, to find out whether or not he makes love well. This is erotic doubt [kāma sanshaya].

24 Because he comes of a good family, she believes he will not behave like a good-for-nothing. This is doubt concerning risks [anartha sanshaya].

She does not know the person who desires her. He has a reputation for being a bad boy, but it is his pride to belong to the royal clan. "Will he make trouble for me?" Not knowing, she has doubts.

Being of a good family, he has no connection with the mob. "Will he make trouble for me or not?" This is doubt concerning risks.

25 Having abandoned the one with whom she had a relationship, he has taken the road to death because he was completely ruined. In this case, does she commit a violation of her duty [adharma]? In this case there appears a doubt as to an evil deed [adharma sanshaya].

They slept together. Being in love, he desired her. She abandons him because he no longer gives her anything. He departs on the way of the dead [the way of the ancestors]. Passing on to another world, it seems he has entered the realm of Yama [the god of death]. She asks herself whether, by leaving him, she has violated her duties. There is a doubt of moral culpability (adharma sanshaya].

26 She has made declarations of love to someone she likes and, not having got him, she wonders whether he lacks temperament or is hostile to her. This is the doubt of enmity [dvesha sanshaya].

Although she has declared her love, no sexual intercourse takes place. Annoyed that the desired relationship has not been established, she does not know whether he would have come up to her expectations, or whether it is a manifestation of hostility on his side.

In either case, it must be considered whether or not there are any grounds for doubt.

27 Now for complex doubts.

Some of these involve contradictions and some do not. The former are described first.

28 Someone whose character is unknown presents himself while an interesting lover is staying with her, or when an important personage is present. Is it reasonable or risky to receive him? This is the doubt.

He presents himself. He arrives. But where does he come from? His character is unknown. Is it reasonable or risky to welcome him?

He is unknown, but it is reasonable to receive a customer who presents himself. However, as compared to the one who is staying with her, or who is present, it is risky. There is a doubt as to what to do.

29 A priest, a chaste student, an initiate, a wandering monk, a Buddhist monk [lingi], etc., having seen her, fall desperately in love with her; or someone else, according to his friends, wants to commit suicide for the same reasons. Sleeping with them is a charitable duty [dharma], yet contrary to their moral law [adharma]. There is doubt between duty and prohibition [dharma-adharma].

An officiating priest, even if married, a chaste student (the first stage of life), an initiate who has made a vow of abstinence for a certain time, a Buddhist monk such as the Tibetans, someone who wishes to die, mad with love, and wants to pass on to the next world, according to what his friends say: is it a virtue or a sin to sleep with them out of charity or goodness? Preventing suicide is a good deed, while breaking their regulations is a fault, hence a sin. In these two cases, how should one manage? These points of view are contradictory.

30 Having formed an idea of someone's merits, according to public opinion, she goes with him without having verified his qualities. The doubt is as to whether there will be love or enmity [kāma-dvesha].

Her decision is based on people's opinion. It is not because she herself has recognized his merits, but only from hearsay. What sort of experience will she have when they have sexual intercourse? Will it involve love or hostility? This is a complex doubt about attraction-rejection.

31 If one's feelings are uncertain, the one as compared to the other, this causes complex doubts [sankīrna sanshaya].
32 If she goes with another for money while living with her steady lover, she gains on both sides.

With the second, she sleeps for money, but she is in love with her steady lover. To speak of going with someone means having physical intercourse for money, which is part of the duties of her state [svadharma]. She never provokes jealousy, however. She sleeps with both and receives money from both. By acting in this way, she attains her goal through uniting with both. Such a union conforms to her interest. In both cases it is a profitable union [artha yoga].

If a prostitute goes with another man for money, her permanent lover may give her even more money to prevent her from doing so. She thus gains in both cases.

33 When she has intercourse at her own expense without earning anything, and her regular lover in fury stops her allowance, she loses on both sides.

In the case in which she sleeps with both, but sleeps with the other at her own expense, without earning anything thereby, the one who is attached to her, with whom she lives, breaks with her because he is furious. The result is a loss. She sleeps with both, for different reasons. Her relationship with both causes her to lose money. She ends by finding herself abandoned by both.
Sometimes there is doubt as to possibilities.

34 When there is some doubt since she does not know whether, in sleeping with another man, she will obtain money, nor whether her steady lover will give her something for living with her, a financial doubt exists in both cases.

Having relations with the one and the other, she does not know what will be the result, nor whether her steady lover, who has no money, will pay her her fee. There is a doubt about money in both cases.

35 She does not know whether her former lover, who kept her, being angry, has become hostile to her and will cause her trouble. Neither does she know whether the new one to whom she has attached herself will lose patience and stop paying her. On both sides there is a doubt about money. Such, according to Uddālaka, is the description of a double relationship.

In this case, she has a double love relationship. She is kept and receives a wage, but she also sleeps with another. The first, to whom she is tied, is against the other. She does not know whether, out of anger, he will do her harm. Since her new lover is jealous of her relations with her former lover, she does not know whether he will take back what he has given her. In both cases, she risks a loss.
Thus ends the subject of keeping double company according to Shvetaketu Auddālaki.

36 Here follows the opinion of the Bābhravyas.

The Bābhravyas also speak of a double union.

37   By sleeping with another, she earns money as well as receiving some from her steady lover, even without intercourse. She gains doubly.

The lover on whom she depends keeps her, even without sexual relations, since "it is said that a kept woman must be treated like a wife." By taking care of the first and sleeping with the other, she receives money from both. This is a profit from both.

38   When she sleeps with a man without a profit, and the one who gives her a pension stops her allowance, she undergoes a loss in both cases.

She goes and sleeps with another, without receiving any fee, which means a lack of earnings. Her steady lover, with whom she does not sleep, turns away from her and leaves her without resource, no longer paying her wage. She suffers a loss on one side and on the other.

39   When she goes with someone without first fixing her rate, not knowing whether he will give her anything and whether her steady lover, even without sleeping with her, will pay her her remuneration, there is a doubt as to her gain in both cases.

40   She is put to the expense of sleeping with someone but, since he is under the influence of his steady mistress, she does not know whether he will pay her. Moreover, she does not know whether her steady lover, with whom she does not sleep, will cut her allowance out of anger. In both cases, she risks a loss.

The above are the four simple questions regarding relations with two lovers. They are simple because they only concern money matters. Complex cases [sankīrna] are contemplated below.

41   In her relations with her two lovers, she must contemplate: the gain on one side, the losses on the other; the gain on one side, uncertain profits on the other; the gain on one side, the risk of losses on the other, to which six cases of complex problems are added.

Besides problems of a single nature [sajāti], the others, involving different orders of values, are of six kinds.
These points are contemplated by the Bābhravyas.

42 By reflecting with the aid of these remarks and considering her assured profits, doubtful gains, and avoiding any great risk, she must decide how to behave.

43 Having determined the relation between duty [dharma] and pleasure [kāma], their relative importance must be considered before establishing relations.

Thus, according to Uddālaka, there are one hundred and ninety-two questions arising with regard to an erotic union and, according to the Bābhravyas, a union is established after having reflected on these problems.
Double relationships are described from three aspects: simple, complex, and multiple. Concerning group sex, it is said:

44 When several profligates gather together to possess a woman, it is called group possession [goshthi parigraha].

Having gathered, come together, having made an agreement, dissolute men, behaving all the same, possess one person: this is called group possession.
Describing these cases of collective sex, or group sex [samantata yoga], he says:

45 Uniting with them, she takes money from each for sexual relations.

She is possessed by several, one after another, sometimes two or more at a time. During these sexual contacts, some of them rub each other reciprocally. She is possessed by one and another in succession, and she asks them for money.
With regard to emulation, it is said:

46 For the spring festival and on other similar occasions, the mother sends messages stipulating that the first to copulate with her daughter will be the one who sends her certain gifts.

During the spring festival and other merrymaking, sensual men are inclined toward sex. Her mother thus seeks to attract them. Since the daughter cannot solicit them directly, her mother makes the arrangements.

The prostitute's mother sends a message to the suitors at the spring festival or the festival of the full moon (Kaumudī), or else at the festival of the god of love (Kāma Mahotsava) and other forthcoming festivals: "My daughter will sleep first with the one who will have brought me such-and-such a thing beforehand."

47 When they argue about sleeping with the girl, she arranges matters to her advantage.

By provoking quarrels, she makes her profit.
She fixes a higher price.
In this connection, he says:

48 At these collective unions, she can earn from one or earn from all, lose with one or lose with all, earn from half and lose with half.

Of those who possess her, she can earn more from one than from all of them, by attempting to arouse their jealousy. Otherwise, in sleeping with all of them, she takes money from all.

49 Even in the case of uncertainty about her profit and about her losses, relations can be performed by taking into account questions concerning ethics or pleasure.

These are the reflections with regard to doubts concerning profits and risks in sexual relations.

In these twelve kinds of union with several men [samantata], account must be taken of profits, losses, morals [dharma] and immorality [adharma], love [kāma] and hostility [dvesha].
This chapter concerns the practice of prostitution [veshya], which is why the various categories of prostitute are mentioned.

50 The various kinds of prostitute are: the water carrier [kumbhadāsī], the servant [parichārikā], the corrupt woman [kulatā], the lesbian [svairinī], the dancer [natī], the worker

[shilpakārikā], the divorcee or widow [prakāshavinashtā], the harlot who lives on her charms [rūpājīvā], and the courtesan [ganikā].

Water carriers are slaves used for humble tasks. Public opinion only contemplates three categories: the water carriers, the courtesans, and the harlots who live by their charms. The others are included in these categories. Female servants are those who look after their master. They are mentioned since they are permanently in contact with him.

The corrupt woman is one who has left her home for fear of her husband and has gone to live in another house, or else a woman who has secret relations with a lover.

The liberated woman, or lesbian, is one who refuses a husband and has relations in her own home or in other houses.

The dancer is a woman of the theater.

The female worker is the wife of a jeweler, a weaver, etc.

The divorcee is one who, having lived virtuously with her husband, whether he is still living or dead, turns to amorous adventures. These are the six kinds, including the one who lives by her charms, which form the social category of prostitutes.

51 Reflections on prostitution include all these categories, comprising those who sleep with them, their assistants, those who are enamored of them, the ways of making love for money, of breaking off, of resuming, special profits, doubts about gains, and the risks of relationships.

Moreover, those who seek them out are studied, including those from whom she expects nothing, the average, or a lot, those who are enamored of her, the rejected lover, resumed relationships, breaking off a stale relationship, the prostitute's profession, the forms of prostitution, suitable behavior for prostitutes. In his work, Dattaka mentions six ways of finding customers, the reasons for intercourse, the limits of love, breaking off, resuming with a former lover, which, added to the eight kinds of relations with prostitutes mentioned by the Bābhravyas, covers the whole subject of prostitution.

Throughout his one hundred years of life, a man must divide his activities into three parts. This is why the sacred books give these teachings, which are also addressed to women.

52 In this connection, a quotation: "Men look for love and women too look for love." The main goal of this treatise is the way to have intercourse with women.

Erotic desire, which is the same for both sexes, is the principal aim of this treatise. According to its teachings, women play the main role in the act of intercourse.

The main objective of relations between men and women is erotic pleasure. The subject of this work is the satisfaction of the erotic pleasure felt by men and women. This is why considerations on the erotic utilization of women have been developed in the chapter on prostitution.

53 Some women look for pleasure, others seek money. The pleasure deriving from amorous relations with prostitutes has been described in connection with prostitution.

Women are of two kinds, those who seek pleasure and those who seek money. At the same time, a description has also been given of men who look for pleasure, who prefer very young girls, who have several wives, who covet other men's wives, who wish to lead a life of pleasure and possess the necessary financial means. As far as relations with prostitutes are concerned, eroticism is tied to money just as much for those women who seek money as for those who frequent them. By sleeping with men, prostitutes gain both pleasure and money.

Some women dream of pure love, but many women desire both pleasure and money. To start with, we have described women who seek pure love, then, in the chapters on prostitutes, a description is given of women who, as well as love and enjoyment, look also for money.

These chapters on prostitution deal with questions of sensuality, immorality, and instability, as well as the prostitute's art of seduction, the ways in which prostitutes have relations with gigolos (vīta), their managers (pīthamarda), and other people of inferior social position, as also with well-born persons of good family. This last chapter particularly includes some considerations on prostitutes' behavior. On reflection, one realizes that a prostitute's behavior is based on three factors: love, sexual impulse, and obstacles. Concerning reasons why people are desirous of sleeping with prostitutes, a simple reply can be found in the *Shishupālavadha* by Māgha (4.17): "When he was weary of eternally drinking the elixir of immortality, Shiva, the creator of the immortals, drank poison." This means that "when the god Shiva, who was immortal due to ceaselessly drinking the elixir of immortality, wearied of it, then the god of gods preferred poison to immortality." This point of view embodies a great truth. When a man has many times enjoyed his devoted wife, who represents nectar, he loses his taste for her and then seeks relations with the prostitute, who is made of poison.

On reflection, from a practical point of view, one can deduce the principle that the desire for change is found among all. By nature, man loves change.

He is attracted by beauty, attracted by novelty. To this, the *Yoga Vāsishtha* (*Nirvāna* 44.2) gives a philosophical reply: "From the moment one has obtained something desired, it is no longer desirable. Who has not had this experience? The desire to obtain something disappears at the moment it is obtained."

In the *Shishupālavadha*, the great poet Māgha says, "The form that renews itself at every moment is the one that attracts." Whether one is dealing with man or woman, prostitute or honest woman, married or unattached people, their actions at every moment evolve according to their impulse. The charms of a condition or situation decline in the long run. This is why the excitation produced by something new causes change.

The *Vishnu Purāna* (I-3, 45–46) explains that "two kinds of feeling or impulse may be born at the same time when pleasure and sorrow, desire and rejection, etc., arise in connection with something. How can it be claimed that this is merely the cause of suffering? At one and the same time, it causes love and gives rise to pain, rejection, satisfaction."

A lover who is infatuated with the beauty of a prostitute may even be insulted and robbed by her, and suffer her blows, but he will not cease from running after her. He cannot bear being apart from her for one moment. In order to explain this, the author of the *Kāma Shāstra* quotes the Scriptures, "In the beloved's absence, one moment seems a year." As a result, prostitutes and those who desire them become dependent on impulses that, at the same time, change from moment to moment. Only weariness puts an end to these stimulations. Weariness appears when, out of boredom, excitation is no longer stimulated. The result is that interest turns elsewhere. So long as interest remains, the individual's heart stays full of enthusiasm. For this reason quarrels start between lovers about matters of their rights.

The author of the *Kāma Sūtra* takes as an example of this kind of conflict, that of the prostitute who leaves her lover in order to take another. Her current lover is deeply wounded. He remains disconsolate, prostrate.

Logically, from a social point of view, this lover should consider the prostitute as a mere sex object. But it is not so. Blinded by desire, he continues to pursue her, run after her. He remains plunged in melancholy and agitation.

In reality, every person has such tendencies: the differences result from the fact that some have higher ideals. People who live in a cultivated society and believe in their ideals always fight such impulses, but those without these advantages fall into the pit of decline.

The last and seventh part of the *Kāma Sūtra* refers to secret and magical techniques, whereas the *Jayamangalā* commentary terminates with the sixth part. From this, some specialists conclude that the seventh part was added later and that Vātsyāyana wrote only six parts. Some scholars assume that the *Jayamangalā* originally contained seven parts and that, for some reason, the last one vanished. From the table of contents at the beginning, it can be deduced that the *Kāma Sūtra* only comprised six parts, which would be why Yashodhara did not write a commentary for the seventh. On the other hand, Yashodhara's phrase "Occult methods (aupanishada vidhi) are explained" proves that the seventh part of the *Kāma Sūtra* is indeed dedicated to secret methods and that it was dealt with in the *Jayamangalā*.

The eulogistic biography of Yashodhara by Pushpikā mentions the suppression of the end of the *Jayamangalā*.

"Grieved by the absence of the lost part, the famous Gurudatta wrote this commentary on the basis of Yashodhara's text." It appears that Yashodhara, after the death of his beautiful wife, had adopted the monastic life, which is mentioned by his disciple Indrapada. However, even after adopting the monastic life, when the pain of separation from his wife had began to lessen, his guru recommended him to write the commentary on the *Kāma Sūtra*. It is highly probable that the name of Yashodhara's wife was actually Jayamangalā.

In the sixth chapter, "Profits and Losses," the problems connected with doubts and the way to remedy them form part of the domain of political art (rājanīti).

In the seventh chapter of the ninth part of his *Artha Shāstra*, Kautilya explains this state of things to the king. In order to halt his enemies' progress, Kautilya points out to the king three things of which he should take care: lack of material, lack of money, and hesitation. These are the same points contemplated by Vātsyāyana for the prostitute when an obstacle arises.

Like Vātsyāyana, Kautilya considers the relation between advantages and disadvantages, both within the amorous relationship and without.

After this, still according to the *Artha Shāstra*, collective profits are described, when money comes from several sides. When earnings are obtained from both sides, the gain is double. Both double and multiple gains are possible. If, by spending nothing or by spending much, profits remain in the black, Vātsyāyana advises the prostitute to go ahead, and Kautilya advises the same thing to the king.

Before finding oneself poverty-stricken, problems must be settled by amassing money. In this chapter concerning profits and losses, Vātsyāyana gives a magnificent example of political intrigue (kuta-nīti).

Here ends the Sixth Chapter
Profits and Losses
and the Sixth Part entitled About Courtesans
of the Kāma Sūtra *by Vātsyāyana*

—— Part Seven ——
Occult Practices
[Aupanishadika]

Chapter One

SUCCESS IN LOVE
[Subhaga]

1   This is an appendix to the *Kāma Sūtra*.

This final part of the Kāma Sūtra *has a double content: magic practices and ordinary procedures.*

The manuscript of Yashodhara's commentary ends here. It is continued according to the reconstruction made by Gurudatta.

2   If the desired results are not obtained by the means described up to this point, occult practices (aupanishadika) must be utilized.

If, through the techniques [tantra] indicated in this treatise, the desired goal is not attained, or one does not find what one is looking for, the procedures indicated in the chapter on occult practices must be contemplated. In connection with success in love, he says:

3   Beauty, qualities, age, and generosity are the causes of success in love.

Beauty depends on the color of the skin and physical fitness. Of these elements, some are permanent while others are subject to decline and are devoured by time. A man's qualities, even if he is not a beauty, embellish him. One must therefore strive to develop them. As far as age is concerned, youth is suited to all kinds of work. One must strive to make it last and preserve it. Growing old is a cause of disaffection, especially for women, which is the reason why practices such as dyeing their hair, etc., should not be neglected.

Generosity makes everyone more likable, whether one is ugly, stupid, or old. He who pays can always have sexual relations.

If physical beauty and other qualities are lacking, the method to be followed is indicated.

4　Physical attractions are improved by anointing the body with a product made of tagara [valerian], kushtha [*Saussurea lappa*], and tālīsha patra [*Flacourtia cataphracta*].

The body should be rubbed with ointments made of tagara. This is made from the roots of a plant from the northern countries and not the one that comes from Nepal.

As far as kushtha [or kūta] (Saussurea lappa or Costus speciosus orarabicus) is concerned, choose the white variety. The leaves of tālīsha patra must be pounded.

This ointment increases sexual attraction.

5　These ingredients, reduced to a fine powder, mixed with lampblack obtained by burning aksha oil [*Terminalia bellerica*], gathered in a human skull, and used as an ointment, have a magical effect.

In a human skull inherited for tantric purposes, the powdered ingredients are lightly mixed with lampblack obtained by burning a cotton wick with aksha oil (or vibhītaka, Myrobalan bellerica), the flame of which is covered. Used as an ointment, it brings good luck.

6　Then, roots of punarnavā [*Boerhavia diffusa*], pāthārachata [*Costus speciosus*, bogweed], sahadevī [dandotpalaka, *Echita pulescens*], sarivā [or sārina, or chitavana, *Hermidermus indicus*], kurantaka [red-flowered piyavansha, yellow amaranth, *Barleria prionitis*] are gathered together with

utpala leaves [water lilies or blue lotus]. These are cooked
and made into a cream for massaging the body.

*Punarnavā is also called gadāpunnā. For sāriva, take utpala sāriva.
Of the lotus leaves, take the inner not the outer part. For the others,
the roots. Cook in oil. Make a cream to use for anointing the body,
which is a source of sexual attraction.*
This product enhances beauty and brings good luck.

7   Add to the same a garland of flowers.

*Beside the cream made of punarnavā and other plants, wear a
necklace of the same flowers, which makes the body attractive.*
One should wear a necklace, made of the flowers mentioned.

8   Crush the flowers of pink lotus [padma] and blue lotus
[utpala], mixed with snake's saffron [nāgakesara, *Mesua
ferrea*]. Let it dry. These ingredients, consumed together
with honey or ghee [butter oil], make one attractive.

*Crush these flowers together with snake's saffron (nāgakesara).
This mixture has a purgative effect. It does not make one immediately
attractive, but improves one's looks after one month.*

9   Adding to it tagara [*Tabernaemontana coronaria*], tālīsha
[*Flacourtia cataphracta*], and tamāla leaves [*Garcinia
pictoria*], smear the body with it.

By rubbing the body with this ointment, one is successful in love.

10   By holding in one's left hand a peacock's or hyena's
eye, wrapped in gold, one finds success in love.

*The peacock's eye should be still fresh, taken when the bird breaks
loose in summer for mating. The same for hyena's eyes. According to
the texts, they should be held in the right hand or the left hand, wrapped
in pure gold leaf, in the spring, when the moon is in the constellation
of Pushya.*
Placing a peacock's eye or hyena's eye in a gold box fixed to the
right arm, beauty and luck are increased.

11 A jewel can also be used, made of a conch winding
from right to left [bādara mani], or a small ball of jujube,
or even an ordinary conch, while chanting the verses of the
Atharva Veda.

*Bādara mani, the jewel of bādara, means the tiny reservoir of sap
taken from the top of the root of the jujuba tree. The pellet of jujuba,
or else the conch winding from right to left, wrapped in gold, is fixed
to the arm. In the* Atharva Veda, *the veda of magic practices, great
importance is attached to the fact of carrying these with one, worn as
a jewel.*

Its usage must be learned as described in the *Atharva Veda.*

12 When a maidservant attains puberty, her master keeps
her for a year in order to teach her the secret techniques
and the art of sexual relations. After this, he gives her hand
in marriage. The girl, thus protected, will be given to which
of her suitors who, attracted by her beauty, will bestow the
most to have sexual relations with her and assure her happiness.

*Once she has learned the secret techniques [tantra], magic words
[mantra], and forms of sexual intercourse [yoga], according to texts
written on birch leaves [bhūrja], it is a matter of setting her up
suitably for a happy union with a young man who will assure her
welfare. Since her childhood, she has only served her master, without
having any relations with other men and, since puberty, has been
protected from sexual relations and sleeps with no one else. Her beauty,
protected by this union from the gaze of lewd men, becomes an in-
finitely desirable object for the covetous desires of libertines. Seized by
passion, they seek amorous relations with this maidservant. Out of
rivalry, they are ready to give much money to procure a love object
that is out of the ordinary, which cannot be obtained without a previous agreement.*

*The practice of giving a girl to someone who desires only to sleep
with her is a common one, especially when one marries a prostitute
with the aim of perfect erotic satisfaction. This is why two kinds of
union are indicated: "A prostitute's marriage is of two kinds, depend-
ing on chance or the man. When by chance, it is the result of the darts
of the god of love; the other, from having slept together."*

In connection with choosing a man, it is said:

13 When a courtesan's daughter reaches puberty, the former summons suitors of good society, saying that he who gives most may marry her and keep her.

When a courtesan has a daughter, she protects her from sexual relations. Then, describing her beauty, she seeks rich men and persons of quality. She summons them to her house to see the girl. From among them, she chooses the one who would desire her and would even have the possibility of keeping her following a religious marriage.

14 The young girl pretends to be in love with the young citizen chosen, ignoring all money matters and her mother's intrigues.

Discreetly, the young girl demonstrates her fondness for the man her mother has chosen. She shows an amorous disposition, pretending that her mother ignores her and that she knows nothing of money matters.

Such demonstrations of love must take into account the conventions of the country and the period.

15 Meetings with her must take place in the music room [gāndharva shālā] where she studies the arts, or at the dwelling of a nun [bhikshukī], or some such place.

The moments chosen are those when she is studying the arts in the music room, where she learns from a dancing and singing master, or else at the house of a nun. She goes to visit a religious who is expert at the arts, and in such places as the temple of the goddess of knowledge, or gardens, etc.

When rich young men, kings, men of well-known families come to a prostitute's house to study the arts, she lets them meet her very young daughter, and the girl, after having met them at home, begins to frequent them. She meets them in the music room, at the house of a nun, wherever she is able to, and thus continues to keep them company.

16 When the mother has received the gifts foreseen from the suitor, she grants him her daughter's hand.

Of those who have shown their desire for the bonds of love, the one who brings the gifts foreseen, gifts agreed upon with the mother, receives in exchange the hand of her daughter, according to local custom.

17   If she does not obtain money from the suitor, the mother places her own money in a given spot and proclaims that she has received it from him.

Not having obtained the agreed compensation, after having given her daughter, she gathers her own assets together in some place, pretending that they are the gifts that had been agreed upon. She proclaims this in order to save her face.

She declares that a certain young man has given all his riches to her daughter.

18   Or else, when the girl is pubescent, she has her deflowered.

Once the girl has attained the age of puberty, her mother has her deflowered in a union for that purpose [daiva vivāha], in order subsequently to be able to give her to all.

As previously explained, the prostitute looks for a young man to break the hymen of her tender daughter.

19   Uniting them secretly, she pretends to know nothing and to have discovered it after the deed. She reports it to the law.

The one she had chosen having secretly deflowered her daughter, she declares she knew nothing about it and discovered it afterward. She informs the justice department, with the aim of obtaining damages for lack of earnings, due to the intercourse that has taken place.

Having united the two young people in secret, the mother informs the judicial authorities of their idyll and starts proceedings against the claimed seducer in order to obtain damages.

If the girl has not been deflowered, what does she do?

20   The courtesan gets rid of her daughter's virginity with the assistance of a female friend or slave, so as to facilitate

her amorous success. Once she has thoroughly studied the practice of sexual relations according to the *Kāma Sūtra,* she liberates her daughter. Such is the ancient custom.

According to ancient custom, with the aid of a female friend or slave, the girl is skillfully freed of her virginity, using a finger, as a boy would do. How will this facilitate her amorous success? She knows the Kāma Sūtra *thoroughly. Properly instructed by her companions, she is expert at practices such as the mare, etc. For this reason, when young, handsome, and shrewd citizens present themselves in order to copulate with her, they find her prepared for her new status.*

Village prostitutes have their daughter's hymen pierced by a female companion or servant and then teach her secretly the forms of sexual intercourse which are part of the trade. Beside her great skill in the arts, a prostitute's daughter acquires much glamour, which she adds to her youthful charm. Judging that her daughter is now perfect for the courtesan's profession, the prostitute gives her her independence.

21   She stays for one year with the man she marries, after which she abandons herself with whoever desires her.

After staying for one year with the man who has married her, who had accepted to take her as wife, she renounces marriage and abandons herself with everyone, according to the ethical rules of the prostitute.

22   The year having gone by, if her husband invites her, the prostitute accepts to spend one night with him, making no profit. Such behavior brings her good luck.

When this time has passed, if she is called by the man she married to spend the night with him, she asks no fee. This brings her luck. Such behavior is called backsliding [punarabhiyāta] in prostitutes' language.
The subject of the prostitute's marriage and her success is terminated.

23   For this, the girl is known as a pleasuremonger [rangopajīvikā].

In theater plays, she is called a pleasure monger.

The practices of dancing and acting are also a part of pleasure.
Girls who practice dancing and acting, which adds to their attrac-
tion, must continue, once married.
On this subject, he says:

24   **Even when married, a woman should practice the four
main arts.**

Of the four arts, music, dancing, etc., dancing is the most attractive.
Dancing and singing help her raise her status.

*The techniques of sympathetic magic [vashīkarana] as a means of
seduction are indicated.*

25   **If a man anoints his penis with datura, black pepper
[maricha], and long pepper [pippalī], crushed and mixed
with honey, its use will allow him to bewitch and subjugate
his partners.**

*Datura seeds are used, crushed and mixed with bees' honey. By
anointing his penis, without the woman's knowledge, she is caught in
his power.*

26   **By crushing and mixing leaves brought by the wind,
the ointment put on a corpse and powdered peacock bone,
one can submit a woman to one's power.**

*With the left hand, catch a leaf brought by the wind, ointments
taken from a corpse, used to anoint the breast, peacock bones from an
old peacock, not from a similar kind of bird. Pulverize them. Anoint
the sex with them. This makes a woman throw herself at a man's feet.*
A woman will fall into a man's power if he takes a leaf brought by
the wind, sandalwood used to anoint a corpse, and powdered peacock's
bone, crushes them together: with this he anoints his penis and makes
love with her.

27   **A person is bewitched if his or her body is anointed
with a paste made of the flesh of a vulture, the bird that
flies in circles, which one has killed oneself, mixed with**

honey and āmalaka juice [*Emblica officinalis,* emblic myrobalan), even if a bath is taken afterward.

A vulture is recognized by the fact that it flies in circles, in a flock, above water. One must kill it oneself.

28 Chop into small pieces a ball of vajrasnuhī [milk hedge, *Euphorbia neriifolia*], sprinkled with manashilā [red arsenic) and powdered fragments of gandhaka [sulphur], let dry seven times, then, mixing with honey, anoint the penis. Its use assures the power of bewitching.

Balls of vajrasnuhī [also known as sāshrī gundakani, thuhāra, sthūna], chopped in pieces and dried seven times.
Anoint the penis with it and enjoy the woman: she will be subjugated.

29 By reducing these ingredients to smoke, during the night, the moon veiled by the smoke assumes the brilliancy of gold.

Gold appears, thanks to this powder. This is explained in the treatises on conjuring.

30 Mixing these powdered ingredients with monkeys' dung, if one sprinkles a girl with it, she will feel no attraction for anyone else.

The droppings to be taken must belong to the species of monkey with a colored face.
Mixing these ingredients with man's or monkey's excrements, the girl who is sprinkled with this substance is entirely subjugated.

31 Make balls of vachā [*Acorus calamus,* orrisroot], coat them with mango oil, and place them in a hole made in the trunk of a shinshapa tree [ashoka, or shishu]. Leave them there for six months, then remove them and use them to anoint the body. It lends a heavenly luster [devakānta], which captivates.

White vachā root is placed in a branch of shishu. The divine
radiance allows one to subjugate. Having extracted the root mixed with
mango from the heart of the tree, one must anoint one's own body,
which will allow one to subjugate but not to bewitch.

32 Small pieces of khadira bark [*Acacia catechu*], torn from
the tree and kept for six months, take on the scent of flowers. Anointing the body with it imparts the radiance of the
heavenly musicians [gandharvakānta], which captivates.

Oil the body with it using the hand. It gives a smell of jasmine.
Apply to the shoulder area and above.

33 Mix priyangu [*Aglaia roxburghiana*] with tagara [vale-
rian, *Tabernaemontana coronaria*] and mango oil [sahakāra].
Make a hole in a nāga tree [nāgakesara, *Mesua roxburghii*]
and leave it there for six months. By anointing the body
with it, one acquires the radiance of the nāgas [the subter-
ranean divinities], which serves to bewitch.

Mix priyangu flowers with tagara, of the kind that resembles
kurantaka [yellow amaranth]. The nāga tree means the nāgakesara.
By anointing one's body thrice with this mixture, one is united with the
heavenly spirits [devagandharva] of the kind known as the nāgas [the
snakes], which are described in other works.
Mix tagara and kākuna (kangunī, *Celastrus paniculata*) with mango
oil, as above. Make a hollow inside a nāgakesara and leave the mixture
there for six months. After this, use it to anoint the body, which allows
one to subjugate women. This ointment gives a radiance like that of the
nāgas.

34 Soak camel's bone in bhringarāja juice [*Vedelia calen-*
dulacea], crush into small pieces, and purify the same in the
fire. Put the cinders into a tube made of camel's bone,
together with antimony [sroto anjana]. Apply to the eyelashes. The person looked at will be bewitched by a single
glance.

Make a powder with crushed camel bone, steep three times, then
burn to make lampblack for the eyes. Keep this eyeblack in a tube made

of camel bone. Mix it with an equal portion of antimony to form a very fine product. Rub on the eyelashes. Upon a single glance, the first person encountered is subjugated. Whoever you throw your first glance at is in your power. This is why it is recommended as a means of seduction.

Put camel bones to soak in bhringarāja juice, together with kohl (suramā), and cook the same packaged in leaves. Then place the product in a makeup box made of camel bone. Apply to the eyes with a small stick of camel bone. The effect of this kohl is bewitching to women.

35 Eyewash may also be prepared with falcon, vulture, or peacock's bones.

In the same manner as for camel bones, the bones of birds such as falcons, vultures, or peacocks may be used.

Even if one manages to subjugate someone, but is unable to consummate the relationship, there will be no result. In order to enhance virility, the science of aphrodisiacs [vrishyā yoga] is described:

36 Mix garlic root with white pepper and licorice. When drunk with sugared milk, it enhances virility.

Take an ordinary root of garlic, commercial white pepper, and licorice. Cook them in cow's milk. Once cooled, add sugar. This beverage increases virility when the member falters.

Virility is strengthened and the flow of sperm increases.

37 Ram's or he-goat's testicles boiled in sugared milk increase sexual prowess.

38 One can take either a ram's or he-goat's testicles and boil them in sweetened milk. This beverage increases virility. Sweet potato roots [vidārī, *Ipomea digitata*], kshīrikā fruits [*Mimusops hexandra*], and svayamguptā roots [*Mucuna pruriens*], crushed and boiled in milk, can also be drunk. These aphrodisiac plants may be utilized together or separately.

Take a root of vidārī, a well-known plant. Kshīrikā, also known as rājādanam or kuili, is a kind of onion. Svayamguptā signifies kapikacchu

(*Mucuna pruriens*). Used either together or separately, these products have an aphrodisiac effect.

39 Similarly, one can also use the seeds of priyāla [piyāla, long pepper, *Buchana latifolia*], morata [*Sanseveriera roxburghiana*] and vidārī [*Ipomea digitata*], and kumharā [*Hedysarum gangeticum*, prickly pear], in milk.

Take one part of priyāla seeds [long pepper] for two parts each of morata and vidārī. In this case, morata means ikshu mula, Aristolochia.

A drink made of chiraunji (piyāla fruit seeds), murahari or morata, and vidārī and kumhara (prickly pear) bulbs, crushed in milk, increases virility.

40 Crush together shringātaka [*Trapa bispinosa*], kaseru [*Gmelina arborea*], and kāmadhulika [mahuā, wild fig], with kshīrakākoli [*Zizyphua napecea*], mixed with sugar and milk. Then cook over a low fire with ghee [clarified butter] in order to make into cakes. He who eats these can sleep with innumerable women, say the ancient masters.

Shringātaka is well known, and should be taken whole. Kaseru [Gmelina arborea] *is a sort of mallikā [jasmine]. Madhulikā [madhuka fruits,* Cassia latifolia*] and licorice [yashtimadhu]. Crush together with kshīrakākoli, a variety of onion found in commerce, and make into small cakes. Eat large quantities of these until replete.*

41 Crumble māshaka beans [*Phaseolus radiatus*], soak in water, and heat in ghee. After softening them, remove and allow to stand. Then cook in cow's milk. Eaten with honey and ghee, this product allows one to possess innumerable women, say the ancient masters.

Crack the māshaka beans and soak in water. Then, remove from the water and allow to dry and stand. Cook in cow's or goat's milk, allow to cool, and mix with equal quantities of honey and ghee before consuming.

These beans must be washed in water and cleaned, and then cooked in ghee until they turn red. After this, leave to stand for some time, then cook in cow's or goat's milk, mixing with equal quantities of honey and ghee. Eaten regularly, these cakes lend the power to enjoy innumerable women.

42   Crush vidārī roots [sweet potatoes] in cow's milk, together with svayamguptā seeds [kauncha, kapikachu, *Mucunia pruriens*], sugar, honey, and ghee. Use it to make biscuits with wheat flour. He who eats them, as many as suits him, can enjoy an unlimited number of women, the ancient masters tell us.

Crush them in small pieces in cow's milk.
By constantly eating these biscuits, one's sperm acquires such force that it is possible to sleep with thousands of women who, in the end, will ask for pity.

43   Dilute chataka [sparrow's] eggs with rice water, cook them in milk, and mix with honey and ghee. Utilized as mentioned above, the same result can be obtained.

The chataka is the common sparrow. Take the juice of their eggs, mixed with rice and cooked in milk, then mix with honey and ghee. When eaten, one's sexual prowess is so enhanced that one can possess an unlimited number of young women, as indicated above.

44   Prepare the juice of sparrows' eggs with husked sesame seeds [tila], shringātaka [*Trapa bispinosa*], kaseruka [kasurika, *Gmelina arborea*], svayamguptā fruits [*Mucunia pruriens*]. Crush all together patiently with wheat and ghee. Cook to make griddle cakes. By eating these, the same result is reached.

To the juice of sparrows' eggs, shelled personally, from which the essence has been extracted, add nishtushā (sesame) seeds and svayamguptā (Mucunia pruriens). Take the fruits, not the roots. Cook these as griddle cakes and eat.
Soak some black sesame (tila), remove the husk, mix it with the liquid sparrows' eggs, then add some sinhādā, kaseru, and kavācha seeds. Mix all together on a board with wheat flour, dilute with ghee, add sugar and milk, and make cakes of it. By constantly eating these sweets unlimited virile strength is acquired.

45   Take two palas [one pala weighs twenty-three grams] each of ghee, honey, sugar, and madhūka [*Cassia latifolia*] flowers, in one karsha [two liters] of palm wine [madhurasa], with one prastha [759 grams] of milk. This elixir made of six ingredients is known to the ancient masters as the elixir of the sages [yuktarasā], which gives sexual power and long life.

Two palas [twenty-three grams] of each ingredient in one karsha [eighty palas] of madhurasa [palm wine], and one prastha [thirty-two palas] of milk. These six ingredients make up one hundred and twenty palas. This pleasant tasting and invigorating elixir facilitates sexual intercourse with women.

46   On the day following the beginning of the spring month [Pushya], drink a cordial made of shatāvari [*Asparagus racemosus*], shvadanshtrā [*Tribulus terrestris*], in red molasses [gudua kashāya], with pippali [long pepper] and licorice paste [madhūkha kalka] cooked in cow's milk and goat's butter. The ancient masters call this the elixir of the sages: it is fortifying, stimulating, and prolongs life.

Shatāvari is well known.
Shvadanshtrā is also called gokshuraka, or mountain gokhuru. Prepare a paste using both, to which is added ghee, pippali [long pepper], and licorice paste, into which cow's milk is poured. Cook at the beginning of the month of Pushya, the day after the sun enters that constellation.

47   Crush together shatāvari [*Asparagus racemosus*], shvadanshtrā [*Tribulus terrestris*], and shrīparnī [kaseru, *Gmelina arborea*], and cook in four times their volume of water. Let the water evaporate. To be taken in the morning. This product assures vigor, erotic strength, and longevity. The ancient masters call it the divine elixir.

Use shrīparnī from Kashmir.

48   Mix together equal quantities of shvadanshtrā [gokhuru] flour and barley flour [yava]. Eat two palas [fifty grams] each morning on arising. This product develops vigor

and sexual power. The ancient masters consider it to be an elixir of the sages.

When it is dry, eat two palas of the mixture each morning. The purpose of what has been said is to acquire an aptitude beyond the norm.

49 Techniques [yoga] favorable to eroticism can also be studied in works on medicine [ayurveda], the *Vedas* (sacred books), scientific treatises [vidyā tantras], and also learned from magicians [mantravādī] and men of experience [āpta].

Study the treatises of ayurveda and with physicians. By Veda, *the* Atharva Veda *is meant. Magicians are those who know magic words. Competent people are those who are expert in the tantras and who are trustworthy.*

Having described the above magic techniques, Vātsyāyana adds:

"Beside these methods (yoga), aphrodisiac formulas should be studied in medical treatises, the *Vedas*, and other works, as well as with competent scholars and experienced physicians."

50 One should avoid the use of products that cause pain, are harmful to the body, risk causing death, or which are not clean.

When a product causes pain, or its use is harmful to bodily health, or its employment can cause death, if it is unhygienic or its use reddens the sperm, it should not be utilized.

Products that cause suffering should never be used as a tonic, nor those that are bad for the health, are mixed with poisons or with unhygienic substances.

51 Utilize only the formulas indicated, according to the procedure recommended by competent persons, Brahmans, or friends who wish you well.

In what has been indicated to obtain the desired results, follow the indications given by those with experience in these practices. Procedures leading to amorous success will not give results without experience. One should follow the advice of those who wish one well.

Following the order of composition of the *Artha Shāstra*, the seventh and last part of the *Kāma Sūtra* is called Aupanishadika (Occult Practices). This chapter is considered an appendix (parishishta) in the table of contents.

The ordinary meaning of the term *Aupanishadika* is "secret," "hidden," or "secret science." An action that remains hidden is called "occult," aupanishadika. Kautilya's *Artha Shāstra* deals with the art of governing. This is why Kautilya, in the chapter headed Aupanishadika, deals with magic practices that surprise, astound, and cause damage to the enemy. With regard to occult means employed in political practice, Kautilya attempts to create difficulties for enemy sovereigns, stir up conflicts, and make their countries ungovernable. Kautilya calls these means aupanishadika, because they always stir up problems that should be avoided inasmuch as they cause damage. When rivalry between kings grows, however, out of a desire to protect the population against and overcome the enemy, a king must use occult means.

Vātsyāyana, taking the same point of view as Kautilya, has collected the various occult means in the last part of the *Kāma Sūtra*. All the means taught here concern eroticism and not political arts.

Like Kautilya, Vātsyāyana considers that such means are to be avoided and condemned. He advises, as a general rule, to renounce them, and to employ them only when other means recommended in the *Kāma Sūtra* have not given the desired result.

As a whole, the *Kāma Sūtra* is divided into two parts from the point of view of content: method (tantra) and the result sought (avāpa). In the first part, Vātsyāyana points out that if, in order to obtain the enjoyment of a body and union of organs, one does not manage to arouse the woman's erotic excitation by such means as caresses and kisses, the techniques described in the part dealing with occult practices should be utilized. This part is divided into two chapters. The first, dealing with amorous success, describes the means of enhancing beauty, bewitchment procedures, and the ways of reaching one's goal. Methods utilizing special ingredients and techniques are then indicated.

From an abstract level of civilization, decency, and worldly hypocrisy, it can be claimed that such practices and methods are base, immoral, barbarous, and condemnable at all points. However, with a view to the aims of human life and the importance of sexual relations, their utility is evident. The aims of human life involve a triple realization on the level of material success, amorous success, and virtue. If one has not succeeded on these levels, success in the final aim, the spiritual life (moksha), is impossible. The raison d'être of the *Kāma Sutra's* composition is based on the realization of these aims.

This is not a personal concept of Vātsyāyana, but a Vedic principle. Long before the *Kāma Sūtra* was composed, with a view to the success of human life and marriage and to make amorous relations pleasant, the *Atharva Veda* indicated such kinds of practice and forms of coupling.

In these chapters, Vātsyāyana indicates the means to amorous success, processes for improving looks, methods for bewitching, and ways of reaching one's goal. The same procedures, the same forms of intercourse and techniques, are described in the *Atharva Veda*.

The *Atharva Veda* says, "Reerecting what is enfeebled, grant me success in love."

The means described in the *Kāma Sūtra* for prolonging life are explained at length in the *Atharva Veda*. Together with the means of erotic success and of prolonging life, Vātsyāyana also describes bewitchment techniques (Vashīkarana Yoga).

These practices include ointments for the body, marks on the forehead, powders sprinkled over the woman and substances she must be made to ingest, the surprising things she must be shown, as well as the means and remedies for subjugating her.

The tradition of bewitchment is very ancient. Important descriptions of methods of bewitchment can be found in the *Vedas* and the *Āgamas*. Bewitchment is practiced with the aid of magic figures (yantras), magic words (mantras), and magic rites (tantras).

Beside the sacred texts, a very widespread usage of mantras is found among the barbarians. In the Muslim religion, the use of yantras, mantras, and tantras is very generalized, and formulas for bewitching are not lacking. Many mantras, however, can be found in the *Atharva Veda*.

The mantras of bewitchment found in the *Atharva Veda* can be used in various ways. In explaining the importance of using the mantra called "Kāma-gāyatrī" for bewitchment, repeating it or meditating on it, the *Agama Tantra* says that one attains the status of the god of love by repeating one hundred and fifty thousand times: "AUM Manobhavāya Vidmahe Kandārshāya dhīmahi Tannah Kāmah prachodayāt."

The *Kuchumāra Tantra* says that, by repeating ten thousand times: "AUM KLIM enam ānaya naya vashatām, AUM, Ksham namah" and by performing ten times the offerings of kadamba (*Anthocephalus indicus*) and palāsha (*Butea frondosa*) flowers, one can succeed in making this mantra effective.

The *Āgama Tantra* indicates how to bewitch by making the person eat betel: "AUM chāmunde hulu hulu chulu vashamānaya āmukhīm svāhā." By giving a woman betel over which this formula has been pronounced seven times, the woman is bewitched.

In order to bewitch through eating betel, one of the shābara (barbarian) mantras is as follows:

> AUM Kāmaru Kamachchhā Kī devī taham baithe
> Ismāīl jogī Ismāīl jogī ne diyā chāra pāna
> ekahi pāna rājī bājī susara pāna viraha
> sanjotī tīsara pāna vyākula
> Kare charon pāna jo mere khāya mere pāsa
> Se Kahin na jāe furo mantra Ishvarovācha
> AUM Tham Tham Tham Tham Thah.

To prevent the power of enjoyment from declining and to maintain it, Vātsyāyana recommends the use of the tonic remedies of ayurvedic medicine. The subject is as per the *Ayur Veda*. The best recipes for tonic treatment are found in medical works. The *Atharva Veda* (6.2) also gives an abundant description of the employment of tonics.

In this chapter, the means indicated for increasing amorous success, for long life, bewitching women, and strength are often methods that have been borrowed from ayurvedic medicine and from the *Tantras*.

Vātsyāyana finds room for these practices because they belong to the subject dealt with and not in order to make profligates immortal, or make studs of them and bewitch other men's wives and daughters. It can happen sometimes, when one finds difficulty in accomplishing one's duty and when questions arise about preserving one's reputation, that it becomes necessary to utilize these procedures. In such cases, however, it is better to employ them after consulting competent and experienced people. This is why, in the end, Vātsyāyana advises that these procedures should only be employed after consulting medical works, the Vedic texts, the *Āgamas, Tantras*, as well as competent and experienced persons, since otherwise one risks adverse results. Thus, in connection with the use of a tonic, the author of the *Kāma Sūtra* says, "Two palas each of ghee, honey, sugar, and mahuā (*Cassia latifolia*)," therefore stating equal quantities, while the wise ayurvedic physicians teach that equal quantities of ghee and honey are a poison. It is thus preferable to leave the decision to an experienced physician, and not prepare the medicines oneself, pounding and crushing the ingredients according to the book. In certain circumstances, the mantras and rites (tantras) are essential. Only the ignorant attempt to learn mantras from books and practice rites according to what they read. It is necessary to follow the instructions of a tantric guru.

End of the First Chapter
Success in Love
of the Seventh Part entitled Occult Practices

Chapter Two

AROUSING A WEAKENED SEXUAL POWER
[Nashtarāga Pratyānayana Prakarana]

The aphrodisiac procedures described above refer to two conditions: organic weakness, or lack of excitation.

At present, these two forms of impotence are contemplated. Whether the condition is natural or acquired, how can impotence be cured?

   1   If one is incapable of satisfying a passionate woman, techniques (yoga) must be used.

To satisfy and bring a sexually aggressive woman to enjoyment, a weakened man must follow treatment involving medicinal plants.

Impotence is of two kinds: natural weakness, or an occasional loss of virility.

In the first case, it is said:

   2   At the outset of copulation, excite the vulva with the hand and, when it becomes damp, practice sexual relations and thus reach orgasm.

At the start of intercourse, at the beginning of the act, although excitation is lacking and his penis stays soft, he wishes to reach orgasm. In such a case, first of all, he excites the vulva with his hand, according to the elephant-hand technique. He stimulates it. The rubbing of his hand on her vulva makes the excited woman start to become moist. He penetrates her with his instrument [yantra] to reach orgasm at the last moment.

For a man who ejaculates before the woman does, if he wishes to share the enjoyment felt by the woman in churning, he must, before intercourse, put his finger into the woman's vulva and penetrate when she becomes moist.

In connection with acquired impotence, it is said:

3 Superior coition [auparishtaka], in the mouth, can arouse passion when, as a result of age or excess, excitation diminishes.

When, although the desire is there, the penis, for lack of ardor, does not erect to undertake intercourse, it can be stimulated by buccal coition. When, as a result of age or excess, the penis deflates, excitation is lacking, and the sex erects with difficulty, sufficient vigor can be found for intercourse with the aid of buccal coition.

When a man is frigid, his body weakened by age or exhausted after repeated intercourse, he must stimulate it with buccal coition, after the manner indicated in the chapter on preliminary practices.

4 Dildos may also be utilized.

Or else one attaches an apparatus [apadravya]. In such a case whether excitation works or not, sexual intercourse is performed by artificial means.

False sexual organs, whether of rubber or wood, may be utilized

5 Some are made of gold, silver, copper, iron, ivory, or horn.

Of these dildos, some are of gold or other materials such as iron horn, or alloys.

6 According to the Bābhravyas, penetration with objects

made of tin [trāpusha] or lead [saisaka] is soft, with the effect of fresh sperm, and they have a pleasant roughness.

Those made of tin alloy or a lead rod are used due to their softness of contact. They are fresh like sperm, during penetration, and have a pleasant roughness that causes greater excitation than those made of wood.

7   However, according to Vātsyāyana, those of wood are more sought after.

They are more appreciated, preferred over any other by some people. Wooden ones should thus be used for penetration.

Master Vātsyāyana therefore recommends penetration using a wooden object, if this satisfies the woman.

In connection with their employment, differences are mentioned.

8   Phallus [linga] size varies greatly, from tiny to enormous.

It is a matter of the size of the artificial phallus and its internal cavity, which may be large or small. If the size of the sex to be inserted does not match that of the artificial phallus, it can be painful.

The artificial phallus must be made according to the size of the man's penis. In order to assuage the woman's itch, the front part of the vulva must be rubbed hard.

9   Some artificial members require two harness attachments [sanghāti].

Some require ties [valaya] or attachments [sandhinī] in three or four places.

Artificial members require two attachments comprising two solid bands, since otherwise they will not stay on.

10   Or else, according to the size, three or more bands [chūdaka] may be necessary.

According to the length of the sex, three or more bands are required. The length of a man's sex ranges from hare to horse.

11   If it is only fixed on one side, there is only one band.

Fixed on one side only, with a rounded shape, made of tin or other material, it forms a covering of the same size as the penis, over its whole length, and is held in place by a single band.

If, according to size, only one side can be covered with a jacket of tin or other material, it is known as a simple band.

12 The sheath [kanchuka] and armor [jālaka] are pierced by two lateral holes at the opening, so that they can be firmly attached to the testicles of the scrotum.

Holes are pierced on both sides of the opening, at the point where the penis is inserted, in order to house the belt string that attaches it firmly to the balls of the scrotum. The sheath [kanchuka], which entirely covers the penis, is thus firmly fixed to the testicles. Double attachments are used for the armor [jālaka]. There are two kinds of sheath, one rough and the other smooth. The one that covers the jewel part [the glans] is a semi-armor, only protecting the jewel. The armor is fixed by its holes to the attachment string, which passes behind the testicles. There are two kinds: perforated as described above, or else, through many holes made in the band [valaya], it is tied by a stretched cord passing between the two testicles, pushing them to either side. The jewel reinforcement is fixed in front, carefully attached according to the size. In both cases, the size of the penis to which it is attached must be taken into account in fixing the armor and the sheath.

An artificial sex, called an armor or sheath, is fixed to the scrotum by a belt with adjustable length and width.

13 In the absence of these instruments, a hollowed-out pumpkin may be used, or bamboo moistened with oil or ointment and attached to the belt, or else a cleaned rod of citron wood [nimbū]. Some men make a rosary of small wooden balls, about the size of an āmalaka fruit, to wind round the penis in order to practice copulation.

If the system described cannot be implemented, a piece of bamboo or something else can be used to take the place of the penis. After cleaning it carefully, it is attached to the belt. In order to obtain the right size, cover it with leather and moisten it. Soften it with oil or ointment before putting it into action. A rosary of small wooden balls of the size of an āmalaka fruit may also be used, with which an irregular necklace is made. When the penis is thus dressed, oil it abundantly.

14 A man experiences no feeling in these ways of copulating.

No enjoyment is felt in utilizing these artificial organs, designed for a form of intercourse for the impotent and for eunuchs.

15 In southern countries, the penis is pierced during childhood, just as one pierces the ears.

Children's ears are pierced. The linga is similarly pierced at the point of the urethra or elsewhere.
The method for piercing is as follows:

16 After piercing the young man's sex with a pointed instrument, it is kept under water as long as the blood is running.

With a pointed tool, pierce the boy's sex. Drawing back the foreskin and pushing it back to free the head [the glans], skillfully pierce obliquely, so that both sides are perforated. Then keep in water to stop the blood running.
To pierce a young man's penis, the foreskin must be lifted and the piercing done crosswise, avoiding the veins, using a sharp instrument. After this, the penis should be kept in water until the blood stops running.

17 To widen, one should exert oneself without stinting the whole night.

To widen the hole and prevent its reclosing, one should exert oneself without restraint by performing coition many times. By doing so, one avoids suffering.

18 Then, with an ointment, clean it every other day.

Clean the wound with ointment made of the five astringents [panchakashāya].
The five astringents are amalatāsa (*Rumex vesicarus*), brāhmī

(*Hydrocotyle asiatica* or *Bracopa monnieri*), kānera (kanikāsa, common oleander), mālatī (jasmine) and shankhapushpī (*Crotalaria varrucosa*).

**19 With a rattan [vetasa] or kutaja [*Holarrhena anti-
ɔyʃenterica*] point, widen it gradually. The opening will
stabilize and the hole get larger.**

**20 Clean it with licorice [yashti madhuka] mixed with
honey.**

If one cleans it with licorice powder mixed with honey, the wound
will heal.

21 Then cover it with a sheet of lead [sīsaka].

Then attach a sheet of lead (sīsaka) to it, since lead will make the
hole wider. Fix the sheet as one would fix a palm leaf. The hole will
rapidly get wider.

22 Moisten with bhallātaka [*Semicarpuʃ anacarɔium*] oil.

Moisten it inside with bhallātaka oil.

23 Into this opening can be inserted any imaginable object.

When the hole has widened, the wound is healed and one no
longer suffers. Accessories can be inserted: long or round, of gold,
wood, terracotta, stone, etc.

**24 According to whim, accessories such as a rounded stick,
a curved stick in the shape of a mortar, an object shaped
like a flower bud, heron's bone, elephant's trunk, octagonal, shaped like a bracelet, shaped like a horn, can be used,
or other accessories that are of use in many erotic activities. They may be flexible or hard.**

*A rounded stick is a simply turned stick [ekatovritta], which one
covers with leather. For the mortar, choose a stick shaped like the moon
in its eighth day, hollow in the middle. Fix it by its narrow part. The
one shaped like a flower is of wood. It has the shape of a lotus bud and
is fixed in the middle. The bracelet is made of a bilva branch [Aegle*

marmelos], *if necessary joining two pieces. The heron's bone is like a square stick.*

A stick of octagonal shape has a square top part.

Other objects can also be used, and other means employed that serve to excite. All these objects should be covered with leather so as not to wound in action. They can be small, medium, or large. The hardest ones must be oiled and handled gently during sexual intercourse.

The artificial aids used according to taste may be round, ring-shaped, curved, in the shape of a lotus bud, irregular like bamboo bark, resembling a heron's bone or elephant's trunk, octagonal, square, horn-shaped. They can be made hard or flexible.

Then is expounded how to increase the size and develop the potential of the penis united with these accessories.

25   Take shūka hairs—the shūka is an insect that lives in trees—mix them with oil and rub the penis with it for ten nights, take it off then put it on again. When a swelling appears, sleep face downward on a wooden bed, letting one's sex hang through a hole.

Other creatures that live in trees are not suitable. Kill the shūka before using its hairs. Take hold of the insect with small pincers and rub it on the sides of the penis. The hairs become detached, torn out by the rubbing. They must then be spread out by massaging with oil. This causes swelling. When the swelling is sufficient, let the penis hang through a hole in the bedboard so that it gets longer.

26   Then with cooling mixtures eliminating the pain, the result is gradually obtained.

Thus, having obtained the desired result, get rid of the pain with a cooling mixture made of the five astringents. This is the way to eliminate the pain caused by the swelling.

27   The swelling caused by the shūka lasts for life.

The swelling produced by the shūka is permanent and lasts for life.

Thus a sensual and erotic man develops the size of his penis in a permanent manner.

28   By rubbing it successively with juice of ashvagandhā
[*Vithania ∂omnifera*], shabara roots [*Rubra cor∂ifolia*, lodhra],
jala shuka [watermelon], brihatī [*Solanum in∂icum*, egg-
plant], buffalo butter, hastikarna [large-leafed castor oil
plant], vajravalli [*Heliothropunum in∂icum*], the penis stays
swollen for one month.

Take the roots of the great lodhra.

29   By boiling these ingredients in oil and rubbing the
penis with them, the effect lasts for six months.

*The effect of using these ingredients, boiled in oil, by rubbing oneself
with the resultant mixture, lasts six months. Erection is sustained.*

30   Take the seeds of dādima [pomegranate], trāpusha
[cucumber], bāluka [*Gi∂ekia pharmaceoide∂*], and the juice
of the brihatī fruits [*Solanum in∂icum*]. Cook over a low
heat. Rub in or sprinkle diluted with oil.

*Take seeds of dādima [pomegranate], trāpusha [cucumber], bāluka
[elabālukā], giant pumpkins [brihatī or kadkabrihati], extract the juice:
knead or sprinkle thoroughly. The increase in size lasts six months.*
Take pomegranate and cucumber seeds, extract the juice of
elabāluka (eluva, *Gisekia pharmaceoides*) and bhatakataiyā (*Solanum indicum*,
eggplant). Cook in oil over a low heat. Use it to massage the penis. It
will remain swollen for six months.

31   All these techniques for increasing size should be
learned from an expert.

Other techniques for developing the penis also exist. They should
be learned from experienced people.

*Beside the means previously described, special techniques [chitra
yoga] are indicated to reach one's goal.*

32   For example, by powdering snuhi thorns [*Euphorbia
neriifolia*, milk hedge], punarnavā [*Boerhavia ∂iffu∂a*,
hogweed], mixed with monkey excrements and lāngalikā

root [*Gloriosa superba*, glory lily], she who receives this mixture on her head will never love another.

Furthermore, to complete this subject, the person whose head is powdered with snuhi thorns will desire none other, remaining entirely dependent on you.

Powder thuhara (snuhi) and punarnavā thorns. Mix them with monkey excrement and karihāri root (indrāyana, glory lily). Crush it all to powder. The woman on whose head this powder is sprinkled will be in your power.

33 In a crucible, prepare a powder of somalatā [*Narcostemia rampant*], avalguja [vākuchī bīja, *Vermonia anthelmintica*], bhringa [bhringarāja, *Vedelia calendulacea*], with powdered iron [loha] and yellow amaranth [upajihvikā]. Make a thick paste by mixing it with the juice of jambu leaves [*Eugenia jambolina*] and vyādhighātaka [golden sephalika, *Rumex vesicarus*]. If this paste is smeared on the woman's vulva, it immediately destroys the excitation of any man who has intercourse with her.

Avalguja are bākuchi seeds. Bhringa is bhringarāja. Take the juice that oozes from the leaves of vyādhighātaka, the sap of the jambu fruit. Make a thick paste. Mere contact destroys desire, the penis will no longer erect. Vyādhighātaka is an anaesthetic. After contact with this product, the penis will no longer erect. Upajihvikā [yellow amaranth] grows on embankments during the rainy season. The whole should be crushed in a crucible.

34 If a women takes a bath in buffalo's milk, in which have been mixed the powder of gopālikā [extract of cow's bile], gurupādikā [rundikā, bahupādikā, fig], and yellow amaranth [jihvikā, *Terminalia tomentosa*], even if she is subsequently showered by the rain, the man who enjoys her becomes impotent.

35 An ointment prepared by crushing nīpa flowers [kadamba, *Anthocephalus indicus*], āmrataka [āmalaka, anvada, *Emblica officinalis*, Java plum], and jambu [jamura, *Eugenia jambolina*, rose apple], brings bad luck.

Nīpa and its flowers are unlucky. A necklace made with these various flowers causes bad luck.

36 Crush kokilāksha [*Aɖteracantha longifolia*] in water. Smeared with this product, the vulva of an elephant woman will narrow in a single night.

The vulva contracts, shrinks, becomes as narrow as a hind woman's. White kokilāksha should be used.

37 Crush the seeds of pink lotus and blue water lily [*Nelubrium ɖpecioɖum*] in honey, together with vajra kadamba [*Anthocephaluɖ caɖamba*], sarjaka sugandha [scented sāla, *Surjea rubrata*]. Applied strongly to a hind woman, this ointment widens her like an elephant woman in a single night.

As small as she may be, when a woman applies it to her vulva, the organ widens.

38 Burn snuhi leaves [*Euphorbia neriifolia,* milk hedge], soma leaves [*Narcoɖtemia*], and arka leaves [*Calotropiɖ gigantea,* madāra]. Mix the ashes with avalguja seeds [vākuchī, globe amaranth] and āmalaka seeds [anvāla, *Emblica officinaliɖ*]. Applied to the head, the blackest hairs become white.

39 Crush the roots of henna [madayantikā, mehandi], kūtajaka [yellow amaranth], dark-flowered anjikā [mountain chameli], girikarnikā [*Clitoria ternatea*], shlakshnapāni [*Teramnuɖ labialiɖ*]. Used to wash the hair, the hair regains its natural color.

Henna is a well-known plant. Kūtajaka is a plant whose fruit produces indrayava seeds. Dark-flowered anjikā and girikarnikā are also well known. For shlakshnapāni, choose the Kashmir variety and take the roots. This product dyes white hair, making it black again.

40 These ingredients must be cooked in oil. Used regularly, its application darkens the hair.

To be applied by oneself every day.

41 Take the sweat from the testicles of a white horse, and dilute in seven volumes of yellow arsenic [ālākta]. Applied to white lips, this mixture makes them become red.

42 By adding Arabian jasmine [madayantī], the effect is reversed.

Applying this product to the lips, they become white again.

43 Extract the juice of the bahupādikā [mint], kushtha [*Saussurea lappa*], tagara [*Tabernaemontana coronaria*], with the leaves of sālīsha [or tālīsha, *Euphorbia antiquarum*], devadāru [cedar, *Pinus deodara*], vajra [*Hygrophila spinosa*], and kandaka [*Dioscorea alata*]. Anoint a reed with it and make a flute. Whoever hears the sound of this flute will be bewitched.

Wholly anoint the outside and inside of the bamboo, which must be thoroughly soaked. The woman who hears the sound of this flute falls into the power of him who plays it.

44 He who takes a drink to which datura seeds have been added becomes mad.

Whether they are eaten or drunk.

45 By taking settled molasses, he returns to his normal state and regains consciousness.

Molasses should be used when it has aged.

46 By rubbing one's hand with the excrements of a peacock, which has been made to take haritāla [yellow myrobalan] and manashilā [red arsenic], everything one touches becomes invisible.

The peacock must be made to swallow haritāla and manashilā after fasting for one month. By rubbing one's hand in the excrements of this peacock, whatever one touches becomes invisible to others.

47 Ash of angāra grass [khasa, vetiver], mixed with oil, makes water like milk.

48 Take haritāla [yellow myrobalan] and āmrataka [*Emblica officinalis*] together with shravana priyangu berries [mālakānguni, *Cardiospermum holocaecabum,* balloon vine], crush the same, and use to coat iron utensils, which take on the appearance of copper.

Cut them into small pieces. Smear the vessels with the same and polish with shravana priyangu, whose berries have been crushed at the same time.

49 Place shravana priyangu in oil in which fragments of snakeskin have been mixed. Soak therein a clean cloth with which lamp wicks are made. Any long piece of wood lightened by the lamp will take on the appearance of a snake.

Whatever is lighted by the said lamp will, due to a magical effect, look like a snake.

50 By drinking the milk of a white cow that has a white calf, longevity and fame are won.

The purity of this milk brings good luck. Its constant use is recommended for well-being, long life, and fame.

51 The same result can be obtained from a Brahman's blessing.

By striving to earn their favor, their blessing is obtained.
It is advisable to follow their teaching as a whole and in detail.

52 Having studied the ancient treatises and observed their applications, I have striven to compose the *Kāma Sūtra* in a succinct fashion.

After studying the ancient treatises, weighing their words and meaning, and having sought confirmation of the same through experience, I have therefore summarized their teachings in this treatise. Among the practices contemplated in this treatise, and in particu-

lar those causing erotic excitation, an indication has also been given of the forms of sexual stimulation that are harmful.

53 Reasonable people, aware of the importance of virtue, money, and pleasure, as well as that of social convention, will not let themselves be led astray by passion.

Whoever knows the profound meaning of the scriptures will observe the rules of virtue and will not let himself be led to misbehave. Worldly conventions denote what is considered civilized or ill-bred.

He who understands the meaning of the *Kāma Sūtra* is drawn to seek virtue, material success, and pleasure, and to respect social conventions. He is not the slave of his passions.

In connection with actions recommended in occult practices that are contrary to ethics, Vātsyāyana says:

54 These strange practices for stimulating eroticism have been described in accordance with the requirements of the subject dealt with, after which each must strive to make a choice.

The subject dealt with requires aphrodisiac procedures to be considered, but having become acquainted with them, a man must strive to find out whether they are to be recommended or forbidden.

In the interest of the treatise everything must be described, both good and bad, followed by an indication of those that can be put into practice and those that may not.

55 One must be able to judge which of the practices illustrated in this treatise refer to anybody. These practices, however, should be performed according to local custom.

56 Vātsyāyana composed the *Kāma Sūtra* according to the rules of holy scripture and in conformity with tradition, inspired by the work of the Bābhravyas.

With due respect for the authority of the Bābhravyas and the ancient masters, he comments on their work according to his own experience and common sense.

In accordance with the meaning of the sūtras of the Bābhravyas and with a more or less complete experience of the works of the *Kāma Shāstra*, Vātsyāyana composed the *Kāma Sūtra* in obedience to the rules of sacred scripture.

He recommends its use, saying:

57 From the beginning to the end, from youthful chastity
to final abnegation, one must succeed in life's pilgrimage
and not live to satisfy one's passions.

*During life's pilgrimage, from youth to the age of renunciation, the
three upper castes must practice marriage and not lead a dissolute life.*
Vātsyāyana's aim is to assure a pleasant and fruitful life for people,
between virginity and final immersion into contemplation. His aim and
his intention comprise neither licentiousness nor passion.
Why should passion not be served?

58 He who wishes to preserve virtue, wealth, and love in
this world and the next must have a thorough knowledge
of this treatise and, at the same time, master his senses.

*The man who knows the essence of this treatise and wishes to
maintain a balance between pleasure, virtue, and social success, seeks
what is appropriate from the point of view of this world and the next.*

59 A shrewd man, expert in one thing and another, considering both ethics and his own material interests, must
not be a sensualist thirsty for sex, but establish a stable
marriage.

*Skilled in several things and knowing the sacred books well, the
sensual man remains moderate so that passion does not become an
obstacle to ethics and prosperity. This is why he makes a marriage.*
*The aim of this treatise is to lead a man to set himself up in society
as a respectable person and not as an unleashed sensualist.*

End of the Jayamangalā *Commentary*
by Yashodhara

In this second chapter, when an incapacity for sexual relations
arises between man and woman, feelings of contempt and indifference
are felt toward each other. In this connection, in the chapter on impotence, Vātsyāyana explains by what means desire and excitation can be
awakened and increased.

The previous chapter dealt with special practices (chitra yoga).
The present one explains astute means for continuing erotic practices.

When a man's sexual power diminishes and copulation is no longer possible, his wife, dissatisfied, becomes alienated from him. Women who, under such circumstances, repress their intense desire for enjoyment, often become ill as a result. They catch diseases such as epilepsy and fainting fits, and their nature becomes unstable. It is women's nature to dissimulate their feelings and repress them. By nature, women always appear to be serious. Unlike men, they are not enterprising and animated.

In copulation, a man remains active from start to finish. This is why, compared to a woman, he is satisfied and ejaculates more quickly. Not being satisfied due to this overrapid ejaculation, the woman remains frustrated, unsatisfied, and discontented and, gradually, problems of health make their appearance. If her desire for enjoyment is not satisfied, a woman does not stay in love with the man. She ceases to admire him. Thus it is that life together becomes cheerless and quarrels arise.

In order to give some spice into the life of a couple that has become dreary and dull, and to bring back passion, the authors of the works of the *Kāma Shāstra* have illustrated highly efficacious means in such texts as the *Kāma Sūtra*, the *Ratirahasya*, the *Ananga Ranga*, the *Nāgarasarvasva*, and so on. The said methods are described very clearly, and from a practical point of view.

Vātsyāyana, in this connection, says something essential: a man who ejaculates prematurely should, using some artificial object, excite and moisten a sensual woman prior to copulation. In so doing, both man and woman experience a simultaneous enjoyment and both are satisfied.

In the *Kāma Sūtra*, Vātsyāyana explains the point at which the waxing of the moon is to be found in a woman, and in which place her eroticism is seated according to the days of the moon. This is the principle of the phases of the moon. If this principle is understood, one knows which part of a woman's body to press in order to make her immediately excited and begin to moisten. Apart from the phases of the moon, a woman's body contains sensitive points that, when touched, make her moisten rapidly. Beside these physical aspects and apart from psychological means, there are also remedies for subjugating. Such remedies, which bewitch and subjugate, have been described in the chapter on occult means. Medical treatises, however, also contain numerous remedies for this purpose.

Utilizing stimulants, however, damages bodily health. The sperm's vivacity and strength disappear, and the nervous system is debilitated. Men who, during copulation, come too quickly, whose capacity for sexual relations and for discharging sperm is weakened, who wish to sustain their excitation, must practice yoga techniques. In the yoga treatises, it is a matter of ashvinī mudrā (the position of the mare). The man who masters this position can enjoy whoever he wants. As long as he keeps separate his respiratory breath and his digestive breath, his seed will not fall.

The ashvinī mudrā is an easy means and can be perfected in a few days. The man who implements this mudrā is a conqueror of women.

Sexual weakness is mainly due to two causes: one is impotence due to mental instability, while the other, which is physical, is due to reasons of frigidity. If one of these causes is present, the man is unsure of himself. His anxiety over his capacity for ejaculation may be such that he is perpetually preoccupied and worried about his sexual success.

He constantly strives to stimulate his sexual power. Weak men of this kind are sometimes unmarried and, in order to try out their sexual prowess, they go to a prostitute and return with lowered head. When impotence is psychological, the man, during intercourse, begins to strain and then to deflate. For such men, in order to remove their mental doubts about their impotence, it must be proved to them through physical experience that their doubts and hesitations are groundless.

Another situation is caused by changes appearing in the nervous system, creating total impotence, which specialists declare they are unable to cure. When the two forms of impotence are found in the same individual, however, and the mental blocks are gradually eliminated, the mental preoccupations being oriented in another direction, the incapacity may disappear.

What ancient concepts knew as desires, impulses, and inclinations, the moderns call eroticism, or sexual appetite, pretending both that the presence of such tendencies should be overcome, and that they form part of man's nature. "That woman must belong to me," or "I want that pretty girl," are the forms in which these appetites manifest themselves.

Indian philosophy stresses the desire for progeny, the desire for a good reputation, and the search for the means of subsistence. These are the three aspects considered. On reflection, the desire for procreation is the basis of eroticism, but sexual intercourse based on considerations of a social order or of respectability are a deviation of this instinct.

Indian philosophy maintains that an individual exaggeratedly attracted to sexuality becomes vagina-dependent. He is like an animal.

On this subject, the lawgivers say: "Food, sleep, and copulation are the same for man and beast. Those who practice ethics are superior; those without are like animals." (*Vishnu Purāna*, 6.5.34)

According to this principle it follows that food and sleep reinforce vigor, fear protects, and copulation depends on vigor and security. Thus the two most important things are food and sexuality.

With this principle in view, Vātsyāyana, in composing the *Kāma Sūtra*, reflects on all aspects of sexuality. The question asked by everyone, "When and in what way does sexual desire manifest itself?" finds an answer in the *Kāma Sūtra*. In this work, Vātsyāyana also strives to explain why, when excitation appears, feeling is also made manifest in the female body.

Why does the desire for copulation appear when a man sees a woman and a woman sees a man? The answer is to be found in the *Kāma Sūtra*. Vātsyāyana tells us that, for a man, woman incarnates the desire for copulation, and it is she therefore who is the cause of sexual desire. Certain parts of a woman's body are centers of copulative desire. By touching, caressing, or even stroking them, the woman's erotic desire is aroused and she begins to become moist. It is for this reason that Vātsyāyana advises men who ejaculate too quickly to caress the woman's sex, to moisten it before enjoying her.

This suggestion of Vātsyāyana's is scientifically proven. Why is the female organ stimulated by being touched? In order to understand, no treatise on sexuality is needed. By touching the penis, by pressing the lower part of the body, by biting the lips, etc., desire for copulation is stimulated. What can one say therefore of that point that is the seat of sexual desire? It follows that sexual need is an impulse, a permanent state of being, which is called "desire" (rati). Desire is a latent state, stimulation causes its arousal, and excitation due to contact is a result. This shows that for every desire, there is an impulse, an aim, an object, and a support.

Vātsyāyana's aim in writing the *Kāma Sūtra* is the interest of society. Society puts a brake on natural instincts and seeks to orient sexual instinct along particular paths. It tries to utilize these instinctive tendencies for social purposes. The principle of society is not to neglect anything, to utilize both small and evil things. Eroticism is a force and, without doubt, a powerful force. Just as man can produce energy by harnessing running water, so he can use to advantage his powerful sexual energy.

Eroticism is a highly important mental activity. Such a force must be used competently. By observing this principle, a man can obtain great material advantages. This is why, since the dawn of humanity, rules of behavior have been devised, an analysis used by society to check and utilize these instincts in the best possible way. Due to these rules, man only realizes certain desires later on. He must be able to control his instincts. Because of these rules, many of man's physical and mental powers remain unused. This truth cannot be ignored. Another result is that mental powers have been divided into categories. If the rules and prohibitions of society admit of no exteriorization and sexuality is repressed, sexual fullness is sacrificed to society.

Society has created an enormous problem by repressing these powerful energies in the depths of man's consciousness. It must be admitted that society has made a great mistake in repressing these terrible energies with its laws, thus imprisoning them within mankind. By preventing these powerful energies from being utilized profitably externally, terrible internal explosions take place in man's mind. Such explosions lead to a lack of balance. Disorders of this kind are not uncommon in society.

The first of society's duties is to orient man's tendencies toward the common good. Whatever hinders the individual's progress is evil. It may be said that civility is good and incivility bad. It is sometimes considered that the satisfaction of natural instincts is uncivilized and its opposite civilized. Civilization as advocated by society consists in preventing the natural instincts from being satisfied, but also in purifying them so that they can be utilized in other useful domains. For Indian civilization, there are two kinds of good: progress and renunciation. According to the *Upanishads*, progress is ambiguous. Progress belongs to the world and allows material success and erotic pleasure to be achieved without difficulty, and if well-being and pleasure are satisfied, society is at peace. No form of disorder or material revolution will spread. The individual is the basis of society, and thus the source of the state's prosperity. The state must therefore always watch over individual well-being. For this reason, it can be said that all the individual's mental capacities are utilized for purposes other than eroticism.

The codes of ethics (*Dharma Shāstra*) and political works (*Nīti Shāstra*) dedicate considerable space to laws and prohibitions.

The sages of old gave instructions that can be considered a condemnation of the overt satisfaction of our tendencies, leaving, however, the possibility of exteriorizing them during festivals such as Holi, the Spring Festival, the festival of light, the festival of the god of love, revolutions, walks in the gardens, etc.

In ancient India, prostitutes were honored as ornaments of the city and the state. They were known as the wives of the city and the state took care of them. To frequent them was a mark of good upbringing and, at a wedding, the blessing of one of the wives of the city was required, as is the case still today. Consorting with prostitutes was not condemned. Men considered their use as a right authorized by the sages.

"Eating meat, drinking wine, making love are not forbidden: they form part of man's inclinations. But to renounce them is of great value." (*Manu Smriti* 5.53)

The *Shrīmat Bhāgavata Purāna* explains that, in this world, all living beings are inclined to eat meat, to drink, to copulate. But society, by forbidding the same, strives to limit them.

"In the world, the prohibition to use meat and wine is not always stringent. At weddings, ritual sacrifices, cups of liquor must not be abandoned." (*Shrīmat Bhāgavata* 11.5, 11)

Vātsyāyana composed the *Kāma Sūtra* with a view to the progress of the individual and of society, for the good of all individuals. In completing his work, Vātsyāyana says, "By compiling the ancient treatises, I have defined practice." This means that he collected the essence of the ancient works and, considering the customs of the various countries, he composed the *Kāma Sūtra*.

Nandi, Shiva's companion, is considered to be the original author of the *Kāma Shāstra*. It is said that the *Kāma Shāstra* counted one thousand chapters. The Bābhravyas summarized Nandi's *Kāma Shāstra* in one hundred chapters. Shvetaketu, Gonardīya, Dattaka, Ghotakamukha, Gonikāputra and other authors divided the *Kāma Shāstra* into various separate treatises. The *Kāma Shāstra* of the Bābhravyas was very large, and the treatises of Shvetaketu and Gonirdīya only dealt with a part. Considering that the work of the Bābhravyas, in its entirety, and the treatises of Shvetaketu, Gonardīya, and others cover merely a part of the subject and are not within the reach of all, Vātsyāyana, for the good of mankind, took what was essential from these various works and, examining the customs of the different countries at his own time, composed the *Kāma Sūtra*.

Describing the contents of his work, the master says that, in this treatise, many subjects were studied from real life. In the practices described, sexual impulses are without any doubt aroused and increased, but at the same time the risks involved are evidenced so that no one may be influenced in an evil manner. Vātsyāyana says that what is written in the sacred books should not be put into practice in all cases. Certain things are described so as not to ignore part of the subject. Their application depends on individual common sense. According to his need, the individual practices good or evil behavior. The duty of the treatise is to explain what is good and what is evil. "This is recommended and this is forbidden." Furthermore, to put men on guard, the master says, "To judge whether something is good or evil, certain elements must be taken into account: place, period, etc."

The teachings contained in the *Kāma Sūtra* should not be considered as a general guide to mankind's behavior. In answer to the question as to why and how the *Kāma Sūtra* has been composed, Vātsyāyana says, "I have listened to, understood, and read the commentaries of the *Kāma Shāstra* of the Bābhravyas and other ancient masters. Furthermore, I have examined and criticized with care the theories expressed. It was only at that point that I wrote the *Kāma Sūtra.*"

In explaining the raison d'être and utility of writing this treatise, the Master says, "The raison d'être of this work is the good state of life and of society. The teachings expressed in this treatise are based on the values of a chaste life. The aim of this treatise is not to spread lust and misconduct."

The man who has assimilated this treatise properly will, without difficulty, achieve virtue, well-being, and pleasure. The master of his senses, he will achieve success and love. Success bows before him. Vātsyāyana affirms that it was after practicing chastity and isolating himself from the world by meditation that he understood the role of sexuality and composed the *Kāma Sūtra* for the good of society and not for the propagation of erotic arts.

Here ends the Second Chapter
Arousing a Weakened Sexual Power
and the Seventh Part entitled Occult Procedures
of the Kāma Sūtra by Vātsyāyana

Appendices

One

TEXTS QUOTED

Abhijñāna Shākuntalam by Kālidāsa
Aitareya Āranyaka
Aitareya Brāhmana
Ananga Ranga by Kalyānamalla
Artha Shāstra by Kautilya
Atharva Veda
Ayur Veda

Bhagavad Gītā
Bhavishya Purāna
Bhoja Prabandha by Vallabha
Brahma Sūtra
Brahmavaīvarta Purāna
Brihad Āranyaka Upanishad
Brihad Samhitā by Varāhamihira

Chanda Vedānga
Chāndogya Upanishad

Daridrachārudatta by Bhāsa
Dashakumāra Charita by Dandin
Dasha Shāyana by Jyotirīshvara
Dharma Shāstra
Dhanur Veda

Gītā Govinda by Jayadeva
Grihya Sūtra, domestic ritual

Harsha Charita by Bāna

Īsha Upanishad

Jyotisha Vedānga

Kādambarī by Bāna
Kāla Vilāsa by Kshemendra
Kalpa Sūtra

Kalpa Vedānga
Kāma Shāstra
Kirātārjuna by Bhāravi
Kāvya Prakāsha by Mammata
Koka Shāstra
Kuchumāra Tantra
Kuttinīmata by Damodara Gupta

Lalita Vistara

Mahābhārata
Mālatī Mādhava by Bhavabhūti
Manu Smriti
Markandeya Purāna by Bhargava
Mīmānsā Darshana
Mitākshara
Mricchakatikā by Shūdraka
Mundaka Upanishad

Naishadīya Charita by Harsha
Nāgarasarvasva by Padmashrī
  (Bhikshu)
Nātya Shāstra by Bharata
Nirukta Vedānga
Nīti Shāstra
Nyāya Sūtra by Gautama

Rasa Manjari by Bhānudatta
Rati Manjari by Jayadeva
Rati Rahasya by Kokkoka

Rig Veda

Sāhitya Darpana
Sāmkhya Darshana
Sarasvatī Kanthābharana
Shikshā Vedānga
Shishupālavadha by Māgha
Shiva Purāna
Shrīmad Bhāgavata Purāna
Shukranīti
Skanda Purāna
Smara Dipikā by Gunākara
Sushruta
Sūtra Vritti by Narsingha Shāstrī
Svapna Vāsavadatta by Bhāsa

Taittirīya Samhitā
Taittirīya Upanishad

Ujjvala Nīlamani by Rūpagosvāmī

Vaisheshika Darshana
Vishnu Purāna
Vivāha Paddhati, marriage ritual
Vyākarana Vedānga

Yājñavalkya Smriti
Yoga Shāstra
Yoga Vāsishtha

Two

Mythical and Historical Characters and Authors Mentioned

Ahalyā, a famous courtesan

Amrapālī, a courtesan

Ashvalāyana, author of the *Āshvalāyana Shrauta Sūtra*

Avimāraka, a hero of savage tribes

Bābharavya, sons of Babhru, authors of the *Kāma Shāstra*

Babhru, father of the Bābharavya

Bali, king of the genies

Bāna, author of the *Harsha Charita* and *Kādambarī*

Bhānudatta, author of the *Rasa Manjari*

Bharata, author of the *Nātya Shāstra*

Bhāravi, author of the *Kirātārjuna*

Bhargava, author of the *Markandeya Purāna*

Bhāsa, poet

Bhavabhūti, author of the *Mālatī Mādhava*

Bhoja, king of the Malvā, patron of the arts

Bhrigu, sage

Bihari, poet

Brihaspati, legendary creator of the *Artha Shāstra*

Charaka, author of a medical treatise

Chārāyana, author of a treatise on eroticism

Damayantī, heroine of a poem by Harsha

Damodara Gupta, author of the *Kuttīnimata*

Dāndakya, author of a work

Dandin, author of the *Dashakumāra Charita*

Dattaka, author of a treatise on eroticism

Draupadī, spouse of the Pandavas in the *Mahābhārata*

Gautama, sage, founder of Nyaya philosophy

Ghotakamukha, author of a treatise on eroticism

Gonardīya, author of a treatise on eroticism

Gonikāputra, author of a treatise on eroticism

Gopikā, author of a treatise on eroticism

Gunākara, author of the *Smara Dīpikā*

Gurudatta Indra, mentor of Yashodhara

Harishchandra, king famous for his virtue

Harsha, author of the *Naishadīya Charita*

Indra, king of heaven

Indrapada, disciple of Yashodhara

Indumatī, sister of Bhoja

Jayadeva, author of the *Gītā Govinda* and *Rati Manjari*

Jīvagosvāmī, commentator of the *Ujjvala Nilamani*

Jyotirīshvara, author of the *Dasha Shāyana*

Karnātaki, famous courtesan

Kautilya, author of the *Artha Shāstra*

Kichaka, general enamored of Draupadī in the *Mahābhārata*

Koka, diminutive of Kokkoka

Kokkoka, author of the *Rati Rahasya* or *Koka Shāstra*

Kshemendra, author of the *Kalā Vilāsa*

Kuchumāra, author of a treatise on eroticism

Lakshmanā, famous courtesan

Māgha, author of the *Shishupālavadha*

Mallanāga, prophet of the Asuras (gods)

Mammata, author of the *Kāvya Prakāsha*

Manu, founder of the *Dharma Shāstra*

Menakā, an apsarās, or nymph, mother of Shakuntalā

Nala, hero of a poem by Kālidāsa

Nandi, creator of the *Kāma Shāstra*

Nārāyana, author of a treatise on eroticism

Narsingha Shāstri, author of the *Sūtra Vritti*

Padmashrī (Bhikshu), author of the *Nāgarasarvasva*

Parāshāra, famous sage, author of *Smriti*

Pingalā, famous courtesan

Prajāpati, god who presides over creation

Pushpikā, author of a biography of Yashodhara

Rāmānuja Āchārya, celebrated philosopher

Rambhā, famous courtesan

Rāvana, demon of the *Rāmāyana*

Rohita, name of Harishchandra

Rūpagosvāmī, author of *Ujjvala Nīlamani*

Sāgara, god of the ocean

Shakuntalā, heroine of the play by Kālidāsa

Shankara Āchārya, famous philosopher and theologian

Shātakarni Shātavāhana, king

Shiva, god

Shivā, goddess

Shūdraka, author of the *Mriccha Katikā*

Shvetaketu Auddālaki, son of Uddālaka, author of a treatise on eroticism

Sītā, heroine of the *Rāmāyana*

Shunahshepa, a mythological character in the *Vedas*

Sugandhā, famous courtesan

Suvarnanābha, author of a treatise on eroticism

Uddālaka, author of a treatise on eroticim, father of Shvetaketu Auddālaki

Urvashī, nymph

Vallabha, author of the *Bhoja Prabandha*

Varāhamihira, author of the *Brihad Samhitā*

Vasishtha, author of the *Yoga Vāsishtha*

Vilāsinī, nymph

Yājñavalkya, author of *Smriti*

Yashodhara, author of the commentary on the *Kāma Sūtra*

Yudhishthira, eldest of the Pandavas in the *Mahābhārata*

Three

WORKS CONSULTED

Apte, V. S. *Sanskrit-English Dictionary*. Bombay: 1924.

Edde, Gérard. *Traité d'Ayurveda*. Paris: Guy Trédaniel, 1987.

Goven, D. V. *Flowering Trees and Shrubs in India*. Bombay: Thacker, 1950.

Gründ. *Arbres et Arbustes*. Prague and Paris: Artia, 1984.

Gupta, K. R. L. *Hindu Practice of Medicine*. New Delhi: 1986.

Raison, Alex. *Harita Samhita, (Nomenclature de médecine ayurvédique)*. France: Institut français d'Indologie, 1974.

Sharma, P. V. *Indian Pharmacology*. Varanasi: 1976.

Sharpe, Elisabeth. *Book of Indian Medicine*. New Delhi: 1985.

Van Hellemont, Jacques. *Compendium de Phytothérapie*. Belgium: Association Pharmaceutique Belge, 1986.

Four

Plants, Herbs, Spices, and Sundry Products

This book is not a work on botanics. We attempted, as far as possible, to identify the plants mentioned. For some of them, however, it was not possible to find out the Latin or English equivalents of the Sanskrit or Hindi names.

In some cases the identification remains uncertain. The reader should therefore use great circumspection in experimenting with the proposed recipes. Synonyms are included in parentheses.

Accharīlā, unknown

Adarakha mircha (ārdraka), *zingiber officinalis*, ginger

Agnimantha, *Premna spinata*

Aguru. *See* **alguru**

Ajamoda, *Pimpinella involucrata*

Aka. *See* **aksha**

Aksha, *Terminalia bellerica*, one of the myrobalans

Alābu (alābuka, kaddu, lauki, or tumbī), pumpkin

Ālākta, yellow arsenic

Alambukhānda, cucumber

Alamodā, unknown

Alguru (shringī, meda shringī), aloes

Ālu (aluka), sweet potato

Āmalaka (amrataka, gulābāsa), *Emblican officinalis,* myrobalan (hogplum, Java plum)

Amalatāsa, *Rumex vesicarnus*

Āmrataka. *See* **āmalaka**

Ancila (kapikacchu, kauncha, kavacha, or svayamguptā), *Mucuna pruriens*

Angāra (bālakoshīraka, khasha), *Saccharum spontaneum*, vetiver

Angur (drākshā), grape

Anjana, *Harwickia binata*

Anjikā, frangipani

Anvadi. *See* āmalaka

Anvala. *See* amālaka

Arani. *See* agnimantha

Ārdraka, ginger

Areca, ingredient of betel

Arishta, *Sapindus nifoliatus* or *Nim margosa*

Arka (madāra, madarat, mandāra, mandarat), *Calotropis procera* or *gigantea*

Ashoka (shishu), *Saraca indica*

Ashvagandhā, *Vithania somnifera*

Avalguja (bākuchī, somarājī), *Vermonia anthelmintica*, globe amaranth

Bādara, *Ziziphus jujuba*, jujube

Baheda. *See* aksha

Bahupādikā (gurupādikā, rundika), mint

Baigana (kapusavarta), eggplant

Bākuchī. *See* avalguja

Bālakoshīraka. *See* angāra

Balamakhira (trāpusha), cucumber

Bālukā. *See* elabālukā

Baragada (gūlara), *Ficus glomerata*

Bhallātaka, *Semicarpus anacardium*, marking nut

Bhantā (kanda, vrintāka), *Chenopodium album*

Bhārgavī (dūrvā), *Cynodon dactilon*, couch grass

Bhatakataiya (brihatī, kanka, or vrihati), *Solanum indicum*, eggplant

Bhilava (bilva, kakadaliya, or vilva), *Aeglo marmelos*, Bengal quince

Bhringa, *Cinnamomum zeylanicum*, cinnamon

Bhringarāja, *Vedelia calendulucea*, marigold

Bilva. *See* bhilava

Bola, myrrh

Brāhmī, *Hydrocotyle asiatica*

Brihatī. *See* bhatakataiya

Champā, *Michelia champaka*

Champakāvalī, frangipani

Chandava, *Santalum album*, sandalwood

Charya, *Piper chaba*, white pepper

Chichinda, *Trichosantes anguina*, snake gourd

Chiraunji (piyala), *Buchanania latifolia*

Chita, *Plumbago zeylanica*

Chitarana. *See* sārivā

Chitavanna (sariva), *Hermidermus indicus*

Chitraka. *See* chita

Choha, unknown

Chuna, lime

Dādima (dālima), *Punica granatum*, pomegranate

Dakha. *See* drākshā

Dālachini (tejapattra, bhringa), *Cinnamonum zeylanicum*, cinnamon

Damanaka, *Artemisia absinthum*, absinthe

Dandotpalaka (sahadevī), *Echita pulescens*
Dantashatha, lemon
Darbha, *Imperata cylindrica*
Dāruhaladī (ghandha palashika), *Berberis asiatica*, turmeric
Dāruharidrā. *See* dāruhaladī
Datura. *See* dhatura
Dauna. *See* damanaka
Devadāru, deodar cedar
Dhaniyā. *See* dhanyāka
Dhanyāka, *Coriandrum sativum*, coriander
Dhatura, *Datura alba*, datura
Drākshā (dakha, hārachūraka, or kāpishāyana), *Vitis vinifera*, grape
Dūrvā. *See* bhārgavī
Dvipautra, *Smilax officinalis*, sarsaparilla

Elā, *Elattaria cardamomum*, cardamom (large)
Elabālukā (bālukā, eluvā, or valuka), *Gisekia pharmaceoides*, kind of red camphor
Eluvā. *See* elābalukā
Enva (kakadi), *Cucumis utilissimus*, cucumber, gourd

Gadāpunnā (purnanavā), *Boerhavia diffusa*, hogweed
Gajapippala (gajapīpala), *Scindapsis officinalis*
Gājara *See* grinjana.
Ghandha palāshikā. *See* dāruhaladī.
Ghandhaka, sulphur
Gavha, carrot
Ghī and ghee, clarified butter

Girikarnikā, *Clitoria ternatea*
Gokhuru. *See* shvadanshtrā
Gokshuraka. *See* shvadanshtrā
Gopālikā, extract of cow's bile
Gorachana, bull's gall
Grinjana (lashuna), *Allium sativum*, garlic
Gudakashāya, red molasses
Gulābāsa. *See* āmalaka
Gulabavasa (gulamsha), *Tinospermum cordifolius*
Gulamsha. *See* gulabavasa
Gūlara. *See* baragada
Gulma, small cardamom
Gundakani. *See* vajrasnuhī
Gurupādikā. *See* bahupādikā

Haldi, turmeric
Hapushā, *Juniperus communis*, juniper
Hārachūraka. *See* drākshā
Haridrā, *Curcuma domestica*, turmeric
Harita, aromatic plants
Haritaka, *Terminalia chebulla*, yellow myrobalan
Haritāla, *Cynodon dactilon*, yellow arsenic
Hastikarna, large-leaved castor-oil plant
Hingu, *Ferula nartex*, asafetida

Ikshamūla (morata, murahari), *Sanseviera roxburghiana*, aristolochia
Ikshu, sugarcane
Ilayachi, cardamom
Indrayana (karihari, lāngalikā), *Gloriosa superba*, glory lily
Irka mūla. *See* ikshamūla

Jala shuka, watermelon

Jambu, *Eugenia jambolana,* rose apple

Japāgulma, China rose

Jātī, *Jasminum grandiflorum,* jasmine

Jau. *See* kalinja

Jihvikā (jīvaka, jīvasa, or upajihvikā), *Terminalia tomentosa,* yellow amaranth

Jīraka, *Cuminum cyminum,* cumin

Jīvaka. *See* jihvikā

Jīvasa. *See* jihvikā

Jūhī, white-flowered ixora

Kadalī, banana

Kadamba (nīpa), *Anthocephalus cadamba* or *indicus*

Kadara, *Acaci suma*

Kadavi, unknown

Kaddu. *See* alābu

Kaitha (kanthā, kapittha), *Feronia elephantum,* wood apple

Kakadaliya. *See* bhilava

Kakadi. *See* enva

Kakantira. *See* konhadu

Kākolī, *Ziziphus napecea*

Kākuna (kangunī), *Celastrus paniculata*

Kakusha mandala. *See* konhadu

Kālaka, *Piper chaba,* pepper

Kali mircha, black pepper

Kalinja (jau), rye

Kāmadhulika (madhūka, mahoa) *Cassia latiflora,* wild fig

Kamala. *See* utpala

Kanda. *See* bhantā

Kandaka, *Dioscorea elata*

Kanera (kanikāsa), *Neruim medicum,* oleander

Kangunī. *See* kākuna

Kanikāsa. *See* kanera

Kanka. *See* bhatakataiya

Kanthā. *See* kaitha

Kapikacchu. *See* ancila

Kāpishāyana. *See* drākshā

Kapittha. *See* kaitha

Kapusavarta. *See* baigana

Karanjā, *Pongamia glabra*

Karihari. *See* indrayana

Kārkati, cucumber

Kārpāsa, cotton

Karpūra, *Camphora officinarum,* camphor

kartika (alābuka), *Lagenaria vulgaris*

Kāsārika (kaseru, shriparnī), *Gmelina arborea*

Kaseru. *See* kāsārika

Kāshmarī *See* khumbari

Kastūrī, musk

Katthā. *See* khadira

Kauncha. *See* ancila

Kaushya, natural silk

Kavacha. *See* ancila

Kesara, saffron

Ketaki, *Pandanus odoratissimus,* screw pine

Khadira (kattha), *Acacia catechu,* catechu

Khasha. *See* angāra

Khumbari (kāshmarī, tilaparni), *Gynandropis pentaphylla,* yellow grape

Kokilāksha, *Asterakantha longifolia*

Konhadu (kakantira, kakusha mandala), unknown

Krimi, silk

Kshauma, vegetable silk

Kshīra kākolī, variety of kākolī
Kshīra vriksha, *Ficus religiosa*,
milk tree
Kshīrikā (kuili, rājādanam),
Mimusops hexandra
Kuili. *See* kshīrikā
Kulaka, gourd, *Trichosanthes dioeca*
Kulattha, *Dolichos biflorus*
Kumāri, aloes
Kumhara, *Hedisarum gangeticum*,
prickly pear
Kunda. *See* sūrana
Kundamalla, unknown
Kunkuma, *Crocus sativus*, saffron
Kurantaka (piyavansha or
priyavansha), *Barleria prionitis
nevara*, yellow amaranth
Kurantika, *Celosia argentea*
Kushmānda, *Benincasa cerifera*,
gourd
Kushtha (kūta), *Saussurea lappa*
Kūta. *See* kushtha
Kūtaja, *Holarrhena
antidysenterica*, wild quince
Kūtajaka. *See* kūtaja

Lāngalikā. *See* indrayana
Lashuna. *See* grinjana
Lauki. *See* alābu
Lavanga, *Caryophillus aromaticus*,
clove
Lodhā. *See* lodhra
Lodhra, *Symplocus racemosa*
Loha, iron

Madāra. *See* arka
Madasinghi or madhashringī,
ginger
Madayantikā (medhi, mehandi),
henna

Mādhavi, fig liquor
Madhu, honey
Madhūka (mahoa), *Madhuca lati-
folia* or *Cassia latifolia*, wild fig
Madhūka kalka, licorice paste
Madhūlikā or madhūka, fruit
Mahoa. *See* madhūka
Maireya, liquor
Mālaka, *Raphorus sativus*
Mālakāngunī. *See* shravana
priyangu
Mālatī, jasmine
Mallikā, *Jasminum sambac*,
jasmine
Manashilā, red arsenic
Mandara. *See* arka
Maraka, *black pepper*
Maratta, unknown
Maricha, *Piper negrum*, black
pepper
Marora, unknown
Marubaka, *Origanum*, marjoram
Māshaka, *Phaseolus radiatus*,
green gram
Māsra parni, (shaksha parni),
Teramus labialis
Meda shringī. *See* alguru
Medhi. *See* madayantikā
Mehandi. *See* madayantikā
Mesha, cardamom (small)
Morata. *See* ikshamūla
Mothā (mustaka, nagara mothā),
Cyperus rotundus, turmeric
Motiya, *jasmine*
Mudga, *Phaseolu mungo*, mungo
bean
Mūlahathi (mūlayashthi), radish
Mūlaka, *Raphanus sativus*,
horseradish
Mūlayashthi. *See* mūlahathi

Mūli. *See* mulaka

Murahari. *See* ikshamūla

Mustaka. *See* mothā

Nāga dhamani, *Artemisia vulgaris*, wormwood, citronella

Nāga kesara, *Mesua ferrea*

Nāga vallī. *See* tāmbūla

Nagara mothā. *See* mothā

Nāgara, ginger

Nandyavarta (kadamba), *Anthocephalus indicus*

Navamālikā, *Plumeria rubra*, frangipani

Nimbū, lemon tree

Nīpa. *See* kadamba

Nishtusha, sesame

Padma, pink lotus

Paishtī, wheat-based wine

Pālaka. *See* paluka

Pālāndra. *See* palāndu

Palāndu (palandra, pilaj), *Allium cepa*, onion

Pālanki, beetroot

Pālankiya, spinach

Palāsha, *Butea frondosa*

Paluka (jūhī), white-flowered ixora

Pāta, *Cannabis sativa*, hemp

Pātala (patalika, patavasa), *Stereospermum suavolens*, lavender

Pātalikā. *See* pātala

Patavāsa. *See* pātala

Pāthā, *Stephania hermandifolia*

Patharachata, *Castus speciosus*, bogweed

Phak (plasha), *Butea frondosa*

Phudina, mint

Pīpala, sacred fig tree

Pippali, *Piper lungum*, long pepper

Piyāj. *See* palāndu

Piyāla (Priyāla), *Buchanania latifolia*, long pepper

Piyavansha. *See* kurantaka

Plasha. *See* phak

Priyangu, *Aglaia roxburthiana*

Punnāga, *Calophyllum inophylnus*

Punarnavā. *See* gadāpunnā

Rājādanam. *See* kshīrikā

Rājavriksha, *Cassia augustifolia*, senna

Rangava, wool

Rasona (ucchatā), *Allium sativum*, garlic

Rātaka, *Emblica officinalis* or *mongiferas*, myrobalan

Rāva, fermented sugar

Rundika. *See* bahupādikā

Sahadevī. *See* dandotpalaka

Sahakāra, mango, mango oil

Sāla, *Shorea robusta*

Sālīsha. *See* tālīsha

Sambhara, rock salt

Sankhapushpī, *Crotalaria verrucosa*

Sapta parna, *Alstonia scholaris*

Sārinā. *See* sārivā

Sārivā (chitavanna, sarjiva), *Hemidesmus indicus*

Sarjaka sugandha, *Surgea rubrata*

Sarjiva. *See* sārivā

Sarshapa, *Brassica campestris*, mustard

Sarvato bhadra (shukanāsa, sonapathā), bignonia

Sāshrī. *See* vajrasnuhī

Sataparna, *Desmodium gangeticum*

Satavara. *See* shatāvari

Sattiva, *Alfalfa*, lucern

Saunpha, mustard

Shabarakanda, *Symplocos racemosa*, Lodhra root

Shahad, honey

Shākhā, pulses

Shaksha parni. *See* māsra parni

Shāli, *Diryza sativa*, rice

Shatapushpā, *Peucedarum graevolens*, fennel

Shatāvari (satavara), *Asparagus racemosus*, asparagus

Shigru, *Molinga pterigosperma*

Shinshapā, *Delbengia sissoo*

Shinghara. *See* shringātaka

Shirīsha, *Albizzia lebeck*

Shishu. *See* ashoka

Shravana priyangu (mālakānguni), *Cardiospermum holocaecabum*, balloon vine

Shringātaka (singhadā, shinghara), *Trapa bispinosa*, water chestnut

Shringī, aloes

Shriparnī. *See* kāsārika

Shūka, hairy insect

Shukanāsa. *See* sarvato bhadra

Shvadanshtrā (gokhuru, gokshuraka), *Tribulus terrestris*, mountain gokhuru

Singhadā. *See* shringātaka

Singhara. *See* shringātaka

Sīsaka, lead

Snuhī (thuhāra), *Euphorbia nerifolia*, milkweed

Soma, *Sarcostemma brevistigma*

Somalatā, climbing *Sarcostemma*

Somarājī. *See* avalguja

Sonapathā. *See* sarvato bhadra

Sora, poisonous root

Sroto anjana, antimony

Sthūna. *See* vajrasnuhī

Supāri, betel nut (areca)

Surā, wine

Suramā, khol

Sūrana (kunda), *Amorphophallus campanulatus*

Svayamguptā. *See* ancila

Tagara, *Tabernae montana coronaria*, valerian

Tāla, *Florassus flabellifer*, palm tree (Palmyra palm)

Tāladala, palm leaf

Tālaka, arsenic

Tālīsha (sālīsha), *Flacoustia cataphracta*

Tālīshapattra. *See* tālīsha

Tamāla, *Garcinia pictoria*, bay leaf

Tāmbūla (nāga vallī), betel leaf (*Piper betel*)

Tejapattra. *See* dālachini

Thuhāra. *See* snuhi

Tila, *Sesamum indicum*, sesame

Tilaparnika, *sandalwood, incense*

Trāpusha. *See* balamakhira

Triphala, the three myrobalans

Tulasī, *Ocimum basilicum*, basil

Tumbī. *See* alābu

Tvach. *See* dālachini

Ucchatā. *See* rasona

Upajihvikā. *See* jihvikā

Utpala, *Nelumbium speciosum*, blue lotus, blue water-lily

Vachā, *Acorus calamus*, orris root
Vajra, *Hydrophila spinosa*
Vajrakadamba. *See* **kadamba**
Vajrasnuhī (gundakani, sāshrī),
  Euphorbia thymifolia, milk
  hedge
Valuka. *See* **elābalukā**

Vilva. *See* **bhilava**
Vrintāka. *See* **bhantā**
Vyādhighātaka, Rumex
  vesicarus, golden sephalika

Yashtimadhu, licorice

Five

Special Terms

Abhimāna, attachment
Abhimāni, amorous games
Abhimāniki, infatuation
Abhiruchi, affection
Abhiyoga, meeting, devotion
Adhorata maithuna, sodomy
Āharyarāga, affection born of habit
Ālingana, embrace, caress
Ānanda, sensual pleasure
Antahpūrikā, gynoecium
Apadravya, dildo
Ārsha, ancestral marriage with gift of oxen
Artha, money, prosperity, material assets
Auparishtaka, superior coition, fellation

Aurasa, bastard
Ayantritarata, sexual activity without limits

Bālā, sixteen-year-old girl
Bhāga, vagina
Bhāgānkura, clitoris
Bhāryā, wife
Bhava, emotional state, mood
Bhāva, feeling, sentiment
Brāhma, priestly marriage, arranged by parents
Buddhā, woman over fifty years old

Chandavega, passionate ardour
Chārsha, sex object
Chitrarata, special tastes

545

Chittavritti, inclinations
Chūta or mango, metaphorically anus

Daiva, astral marriage with the officiating priest
Dashana cheda, bites
Dharma, virtue
Dūta, go-between

Gāndharva, angelic marriage, by elopement or mutual agreement
Gāndharva shālā, music room
Ganikā, courtesan
Goshthi parigraha, group sex
Guda, anus

Hāva, seduction
Hela, fondness
Hijrā, male prostitute

Ichchā, desire

Jaghana, ass, vagina
Jālaka, armor, artificial sex organ
Janakhāpana, homosexuality

Kāla, destiny
Kāma, Eros, eroticism, love
Kāma vivāha, love marriage
Kanchuka, sheath, artificial sex organ
Kanyā, seven-year-old girl
Khalarāga, degrading love
Kritrimarāga, feigned love
Kshema shiras, sect of magicians
Kulatā, nymphomaniac
Kumbhadāsī, female waterbearer

Latāveshtitaka, to entwine like a liana, posture
Laukāyitaka, materialists, system of philosophy
Launda, transvestite prostitute
Linga, phallus, male sexual organ

Maithuna, copulation
Matkārya, female masturbation
Meha, sexual organ
Mohana, to be bewitched, seduce
Mūla vāsanā, basic desire

Nakharadāna, to scratch
Napunsaka, impotent, eunuch
Nārāyitam, homosexuality
Nīvī, fold of clothing between the legs

Pāyu, anus
Pīthamarda, manager, steward
Potārata, neutral sex
Prahana, to strike, slap
Prājāpatya, royal marriage, arranged without counterpart
Pramadā, young girl
Praudhā, ripe woman (from thirty to fifty years old)
Prīti, sexual attraction, love, affection
Purushāyita, virile behavior by a woman
Purushopasripta, sodomy, to possess a man
Putāputa yoga, magical practices

Rāgavat, love, passion
Raha, being alone together
Rākā, menses
Raktāvāsa, chamber of love
Rangopajīvikā, tart
Rasa, taste, pleasant feeling
Rasika, sensualist, lover of sex
Rata, copulation, desire
Rati, pleasure, sexual desire
Rati-āvāsa, chamber of love
Rūpājīvika (also rūpājīvā), girl living on her charms
Rūshya, ejaculation

Sahāya, pimp
Samāgama, sleeping together
Sambādha, vulva
Sambhoga, enjoyment, copulation
Samprayoga, amorous approaches
Samputa, the box, sleeping face to face
Samvega, sexual impulse, excitation
Samyoga, union
Sanghātaka, group sex
Sanveshana, penetration, coition, sexual union
Shayana, sleeping together
Shringāra rasa, loving feeling
Sītkāra, sigh
Simhākrānta, "seizing the lion," to masturbate
Skhalana, ejaculation
Sphutaka, erection
Surata, successful copulation
Svadharma, individual ethics
Svairinī, lesbian
Svayamvara, free choice of a suitor

Tarunī, young woman (from sixteen to thirty years old)
Trishna, thirst, desire
Tritīya prakriti, third nature (homosexuality)

Uddhapana, erection, excitation
Upagahana, hugging, clasping
Upasarga, ejaculation
Upastha, sexual organ

Vādavā, vulva
Varāngaushtha, labia of the vulva
Vāsanā, affection
Vashīkarana, bewitching, magical practices
Vedanā, feeling
Vega, ardor
Vesha, prostitution
Veshyā, prostitute
Vidūshaka, confidant, jester, facetious secretary
Vilāsa, pleasure
Vishaya, beloved
Vishayātmika, venal love
Vita, gigolo
Vrikshādhiruraka, climbing the tree, posture
Vrishyā yoga, preparation of aphrodisiacs
Vyavahitarāga, love by substitution

Yantra, instrument, male sexual organ
Yauna, coupling
Yoga, sexual union
Yoni, vagina

INDEX

ABOUT THE TRANSLATOR

Born in Paris on October 4, 1907, Alain Daniélou displayed artistic and musical talent from an early age. While attending school in the United States he exhibited his paintings and played piano for silent movie theaters. After returning to France, he studied dance with Nicholas Legat (Nijinski's master), as well as singing and composition. Between 1927 and 1932 he was active in the Parisian art world, where he was associated with Jean Cocteau, Jean Marais, Serge Diaghilev, Igor Stravinsky, Max Jacobs, and other creative artists of that remarkable time and place.

A great sportsman, canoeing champion, and an expert driver of racing cars, he explored the Afghan Pamir in 1932 and performed an endurance test by car from Paris to Calcutta in 1934. He traveled in North Africa, the Middle East, India, Indonesia, China, and Japan with the Swiss photographer Raymond Burnier and described these adventures in his memoir *Le tour du monde en 1936* (Flammarion, 1987).

Daniélou eventually established himself in India, where Rabindranath Tagore appointed him director of his school of music at Shantiniketan. Later, at Banaras, Daniélou became gradually initiated into the traditional culture of India. For fifteen years he studied classical Indian music with the most prestigious masters, and he plays the vīnā like a professional. He also studied Sanskrit, philosophy, and Hindi, which he speaks and writes as fluently as his mother tongue. Swami Karpatri, the famous *sannyāsi*, initiated him into the rites of Shaivite Hinduism, under the name of Shiva Sharan, which means "protected by Shiva."

In 1949 Daniélou became the director of the College of Indian Music at the Hindu University of Banaras. Greatly interested in the symbolism of Hindu architecture and sculpture, he made expeditions to many important sites in central India and Rajputana. He then became the director of the Adyar Library of Sanskrit manuscripts and editions at Madras in 1954. Two years later he was made a member of the Institut Français d'Indiologie at Pondicherry, and subsequently of the Ecole Française d'Extrême-Orient, of which he had been an honorary member since 1943.

A close friend of the Nehru family, Daniélou was sympathetic to the independence movement. Yet when the new government attacked orthodoxy, it was suggested that his role would be more useful in presenting the true face of Hinduism to the West. He returned to Europe and in 1963, with the help of the Ford Foundation, created the International Institute for Comparative Music Studies, based in Berlin and Venice. By organizing concerts for the great musicians of Asia and through the publication of recorded collections of traditional music under the aegis of UNESCO, Daniélou was a key figure in the rediscovery of Asian art music in the West.

Because of his immersion in two cultures, Alain Daniélou has been able to view both East and West from a unique perspective. In a career spanning six decades, he has written over twenty books on Hindu religion, society, music, sculpture, and architecture, in addition to translating such Indian classics as the *Kāma Sūtra* and the Tamil novel *Manimekhalai*. Two of his books, *Gods of Love and Ecstasy* and *While the Gods Play*, deal with the problems of a Western culture that has lost its own traditions, taking humankind away from both nature and the divine. A true Renaissance man, Alain Daniélou has distinguished himself both as a leading Orientalist and as a profound critic of the Western condition.

The Myths and Gods of India
The Classic Work on Hindu Polytheism
From the Princeton Bollingen Series

ISBN 0-89281-354-7 • $19.95 illustrated paperback

This thorough study of Hindu mythology explores the significance of the most prominent Hindu deities and reveals the message of tolerance and adaptability that is at the heart of this ancient religion.

"The style is lucid; the lack of polemic is particularly attractive. The total result is a volume that is a pleasure to behold and an invigorating experience to read."
American Anthropologist

Yoga
Mastering the Secrets of Matter and the Universe

ISBN 0-89281-301-6 • $10.95 paperback

In this book, Daniélou gives an account of the principles and practice of yoga, compiled from the teachings of many of its living exponents and from published and unpublished Sanskrit sources. It is fully authentic in its presentation of the aims, methods, and different forms of yoga, explaining the technical processes by which, according to the doctrines of yoga, the subconscious may be brought under control, the senses overpassed, and modes of perception obtained, which can lead to remarkable achievements, both spiritual and intellectual.

Virtue, Success, Pleasure, and Liberation
The Four Aims of Life in the Tradition of Ancient India

ISBN 0-89281-218-4 • $14.95 paperback

Daniélou here explores the four aims of life in traditional Hindu culture. He shows that, while differing profoundly from accepted social order in the West, the structure of Hindu society served as a model for the self to actualize its full potential.

While the Gods Play

Shaiva Oracles and Predictions on the
Cycles of History and the Destiny of the Universe

ISBN 0-89281-115-3 • $12.95 paperback

According to the early writings of the Shaiva tradition—still alive in India and dating back at least 6,000 years—the arbitrary ideologies and moralistic religions of modern society signal the last days of humanity. This prediction is only a fragment of the vast knowledge of Shaivism, the religion of the ancient Dravidians. An initiate of this wisdom, Daniélou here revives the essential concepts of the Shaiva philosophy and its predictions, and reflects on what action can be taken to consciously and creatively influence our own destiny.

"These revelatory books are remarkable for their clarity, scholarship, and uninhibited celebration of mystical ecstasy." Interview Magazine

Gods of Love and Ecstasy

The Traditions of Shiva and Dionysus

ISBN 0-89281-374-1 • $12.95 paperback

Drawing on the earliest sources of the traditions of Shiva and Dionysus, Daniélou reconstructs religious practices which were observed from the Indus Valley to the coasts of Portugal nearly 6,000 years ago. These are the ancient Hindu and Greek gods of ecstatic sexuality, of magical power, intoxication and transcendence, through whom we can participate in the joy of creation.

❖

These and other Inner Traditions titles are available at many fine bookstores or, to order directly from the publisher, send a check or money order for the total amount, payable to Inner Traditions, plus $3.00 shipping and handling for the first book and $1.00 for each additional book to:

Inner Traditions
One Park Street
Rochester, VT 05767

Be sure to request a free catalog.